PLATINUM-BASED DRUGS IN CANCER THERAPY

Cancer Drug Discovery and Development

Beverly A. Teicher, *Series Editor*

Tumor Suppressor Genes in Human Cancer, edited by *David E. Fisher,* 2000

Matrix Metalloproteinase Inhibitors in Cancer Therapy, edited by *Neil J. Clendeninn and Krzysztof Appelt,* 2000

Prenyltransferase Inhibitors in Cancer and Cardiovascular Therapy, edited by *Said M. Sebti and Andrew Hamilton,* 2000

Platinum-Based Drugs in Cancer Therapy, edited by *Lloyd R. Kelland and Nicholas P. Farrell,* 2000

Signaling Networks and Cell Cycle Control: *The Molecular Basis of Cancer and Other Diseases,* edited by *J. Silvio Gutkind,* 1999

Apoptosis and Cancer Chemotherapy, edited by *John A. Hickman and Caroline Dive,* 1999

Antifolate Drugs in Cancer Therapy, edited by *Ann L. Jackman,* 1999

Antiangiogenic Agents in Cancer Therapy, edited by *Beverly A. Teicher,* 1999

Anticancer Drug Development Guide: *Preclinical Screening, Clinical Trials, and Approval,* edited by *Beverly A. Teicher,* 1997

Cancer Therapeutics: *Experimental and Clinical Agents,* edited by *Beverly A. Teicher,* 1997

Platinum-Based Drugs in Cancer Therapy

Edited by

Lloyd R. Kelland

*CRC Centre for Cancer Therapeutics,
The Institute of Cancer Research, UK*

and

Nicholas P. Farrell

*Department of Chemistry,
Virginia Commonwealth University*

Humana Press
Totowa, New Jersey

999 Riverview Drive, Suite 208
Totowa, New Jersey 07512

For additional copies, pricing for bulk purchases, and/or information about other Humana titles, contact Humana at the above address or at any of the following numbers: Tel.: 973-256-1699; Fax: 973-256-8341; E-mail: humana@humanapr.com or visit our Website: http://humanapress.com

---

This publication is printed on acid-free paper. ∞
ANSI Z39.48-1984 (American National Standards Institute) Permanence of Paper for Printed Library Materials.

Cover design by Patricia F. Cleary.

Printed in the United States of America. 10 9 8 7 6 5 4 3 2 1

Library of Congress Cataloging-in-Publication Data

Platinum-based drugs in cancer therapy / edited by Lloyd R. Kelland and Nicholas P. Farrell
p. cm. —(Cancer drug discovery and development ; 7)
Includes bibliographical references and index.
ISBN 0-89603-599-9 (alk. paper)
1. Cisplatin. 2. Platinum compunds—Therapeutic use. 3. Cancer—Chemotherapy. I. Kelland, Lloyd R. II. Farrell, Nicholas, 1948— . III. Series.
[DNLM: 1. Antineoplastic Agents. 2. Cisplatin. 3. Neoplasms—drug therapy. 4. Platinum Compounds—therapeutic use. QV 269 P7163 2000]
RC271.C55P56 2000
616.99'4061—DC21 99-32239
DNLM/DLC CIP
for Library of Congress

PREFACE

It all started with an accidental discovery in the laboratory of Dr. Barnet Rosenberg at Michigan State University in the mid 1960s. Now, thirty years from the landmark publication of the anticancer activity of cisplatin, this volume follows in the wake of the 8th International Symposium on Platinum and Other Metal Coordination Compounds in Cancer Chemotherapy, held in Oxford, UK, in March 1999. From small beginnings, this quadrennial Symposium now attracts several hundred laboratory and clinical scientists from all corners of the world.

Although the chemical structure of the inorganic square planar platinum-based coordination complex had been known for over 100 years prior to Rosenberg's studies, the medical oncology and, indeed, the scientific community at large were unaware of the dormant giant that lay waiting to be discovered. From the beginning of its clinical trials in the early 1970s, cisplatin made an immediate impact in the treatment of a variety of cancers (especially testicular and ovarian), but there were also significant problems in terms of inducing severe side-effects (especially kidney damage and nausea/vomiting). At the preclinical level, the next 10 years or so saw the emergence of a band of scientists who began to put in place the multidisciplinary approach essential to modern anticancer drug discovery. Notable from those early days were Joe Burchenal, Mike Cleare, Tom Connors, Ken Harrap, Jim Hoeschele, Yoshinori Kidani, John Roberts, and the National Cancer Institute (NCI).

Initial efforts focused on understanding the chemistry and biochemistry necessary to produce improved (less-toxic) analogs and elucidate the mechanism by which cisplatin exerted its antitumor effects. During the 1970s and 1980s, hundreds of new platinum-containing agents were synthesized, the focus being largely on reducing side-effects while retaining the antitumor activity of the parent molecule. One of the most important collaborations was established between the Johnson Matthey Company and academia, at The Institute of Cancer Research in Sutton UK, which resulted in the discovery of several key agents for clinical testing, including JM8 (carboplatin) and JM9 (iproplatin). From these trials, carboplatin (Paraplatin®) emerged as a significant new platinum-based anticancer drug in being broadly equivalent to cisplatin in terms of its spectrum of antitumor activity, but producing markedly less patient morbidity. Carboplatin remains the only cisplatin analog to be widely registered for clinical use.

For the last 10 years, the major focus of platinum drug development has been on the critical clinical need to broaden the number of tumor types that respond to this class of drug. Laboratory-based studies have shed light on the mechanisms by which tumors are, or become, resistant to the effects of cisplatin, thus allowing for the rational design of improved analogs. Several interesting new classes of platinum agents have been identified, including active *trans* isomers, orally active platinums, improved diaminocyclohexane (DACH) platinums, and bi- and tri-nuclear platinums. In total, approximately 30 platinum-based drugs have entered clinical trial. Importantly, their structural diversity continues to expand and many important trials are still ongoing.

Some 30 years on from the discovery of cisplatin, it is pertinent to ask "Where do we go from here?" The multidisciplinary approach of anticancer drug research involves synthetic chemists, molecular biologists, pharmacologists, and clinical oncologists. This volume brings together all of these and provides a comprehensive state-of-the-art appraisal by a panel of international contributors on:

(1) Platinum Chemistry. This section includes information on the chemistry of cisplatin in aqueous solution, the molecular interaction of platinum drugs with DNA, and transplatin-modified oligonucleotides.

(2) Platinum Biochemistry. Herein, there is particular emphasis on the burgeoning new areas of DNA mismatch repair, replicative bypass, and apoptosis, as well the important issue of how platinum drugs are transported into tumor cells.

(3) Clinical Antitumor Activity and Toxicology. This part covers an overview of the clinical experience with cisplatin and carboplatin, the exciting recent studies combining platinum drugs with taxanes, and clinical experience with DACH-based platinum drugs, particularly oxaliplatin. Moreover, an appraisal of the toxicological aspects of platinum drugs from both a clinical and a regulatory perspective is provided.

(4) New platinum drugs of the future. The volume concludes with an ongoing and futuristic look at new platinum drugs, including orally active drugs (JM216, ZD0473) and novel polynuclear charged platinums, such as BBR3464, which take the field into a new paradigm.

We are no longer completely in the dark as to how cisplatin exerts its antitumor (and toxicological) effects and how tumors acquire resistance; the considerable challenge is to exploit this knowledge to the further benefit of cancer sufferers. The field is poised at an especially exciting phase, the essence of which is captured in these chapters.

We wish to thank each of the contributors to *Platinum-Based Drugs in Cancer Therapy.* We are indebted to the time and effort each has provided to both the overall field of platinum anticancer drug development in making platinum-based chemotherapy more efficacious and more "patient-friendly" and for their particular input into this volume.

Lloyd R. Kelland
Nicholas P. Farrell

CONTENTS

CONTRIBUTORS

PAUL A. ANDREWS • *Division of Oncology Drug Products, Food and Drug Administration, Rockville, MD*

TREVOR G. APPLETON • *Department of Chemistry, University of Queensland, Brisbane, Australia*

JULIE G. BEITZ • *Division of Oncology Drug Products, Food and Drug Administration, Rockville, MD*

SUSAN J. BERNERS-PRICE • *School of Science, Griffith University, Brisbane, Australia*

VIKTOR BRABEC • *Institute of Biophysics, Academy of Sciences of the Czech Republic, Brno, Czech Republic*

ROBERT BROWN • *CRC Department of Medical Oncology, CRC Beatson Laboratories, Glascow, UK*

A. HILARY CALVERT • *Cancer Research Unit, University of Newcastle upon Tyne, Newcastle-upon-Tyne, UK*

STEPHEN G. CHANEY • *Department of Biochemistry and Biophysics, University of North Carolina, Chapel Hill, NC*

DIANA L. CLARK • *Division of Oncology Drug Products, Food and Drug Administration, Rockville, MD*

JOSEPH J. DEGEORGE • *Division of Oncology Drug Products, Food and Drug Administration, Rockville, MD*

NICHOLAS P. FARRELL • *Department of Chemistry, Virginia Commonwealth University, Richmond, VA*

DANIEL FINK • *Department of Obstetrics and Gynecology, University of Zurich, Switzerland*

MARIE-JOSEPHE GIRAUD-PANIS • *Centre de Biophysique Moleculaire, CNRS, Orleans, France*

MARTIN GORE • *Royal Marsden Hospital NH Trust, London, UK*

MARTIN S. HIGHLEY • *Cancer Research Unit, University of Newcastle upon Tyne, Newcastle-upon-Tyne, UK*

STEPHEN B. HOWELL • *Cancer Center, University of California at San Diego, La Jolla, CA*

STEVEN W. JOHNSON • *University of Pennsylvania Cancer Center, Philadelphia, PA*

ROBERT L. JUSTICE • *Office of Review Management, Food and Drug Administration, Rockville, MD*

Lloyd R. Kelland • *CRC Centre for Cancer Therapeutics, Institute of Cancer Research, Sutton, Surrey, UK*
Vladimír Kleinwächter • *Institute of Biophysics, Academy of Sciences of the Czech Republic, Brno, Czech Republic*
Marc Leng • *Centre de Biophysique Moleculaire, CNRS, Orleans, France*
Mark J. McKeage • *Department of Pharmacology and Clinical Pharmacology, University of Auckland, New Zealand*
Peter J. O'Dwyer • *University of Pennsylvania Cancer Center, Philadelphia, PA*
Francisco Sapunar • *Royal Marsden Hospital NH Trust, London, UK*
Annie Schwartz • *Centre de Biophysique Moleculaire, CNRS, Orleans, France*
D. D. Smith • *Division of Biometrics, Food and Drug Administration, Rockville, MD*
James P. Stephenson • *University of Pennsylvania Cancer Center, Philadelphia, PA*
Alexandra Vaisman • *Department of Biochemistry and Biophysics, University of North Carolina, Chapel Hill, NC*
Michelle Vaughan • *Royal Marsden Hospital Trust, London, UK*

I PLATINUM CHEMISTRY

1 The Chemistry of Cisplatin in Aqueous Solution

Susan J. Berners-Price and Trevor G. Appleton

CONTENTS

1. INTRODUCTION

The antitumor properties of platinum-containing drugs are attributable in large measure to the kinetics of their ligand displacement reactions. As is discussed at length in other contributions to this volume, their primary target is believed to be nitrogen donor atoms in the nucleobases of DNA. The bonds formed between the metal ion and these atoms must be sufficiently long-lived to interfere with the process of cell division, or to trigger the intracellular mechanisms that recognize irreparable damage to a cell. Bonds between the nucleobase nitrogen atoms and platinum(II) clearly fulfil this requirement. Metal ions that form labile bonds with the nucleobase nitrogen atoms cannot act in a similar way and do not give active compounds *(1)*. On the other hand, the metal-based drug that is injected must undergo in a relatively short time a sequence of reactions that allows the "leaving groups" on the initial compound

From: *Platinum-Based Drugs in Cancer Therapy*
Edited by: L. R. Kelland and N. Farrell © Humana Press Inc., Totowa, NJ

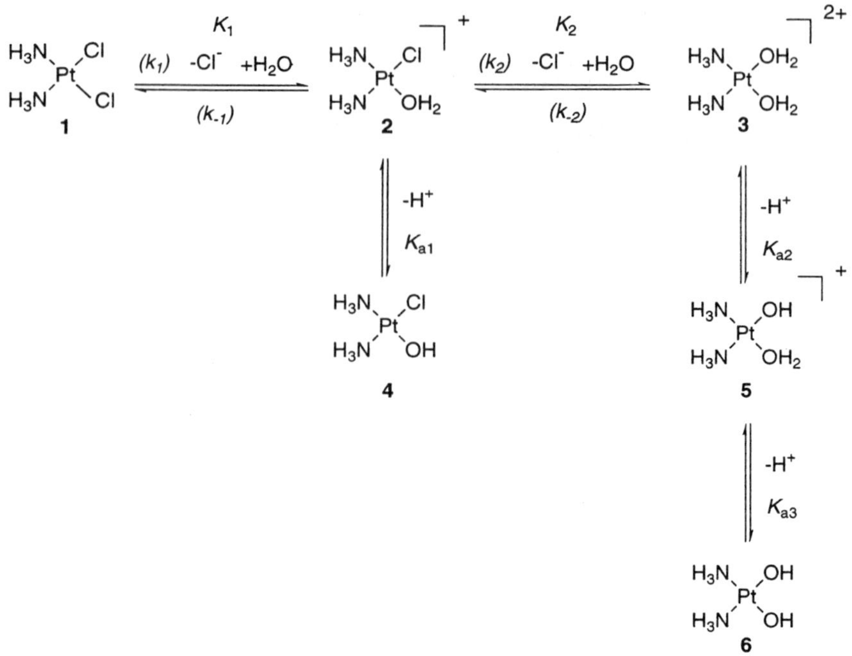

to be replaced by the DNA base nitrogen atoms. Compounds that are totally inert are also inactive *(1)*.

Cisplatin, *cis*-$[PtCl_2(NH_3)_2]$ **(1)** is a relatively unreactive molecule. It does not react directly with any of the molecules present in biological systems that will bind to the platinum through nitrogen or oxygen donor groups, including nucleobases *(2,3)*. In aqueous solution, however, the chloro ligands of cisplatin may be replaced in a stepwise manner by water to form *cis*-$[PtCl(H_2O)(NH_3)_2]^+$ **(2)** and *cis*-$[Pt(H_2O)_2(NH_3)_2]^{2+}$ **(3)**. Depending on the pH of the solution, the bound water molecules may deprotonate to give hydroxo complexes **4, 5,** and **6** (Scheme 1). The Pt-OH_2 bond is much more reactive than Pt-Cl. The aqua complexes therefore react readily with N-donor ligands, such as DNA nucleobases. Hydrolysis of cisplatin is therefore usually considered to be a necessary prelude to its reaction with DNA *(2)*.

The aqua complexes also react more readily than cisplatin with molecules present in vivo other than target DNA. They therefore are involved in reactions that lead to toxicity. The bound water molecules of *cis*-$[Pt(H_2O)_2(NH_3)_2]^{2+}$ **(3)** are very labile, so that this species reacts nondiscriminately with many biologically important molecules. It is therefore very toxic *(1)*.

Carboplatin **(7)** is less toxic than cisplatin but also has less antitumor activity on an equal-dose basis. These properties are correlated with its much lower tendency to undergo hydrolysis reactions—indeed, the rate of hydrolysis is

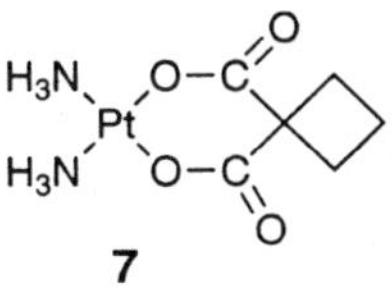

7

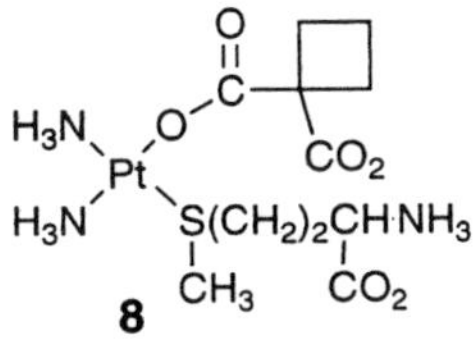

8

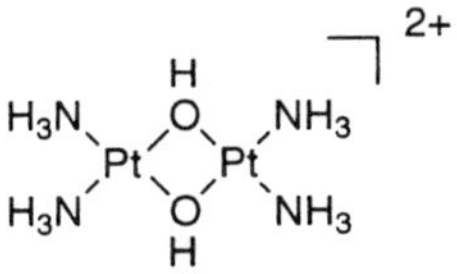

9

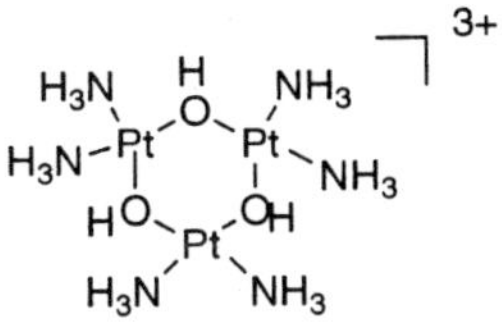

10

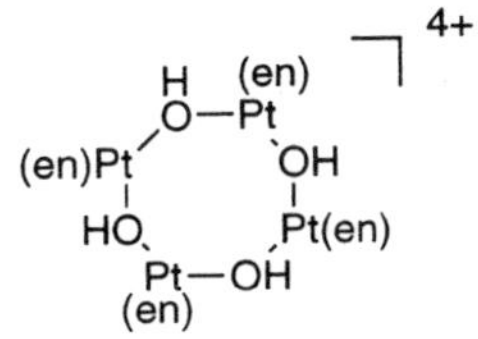

11

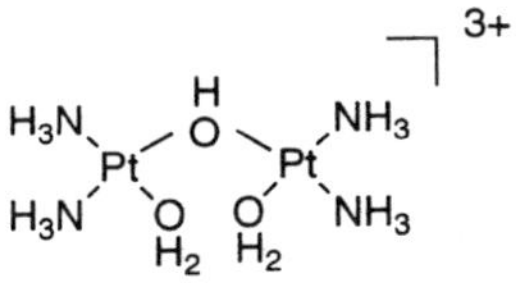

12

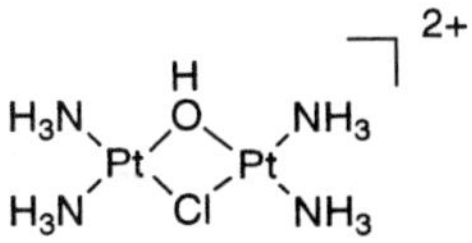

13

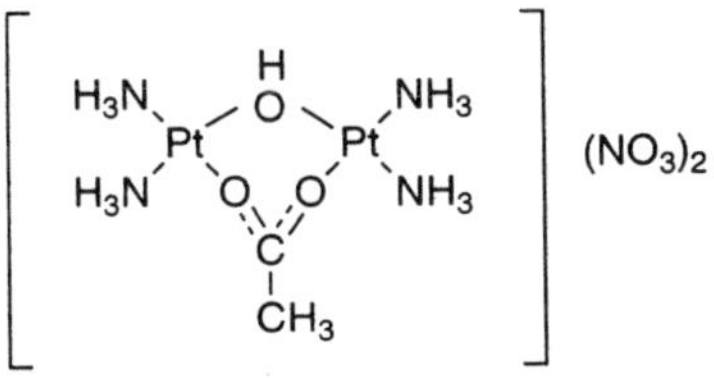

14

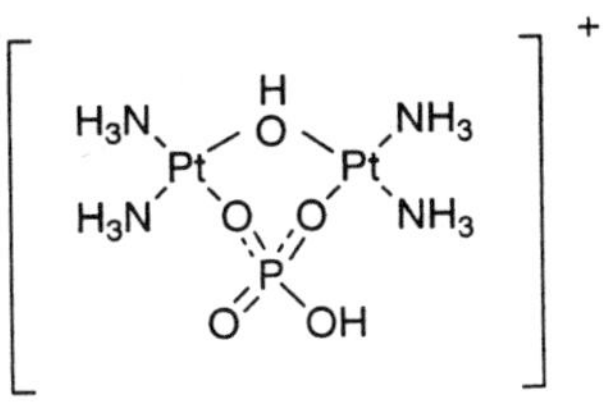

15

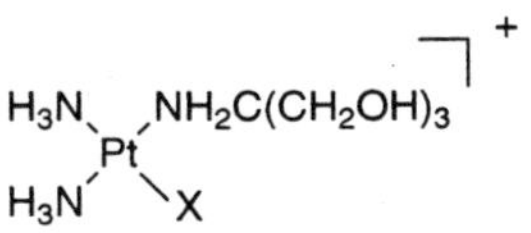

$X^- = Cl^-, OH^-$

16

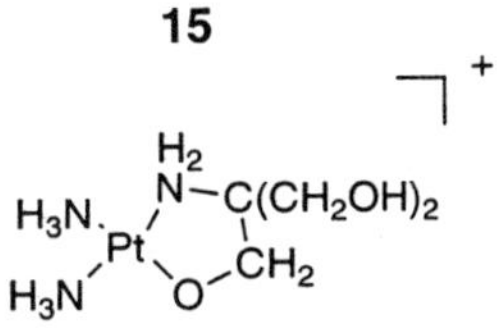

17

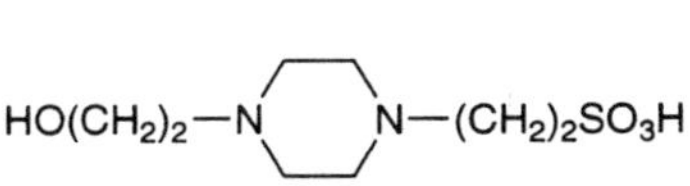

hepes

18

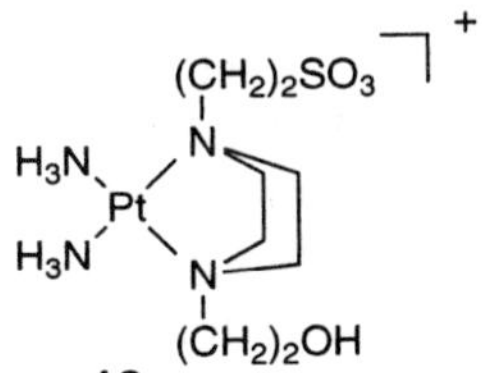

19

negligibly slow under physiological conditions *(4)*. Carboplatin does react directly with guanosine monophosphate, but only slowly *(4)*.

Cisplatin and carboplatin do react directly with sulfur-containing ligands (e.g., methionine, cysteine) without the need for prior hydrolysis *(5–8)*. With methionine, for example, carboplatin gives the relatively long-lived species **8**, in which both methionine and the dicarboxylate ligand are bound monodentate *(5)*. Since thioether ligands bound monodentate through sulfur may in some cases be displaced by guanosine nitrogen *(7)*, it has been suggested *(7,9)* that such thioether complexes may be major intermediates in DNA platination, bypassing the hydrolysis route. This possibility remains the subject of extensive experimentation, and a detailed consideration is beyond the scope of this chapter. Whatever the role of such mechanisms may be, it remains true that the hydrolysis chemistry of cisplatin (and of compounds *cis*-$[PtCl_2(amine)_2]$ generally) is an important factor in the antitumor activity, metabolism, and toxicity of these platinum-based drugs.

2. HYDROXO COMPLEXES

At high pH (>9), all coordinated water molecules will be deprotonated, to give hydroxo complexes, such as *cis*-$[PtCl(OH)(NH_3)_2]$ **(4)** and *cis*-$[Pt(OH)_2(NH_3)_2]$ **6**. The Pt-OH bond is quite inert, so that, for example, **6** does not react with glycine *(10)*. Since the Pt-OH_2 bond is much more reactive, reactions can begin to occur slowly with N-donor ligands via traces of aqua complexes if the pH is decreased to less than 2 pH units above the pK_a value for deprotonation of the aqua complex. If the pH is in the range p$K_a \pm 2$, however, so that appreciable proportions of both aqua and hydroxo complexes are present together in solution, hydroxo-bridged oligomers form readily if the concentration of diammineplatinum(II) species is not extremely small.

Thus, under conditions in which *cis*-$[Pt(OH)(H_2O)(NH_3)_2]^+$ **(5)** is present in solution, the hydroxo-bridged complexes $[\{Pt(NH_3)_2(\mu\text{-}OH)\}_n]^{n+}$ are formed [n = 2 **(9)**, 3 **(10)**]. Crystal structures have been determined of salts of these oligomers [n = 2 *(11,12)*, 3 *(13)*] and characterized by ^{195}Pt nuclear magnetic resonance (NMR) (*see* Section 7.2). Analogous species are formed in other *cis*-diamine systems [e.g., with isomers of 1,2-diaminocyclohexane (DACH) *(14,15)*]. A tetrameric species, $[Pt(en)(\mu\text{-}OH)\}_4]^{4+}$ **(11)**, en = 1,2-diaminoethane) has been characterized crystallographically *(16)*. Its formation is probably facilitated by reduced steric interaction between the hydroxo ligands and the amine, because the "bite angle" of chelated ethylenediamine is <90°. Even so, the dimer and trimer appear to be the major species in solution *(17)*.

It has been claimed that the hydroxo-bridged diammine complexes (9) and (10) are toxic, but that the DACH analogs are nontoxic *(14)*. Once formed, **9** and **10** persist in mildly acidic solution. At pH 3, the oligomers are decomposed, but **12**, with a single hydroxo bridge, persists in solution *(18)*.

In the presence of other ligands, compounds may be obtained that contain bridging hydroxide and a second bridging ligand. For example, when both *cis*-$[PtCl(H_2O)(NH_3)_2]^+$ (**2**) and *cis*-$[PtCl(OH)(NH_3)_2]$ (**4**) are present in solution (i.e., when the pH is close to the pK_a of **2**), $[\{$*cis*-$Pt(NH_3)_2\}_2(\mu\text{-}Cl)(\mu\text{-}OH)]^{2+}$ (**13**) is formed *(19)*. Addition of acetate to a solution *cis*-$[Pt(H_2O)_2(NH_3)_2](NO_3)_2$ causes slow crystallization of $[\{$*cis*-$Pt(NH_3)_2\}_2(\mu\text{-}CH_3CO_2)(\mu\text{-}OH)](NO_3)_2$ (**14**), whose crystal structure has been determined *(20)*. This is not a major species in solution *(18)*, but analogous compounds are formed near pH 5 when longer-chain amino acids $^+NH_3(CH_2)_nCO_2^-$ (n = 2,3) are added to a solution of *cis*-$[Pt(H_2O)_2(NH_3)_2]^{2+}$ *(21)*. A compound **15** containing bridging phosphate as well as hydroxide has been characterized by NMR *(18)*. Analogous compounds are formed with aminoalkylphosphonate ligands *(22)*.

If a mononuclear diammineplatinum complex were injected in vivo, the concentration would be too low for dimerization to occur. However, if the solution injected already contained a hydroxo-bridged oligomeric species, it would be likely to persist in vivo.

3. ACID DISSOCIATION CONSTANTS FOR AQUA COMPLEXES

As Pt-OH_2 bonds are more reactive toward DNA and other biomolecules than Pt-OH (or Pt-Cl) bonds, it is important to know the pK_a values of the coordinated water molecules in the cisplatin hydrolysis products **2** and **3** to establish the relative proportions of hydroxo species **4**, **5**, and **6** (Scheme 1) that are likely to be present under physiological conditions (pH 7.4). It is difficult to obtain reliable experimental determinations of these acid dissociation constants from potentiometric measurements because the interpretation of titration curves is complicated by the further hydrolysis of *cis*-$[PtCl(NH_3)_2(H_2O)]^+$ (**2**), and its competing anation by Cl^- during any potentiometric titration, as well as the formation of hydroxo-bridged oligomers **9** and **10** in solutions containing moderate concentrations of *cis*-$[Pt(NH_3)_2(OH)(H_2O)]^+$ (**5**) (see above). The work of Green and co-workers *(23)* has also demonstrated that for pK_a measurements of the diaqua complex **3**, the choice of counter-anion has a significant effect. Their measured values for pK_{a1} were slightly lower for the noncoordinating anions triflate and perchlorate than for nitrate, which, though a poor ligand, can bond weakly at the fifth and sixth coordination sites.

The pK_a of **2** has been determined recently by an indirect method that probed the influence of pH on the reaction between **2** and chloride ion *(24)*. However, the results may be complicated by the use of HEPES buffers, which are known to interact with cisplatin hydrolysis products *(25,26)* (*see* Section 6).

The pK_a values of species in mixtures can be determined by NMR spectroscopy provided they have suitable resonances that can be monitored as a function of pH. If ^{15}N-substituted ligands are used, the individual Pt-NH_3 complexes can be distinguished by ^{15}N NMR since both the ^{15}N chemical shift and the ^{195}Pt-^{15}N cou-

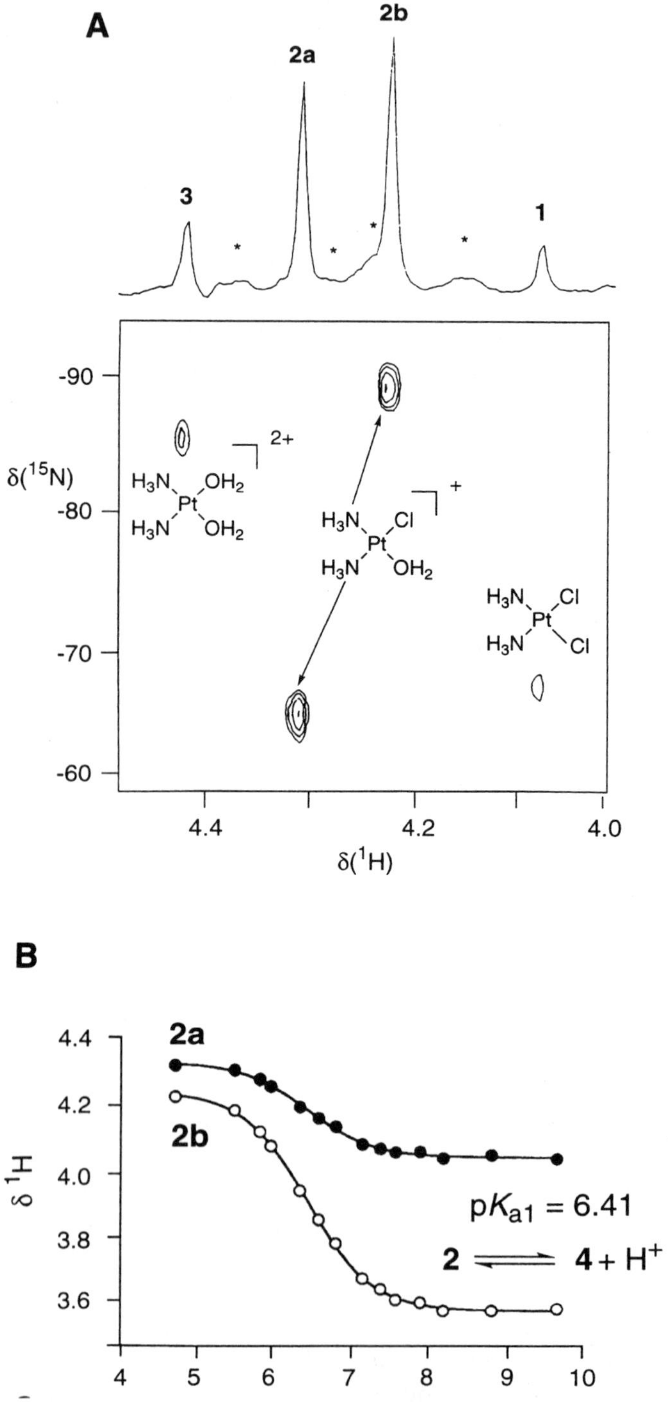
A
2b
2a
3
1
-90
-80
-70
-60
δ(15N)
H3N OH2 Pt H3N OH2 2+
H3N Cl Pt H3N OH2 +
H3N Cl Pt H3N Cl
4.4
4.2
4.0
δ(1H)
B
2a
2b
4.4
4.2
4.0
3.8
3.6
δ 1H
pKa1 = 6.41
2 ⇌ 4 + H+
4
5
6
7
8
9
10

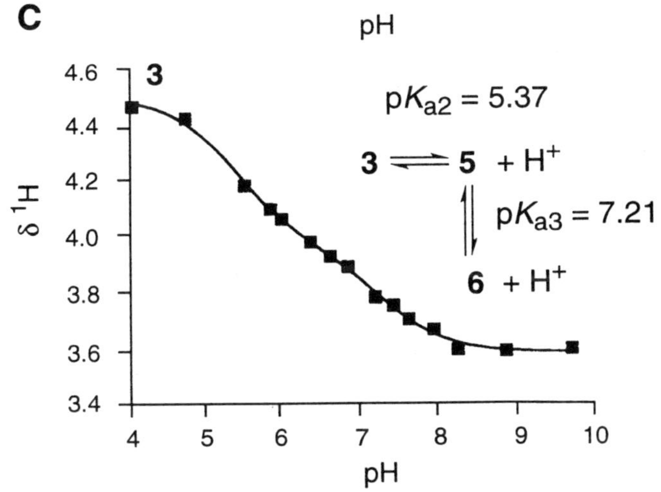

Fig. 1. [^{1}H, ^{15}N] NMR spectrum (**A**) of a 5 m*M* solution containing ^{15}N-cisplatin (**1**) and the hydrolysis products *cis*-[PtCl(H_2O)($^{15}NH_3$)$_2$]$^+$ (**2**) and *cis*-[Pt(H_2O)$_2$($^{15}NH_3$)$_2$]$^{2+}$ (**3**) in 95% H_2O-5% D_2O at pH 4.72. The assignments are based on the ^{15}N-shifts, which are diagnostic of the ligands *trans* to each NH_3-Pt group (Fig. 4). ^{195}Pt satellites are marked with an asterisk. Plots of the Pt-NH_3 ^{1}H NMR chemical shifts vs pH for (**B**) complex **2** and (**C**) complex **3** allowed direct determination of the acid dissociation constants pK_{a1}, pK_{a2} and pK_{a3} (Scheme 1). (Adapted from ref. 27.)

pling constant are sensitive to the ligand *trans* to the ammine (Section 7.2). Appleton et. al.*(19)* used this approach to obtain the first direct measurements of the pK_as of the cisplatin hydrolysis products. However, polymerization was still a problem at the high concentrations of Pt (*approx* 100 m*M*) needed for direct observation of ^{15}N and the measurements had to be carried out at 5°C.

The use of indirect [^{1}H,^{15}N] NMR methods (Section 7.2) has recently allowed the rapid and reliable determination of the pK_a values directly at low (millimolar) concentrations *(27)*. Since all hydrolysis products can be distinguished in the [^{1}H,^{15}N] NMR spectrum (Fig. 1), the problems associated with other methods are overcome.

Table 1 compares the pK_a values obtained by the different methods. The acid dissociation constants of **2** and **3** are such that, under physiological conditions the hydrolysis products will be predominantly, but not totally, in the hydroxo forms **4** and **5**.

4. KINETICS AND EQUILIBRIA IN THE HYDROLYSIS OF CISPLATIN

The popular model for the mechanism of action of cisplatin assumes that in extracellular fluid cisplatin is present as the intact drug since the high chloride con-

Table 1
Acid Dissociation Constants for Cisplatin Hydrolysis Products 2 and 3 (Scheme 1)

pK$_a$	*Temperature (°C)*	*Method*	*Ref.*
cis-$[PtCl(H_2O)(NH_3)_2]^+$(**2**)			
pK_{a1}			
6.41	27	$[^1H, ^{15}N]$ NMR	*27*
6.85	25	^{15}N NMR	*19*
6.56	37	Indirectly by studying influence of pH on reaction between **2** and Cl^-	*24*
6.3	20?	Estimate based on potentiometric data of Jensen *(29)* for **3**	
cis-$[Pt(H_2O)_2(NH_3)_2]^{2+}$(**3**)			
pK_{a2} pK_{a3}			
NO_3^- salt			
5.37 7.21	27	$[^1H, ^{15}N]$ NMR	*27*
5.93 7.87	5	^{15}N NMR	*19*
5.56 7.32	20	Potentiometry	*29*
5.52 7.10	20	Potentiometry	*82*
5.02 6.93	37	Potentiometry	*23*
5.55 7.33	20		
$CF_3SO_3^-$ salt			*23*
4.99 6.84	37		
5.24 7.10	22		
ClO_4^- salt			*23*
5.24 7.42	22		

centration (103 m*M*) prevents hydrolysis of the chloro ligands. Once inside the cell the drug is activated by the low intracellular Cl^- concentrations which shift the equilibrium to favor the aquated species that are more reactive toward nucleophiles (e.g., DNA, proteins). Estimates of the relative proportions of cisplatin and aquated species present at physiological pH, and under different Cl^- concentrations require accurate estimates of the rate and equilibrium constants for the first and second hydrolysis steps (Scheme 1), together with the acid dissociation constants pK_{a1}, pK_{a2} and pK_{a3} (see above). Until recently, estimates of the relative proportions of species present under different biological conditions *(28)* were based on pK_a values derived from the early potentiometric titration data of **3** by Jensen *(29)* and estimated values for the pK_a of the mono-aqua complex **2** *(28)*. Calculations have normally assumed an intracellular chloride concentration of

Table 2
Rate and Equilibrium Constants for the Hydrolysis of Cisplatin (Scheme 1)

Parameter	*Value*	*Condition*
k_1	$5.18 \times 10^{-5}\ s^{-1}$	25°C, I = 0.1 *M*
k_{-1}	$7.68 \times 10^{-3}\ M^{-1}\ s^{-1}$	25°C, I = 0.1 *M*
pK_1	2.17	25°C, I = 0.1 *M*
	2.07^a	37°C, I = 0.1 *M*
k_2	$2.75 \times 10^{-5}\ s^{-1}$	25°C, I = 1.0 *M*
k_{-2}	$9.27 \times 10^{-2}\ M^{-1}\ s^{-1}$	25°C, I = 1.0 *M*
pK_2	3.53	25°C, I = 1.0 *M*

[a]From ref. 33.
Data from ref. 34.

4 m*M* (the value widely cited in the cisplatin literature), but a recent study by Jennerwein and Andrews *(30)* has shown that in cancer cells chloride levels are much higher than this (e.g., 22.7 m*M* in 2008 human ovarian carcinoma cells).

Values for the rate constants (k_1, k_{-1}, k_2, k_{-2}) and equilibrium constants (K_1 and K_2) have been obtained from the careful work of House and co-workers *(25,31–34)* who, in a series of recent papers, have described a complete speciation profile for cisplatin in aqueous solution. Their studies have been carried out under stringent controls of reaction conditions so that the nature of the hydrolysis products is well defined. Buffer components that can potentially coordinate to Pt(II) have been avoided. Their most recent values for these parameters are tabulated in Table 2.

There are important differences in the hydrolysis kinetics of cisplatin that occur in acidic *(31)* and basic *(32)* solution. In an acidic aqueous solution of cisplatin (pH < 5), one of the bound chloride ions dissociates to give **2** until an equilibrium is established between **1**, **2** and the liberated chloride ion (Scheme 1). The reaction does not proceed further to produce significant amounts of **3**, as the small value for K_2 effectively prevents further chloride ion release. The rate is independent of H^+ concentration and ionic strength, and the extent of the reaction is suppressed by added chloride *(31)*. On the other hand, in basic solution (pH > 9) irreversible hydrolysis of cisplatin occurs, and both chloro ligands are lost to give the dihydroxo complex **6**. The rate is independent of the background chloride ion concentration, the hydroxide ion concentration and the ionic strength *(32)*. To assess whether base hydrolysis was likely to occur under physiological conditions, by use of a combined pH-stat/spectrophotometric technique, Miller and House *(25)* investigated the rate and extent of hydrolysis of cisplatin in non-buffered aqueous solution in the pH region 4.0–8.5, both with and without added chloride ion. Based on these results and using estimates for the equilibrium constants and acid dissociation constants available at the time *(19,31,32)*, they calculated that at

Table 3
Estimates of the Relative Proportions of Cisplatin and Aquated Species Under Physiological Conditions

Ref.	pH	$[Cl^-]$ (mM)	mol fraction (%) Cl/Cl (1)	Cl/H_2O (2)	H_2O/H_2O (3)	Cl/OH (4)	OH/H_2O (5)	OH/OH (6)	Comments
25	7.5 (25°C)	100	68	7	<1	24	<1	<1	Based on K_1 and K_2 values from refs. *31* and *32* and pK_a values from ref. *19*
30	7.2	22.7 1.5	59.2 2.5	4.6 3.1	0.06 0.6	28.6 18.9	3.8 37.9	3.7 37	Based on K_1 and pK_a values from ref. *27* and K_2 from refs. *32* and *33*
27	7.4	4	—[a]	5	0.1	—[a]	15	—[a]	Based on species observed at equilibrium by [^{1}H, ^{15}N] NMR
83	7.5	4	31	28	<1	32	7	<1	Based on old equilibrium constants, but data are in agreement with more recent estimates *25*
84	7.4	103 4	84 9.2	3.5 10	0.06 4.6	3.5 10	3.9 29.2	4.9 36.6	Old estimates based on *K* values from ref. *85*, pK_a values from ref. 86, and an estimate of pK_{a1}

[a]Not reported.

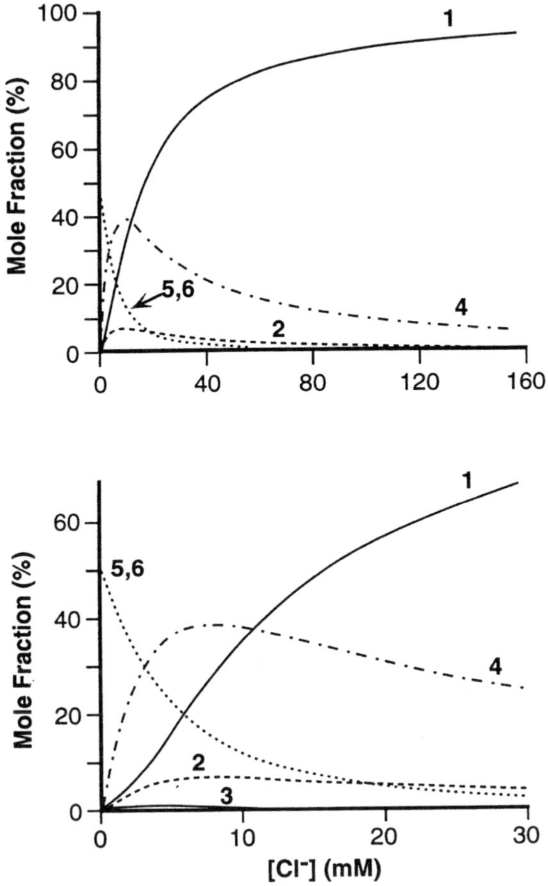

Fig. 2. Mole fraction of Pt(II) complexes vs Cl^- concentration at pH 7.2, from the work of Jennerwein and Andrews *(30)*. The structures of the different species (**1-6**) are shown in Scheme 1. The values were calculated based on recent values for equilibrium constants and acid dissociation constants: K_1, pK_{a1}, pK_{a2} and pK_{a3} from ref. *27* and K_2 from refs. *32* and *33*. The lower plot is an expansion of the upper plot for Cl^- concentrations between 0 and 30 m*M*. (Adapted from ref. *30*.)

physiological pH and extracellular chloride ion concentration an equilibrium involving **1** (68%), **2** (7%), and **4** (24%) is produced in about 6 h. At a concentration of 4 m*M* Cl^- they calculated almost complete hydrolysis of cisplatin will occur (half-life of approx 2 h at 37°C) to give a 50:50 mixture of **2** and **4**.

Table 3 summarizes the calculated equilibrium distributions of cisplatin and hydrolysis products that have been calculated to exist under physiological conditions, based on various equilibrium constant data available in the literature. Figure 2 shows distribution plots vs chloride concentration from the recent paper by

Jennerwein and Andrews *(30)* based on the most reliable recent pK_a values *(27)*. It is important to note that all these calculations pertain to equilibrium conditions that are never attained under biological conditions. Reactive aqua species removed by reaction with nucleophiles will be replaced immediately by protonation of the respective hydroxo species to maintain the equilibrium concentration as dictated by the pK_as. Inert hydroxo species can be considered therefore as mobile reservoirs of reactive platinum. Also, the ready reactions of platinum(II) aqua complexes with phosphate (*see* Section 6) suggest that the popular model assuming that cisplatin, once inside the cell in a low-chloride environment, simply loses chloride to give aqua/hydroxo complexes is probably an over simplification.

The data based on recent equilibrium constants show that the diaqua complex **(3)** will not be present at significant concentrations in either aqueous solutions of cisplatin, or under physiological conditions in vivo. Thus data in the literature that suggest experimental evidence for **3** under these conditions (e.g., ref. 35) should therefore be viewed as unreliable.

5. PREPARATION AND PURITY OF PLATINUM DRUGS

5.1. Preparation of Cisplatin

Early preparations of cisplatin and other complexes *cis*-$[PtCl_2L_2]$ (L = amine ligand) directly from $K_2[PtCl_4]$ and ammonia and L were slow, produced relatively low yields, and gave products contaminated by "Magnus salt" products $[PtL_4][PtCl_4]$ *(36)*. The "Magnus salts" could be removed from a mixture with *cis*-$[PtCl_2L_2]$ by reaction with a silver salt ($AgNO_3$ or $AgClO_4$). The bound chloride is abstracted from *cis*-$[PtCl_2L_2]$ to give solid AgCl and *cis*-$[Pt(H_2O)_2L_2]^{2+}$ *(37)*. In this reaction, $[PtL_4][PtCl_4]$ gave solid $Ag_2[PtCl_4]$, and left $[PtL_4]^{2+}$ in solution. Addition of hydrochloric acid to the solution of *cis*-$[Pt(H_2O)_2L_2]^{2+}$ causes precipitation of *cis*-$[PtCl_2L_2]$ with any contaminating AgCl removed from the solid by washing with dilute aqueous ammonia *(38)*. In 1970, Dhara *(39)* published a new procedure (Scheme 2), which, with minor modifications *(40)*, quickly became the standard method for preparation of cisplatin and other complexes *cis*-$[PtCl_2L_2]$, usually with good purity, and in high yield. Because of the high *trans* effect of iodide, *cis*-$[PtI_2L_2]$ is formed cleanly, without any significant tendency for $[PtL_4]^{2+}$ to form. The following comments on the procedure are based on the experience of the authors. A difficulty can occur if the solution in the initial reaction of $[PtCl_4]^{2-}$ with iodide is heated for too long, as this results in precipitation of black PtI_2, which reacts only slowly with L. The *cis*-$[PtI_2L_2]$ formed as the initial product may not be absolutely pure. There may, for example, be some contamination with chloro complexes. If the iodo complex is desired, it is therefore best to prepare a solution of *cis*-$[Pt(H_2O)_2L_2]^{2+}$ and add iodide to it, with warming. A small excess of iodide, with warming and stirring, is required to guard against contamination of *cis*-

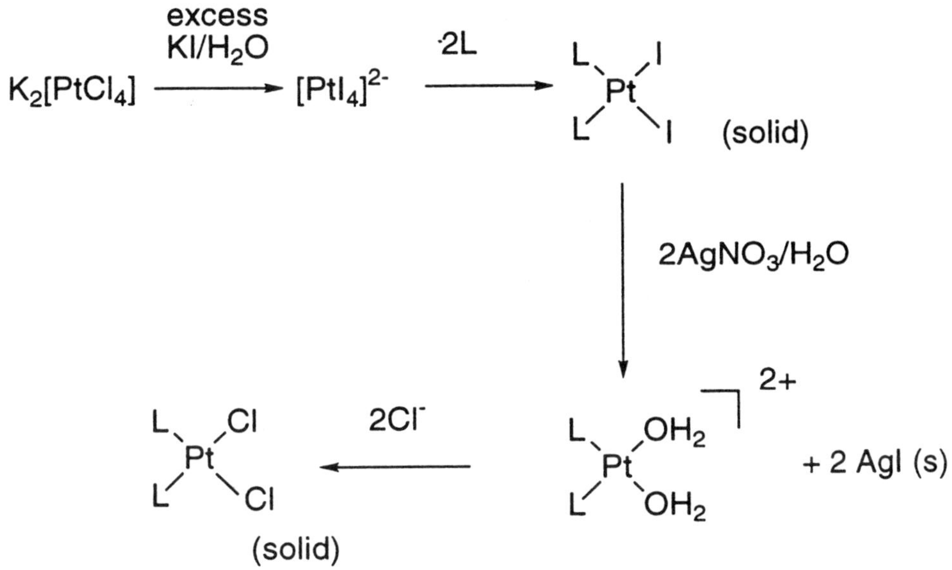

$[PtI_2L_2]$ by species such as $[\{PtL_2(\mu\text{-}I)\}_2](NO_3)_2$, which tend to be sparingly soluble *(19,41)*. The reaction of *cis*-$[PtX_2L_2]$ (X = Cl, I) with $AgNO_3$ solution proceeds well with gentle heating (up to approx 60°C), but care must be taken to avoid boiling the mixture, as this destroys all the desired product. (It is still not clear just what the chemical transformations are.)

5.1. Preparation of Cisplatin Hydrolysis Products

Solid *cis*-$[Pt(ONO_2)_2(NH_3)_2]$ is a useful starting material in the preparation of solutions containing *cis*-$[Pt(H_2O)_2(NH_3)_2]^{2+}$ (**3**). It may be obtained by removing solvent water from a solution of *cis*-$[Pt(H_2O)_2(NH_3)_2](NO_3)_2$ *(42)*. Its crystal structure has been determined *(42)*. With gentle warming and stirring, it redissolves in water to give predominantly *cis*-$[Pt(H_2O)_2(NH_3)_2](NO_3)_2$. Depending on concentration, there may be a small proportion of *cis*-$[Pt(ONO_2)(H_2O)(NH_3)_2]^+$ present *(18)*. If the amount of silver nitrate used in the preparation is slightly greater than that required to react with the halide bound to platinum, the dinitrato complex may be contaminated with silver nitrate. If the platinum complex is in slight excess in the reaction, the product may be contaminated with a small amount of chloro complex. Although, in principle, the initial *cis*-$[PtI_2(NH_3)_2]$ from the Dhara preparation could be used in the preparation of *cis*-$[Pt(ONO_2)_2(NH_3)_2]$, this is not usually advisable because the lack of purity often found in this product leads to uncertainty in the stoichiometry of the reaction. The dinitrato complex has some surface sensitivity to light, and therefore should be stored in the dark. Very similar chemistry occurs with other amines L.

cis-$[Pt(H_2O)_2(NH_3)_2](ClO_4)_2$ may be prepared in solution by analogous reactions using silver perchlorate *(37)*. There are no detectable perchlorato complexes present in solution *(18)*. The lack of an easily handled air-stable solid comparable to the nitrato complex makes the perchlorate less convenient when stoichiometry of reactions needs to be carefully controlled.

Sulfato complexes have also been used as sources of the diaqua complex when dissolved in water. However, their use is complicated by the existence of two types of compound. Reaction of *cis*-$[PtX_2(NH_3)_2]$ with Ag_2SO_4 gives a solution containing predominantly *cis*-$[Pt(H_2O)_2L_2]SO_4$, with a small amount of *cis*-$[Pt(OSO_3)(H_2O)(NH_3)_2]$ present *(18)*. Removal of solvent water at 25°C gives *cis*-$[Pt(OSO_3)(H_2O)(NH_3)_2]$ as a solid that readily redissolves in water. However, crystallization of the sulfato complex from aqueous solution at higher temperatures gives anhydrous $[Pt(SO_4)(NH_3)_2]$, which redissolves only with great difficulty. The two forms may be distinguished by infrared (IR) spectroscopy *(18)*. Analogous chemistry appears to occur with other ligands L, and the crystal structure has been determined for $[Pt(OSO_3)(H_2O)$(*N,N'*-dimethylethylenediamine)] *(43)*. McAuliffe and colleagues *(44)* have advocated a general preparative method for preparation of *cis*-(diamine)platinum(II) complexes with leaving group Z^-, *cis*-$[PtZ_2L_2]$, by reaction of a solution of *cis*-$[Pt(H_2O)_2L_2]SO_4$ with the barium salt of Z, BaZ_2. This produces a precipitate of $BaSO_4$, leaving in solution *cis*-$[PtZ_2 L_2]$ to be isolated by removal of solvent.

Unlike *cis*-$[Pt(H_2O)_2(NH_3)_2]^{2+}$ (**3**), for which the dinitrato complex is a convenient solid precursor, there is no solid compound that may be conveniently used as a source of *cis*-$[PtCl(H_2O)(NH_3)_2]^+$ (**2**). A solution of **2** cannot be obtained by reaction of solid *cis*-$[PtCl_2(NH_3)_2]$ (**1**) with an aqueous solution of 1 mol equivalent of a silver salt—such attempts produce **3**, leaving half of the initial solid **1** unreacted. However, **1** is soluble in dimethylformamide (DMF), and reaction of a solution in DMF with 1 mol equivalent of $AgNO_3$ gives a solution containing approx 80% *cis*-$[PtCl(NH_3)_2$(DMF-*O*)](NO_3), with smaller proportions of **1** and *cis*-$[Pt(NH_3)_2$(DMF-*O*)$_2](NO_3)_2$ *(2)*. Dilution of such a solution with water gives a solution containing predominantly **2**, although **1** and **3** will also be present, as well as some DMF in the solvent, which may have some effect on kinetics and equilibria. Careful addition of NaCl solution (1 mol equiv.) to a solution of **3** gives a solution containing predominantly **2**, with smaller amounts of **1** and **3** *(19)*. With care and patience, this method may be used to give a solution containing >90% **2** *(45)*. Gonnet et al. *(46)* have reported the preparation of a sample containing pure **2** in a $NaClO_4$ solution by semipreparative high-performance liquid chromatography (HPLC), with a cation exchange column as the stationary phase, and elution with $NaClO_4$ solution. Only relatively small quantities may be prepared, but this is the only method available to date that produces a solution of **2** quite uncontaminated by **1** and **3**.

A solution of **2** is thermodynamically unstable with respect to chloride redistribution reactions, which would produce, eventually, an equilibrium mixture of **1**, **2**, and **3** (Scheme 1). These reactions occur rapidly if a solution containing predominantly **2** is concentrated *(19)*. From experiments carried out by the authors, a dilute solution containing 90% **2** remains stable for approximately 4 h, after which chloride redistribution reactions become significant. Storing a solution in the refrigerator accelerates the redistribution reaction, as does a freeze-thaw cycle.

5.2. Purity of Platinum Drugs

The use of aqua complexes in preparative procedures (see above) raises the possibility that small amounts of aqua or hydroxo complexes may contaminate the products. Because these hydrolysis products are frequently very active against tumors, it is important that potential new drugs be known to be pure, and, especially, free from such impurities, before any biological testing occurs. For example, the complexes [Pt(Rida)(*R,R*-DACH)], where DACH = 1,2-diaminocyclohexane, and Rida is an iminodiacetate with substituent R on nitrogen, were initially reported to have high antitumor activity, with *O,O′*-coordination of the ligand *(47)*. It was subsequently shown *(48)* that the ligand coordinated *N,O*, as in analogous diammine complexes *(10)*, and that the pure compounds had negligible antitumor activity. A number of aminomalonate complexes prepared by Gandolfi et al. *(49)* were assigned structures with *O,O′*-coordination of the ligand, and high antitumor activity was reported. Gibson et al. *(50)* subsequently showed that the compounds contained *N,O*-chelate rings, the most stable coordination mode thermodynamically *(51)* and had no antitumor activity when purified. In a similar way, samples of [Pt(aspartate-*N,O*)(DACH)] with different DACH isomers showed antitumor activity, which disappeared when the compound was purified *(52)*.

As a general rule, every compound that is to undergo biological testing, or that is to be used clinically, should be checked for purity using all available spectroscopic and analytical techniques—especially HPLC under conditions that will detect likely impurities.

6. REACTIONS OF CISPLATIN HYDROLYSIS PRODUCTS WITH COMPONENTS OF BUFFER SOLUTIONS

The cisplatin hydrolysis products **2** and **3** react with many substances that might be used to buffer solutions, especially at pH values near 7.

In 1972, Shooter et al. *(53)* discovered that solutions of *cis*-[$PtCl_2(NH_3)_2$] (**1**) or [$PtCl_2$(en)] in phosphate buffer at 37°C slowly turn blue. Wood et al. *(54)* and subsequently Appleton et al. *(18)* studied the reactions of *cis*-[$Pt(H_2O)_2(NH_3)_2]^{2+}$ (**3**) with phosphate by multinuclear NMR. A number of phosphate-containing species were characterized, including *cis*-[Pt(-OPO_3H)(H_2O)($NH_3)_2$] and [{$Pt(NH_3)_2\}_2(\mu\text{-}PO_4H)(\mu\text{-}OH)]^+$ (**15**). Similar reactions occur with other amines, including ethylenediamine *(55)*. The blue colors that develop appear to be due to oligomeric phosphato-bridged compounds containing platinum in mixed II/III oxidation states *(56)*.

Prenzler and McFadyen *(26)* have studied the reactions of **1** and its hydrolysis products with the common buffers Tris, $NH_2C(CH_2OH)_3$, and HEPES (**18**). In the reaction of Tris with *cis*-$[Pt(OH)_2(NH_3)_2]$ (**6**) at pH 10, the initial complex was (**16**)(X = OH) with Tris bound monodentate through nitrogen, with the ultimate product the chelate complex **17**. In reaction with **1** at pH 7, Tris formed the *N,O*-chelate complex **17**, presumably via an intermediate **16** (X = Cl). Reaction of HEPES with *cis*-$[Pt(H_2O)_2(NH_3)_2]^{2+}$ (**3**) at pH 5 ultimately gave the chelate complex (**19**) in which HEPES is bound through both nitrogen atoms. Intermediate complexes were observed in which HEPES was bound through one nitrogen atom only, with no discrimination between the different nitrogen atoms. The reaction of cisplatin (**1**) HEPES at pH 7 (40°C) was slow, very much slower than the reaction with Tris, but, after 19 h, still producing 60% of the platinum as the chelate complex **19.**

To our knowledge, there is no buffer that can safely be considered to be unreactive toward cisplatin and its hydrolysis products under physiological conditions. Unless account is taken of the reactions of these compounds with the buffers, it is safer to control pH by careful additions of acid or base. These considerations may not apply to other platinum compounds that are kinetically more inert.

7. TECHNIQUES FOR CHARACTERIZING CISPLATIN HYDROLYSIS PRODUCTS AND METABOLITES IN BODY FLUIDS

7.1. HPLC

HPLC methods provide a convenient high-sensitivity method for detection and monitoring of cisplatin and its hydrolysis products in a variety of media, including biological fluids. Most systems have used a form of reversed-phase HPLC. In a typical reversed-phase experiment, in which the separation of cationic species is desired, a stationary phase is used consisting of silica particles with a hydrocarbon (C_8 or C_{18}) surface. Elution is with an aqueous solution, usually containing an organic modifier such as methanol, isopropanol, or acetonitrile, to adjust polarity. An "ion-pairing" agent is usually used in the mobile phase, such as sodium dodecylsulfate (SDS) or hexanesulfonic acid. These may function by adsorption onto the hydrocarbon surface of the stationary phase, giving it some ion-exchange character, by forming an ion-pair complex with cations, effectively rendering them into less polar species with reduced charge, or by a combination of these effects. For species with ionizable protons, it is also necessary to control the pH of the solution.

In a number of the attempts that have been used to apply reversed-phase HPLC to the monitoring of cisplatin hydrolysis products, insufficient account has been taken of the reactivity of these compounds with potential ligands. Thus, a number of authors have used phosphate, or phosphate-borate buffers in the mobile phase *(57–59)*. As mentioned above, phosphate is a very good ligand for platinum(II) and readily displaces coordinated water. Not surprisingly, therefore, De Waal et al. *(60)* and Heudi et al. *(61)* have found that on-column reactions occur between phosphate and cisplatin hydrolysis products. Acetonitrile has been used as an organic modifier *(62)*, although it binds well to platinum(II) and reacts readily with the aqua complexes **2** and **3** under the conditions used in chromatography *(45)*. Carboxylic acids have also been used in the mobile phase, with the functions of adjusting pH and acting as an organic modifier *(63)*. Heudi et al. *(61)* did not detect interaction between formic acid and **2** and **3**. However, acetate ion is a good ligand for platinum(II) and readily displaces coordinated water *(18)*. Acetic, formic, and trifluoroacetic acids all react with the platinum(II) aqua complexes in aqueous solution *(45)*.

The presence in a mobile phase of species that can bind to the platinum aqua complexes is clearly undesirable, and can lead to conclusions that are erroneous.

Neither of the "ion-pairing" agents SDS or hexanesulfonate reacts significantly with platinum aqua complexes in aqueous solution *(45)*. However, commercial SDS contains sufficient chloride impurity to affect results. This chloride should be removed before this agent is used *(45)*.

A mobile phase that does not contain any components that will bind to platinum(II) under the elution conditions has been proposed *(45)*: an aqueous solution containing 3% methanol (v/v) as an organic modifier, purified SDS, with pH adjusted to 2.5 with trifluoromethanesulfonic ("triflic") acid. Neither triflate ion nor methanol bind to platinum(II) in this aqueous solution. SDS gives better separation of the peaks from **1**, **2**, and **3** than hexanesulfonate, with the separation increasing as SDS concentration is increased from 0.05 to 0.5 m*M*.

It should be mentioned that the presence of reactive species in the mobile phase may not cause difficulty if the platinum compounds being separated are more robust than the aqua complexes for example, if the only compounds of interest are methionine chelate complexes.

Gonnet et al. *(46)* used an anion exchange resin as the stationary phase, and elution with $NaClO_4$ solution to prepare solutions of *cis*-$[PtCl(H_2O)(NH_3)_2]^+$ (**2**). This method could also be used to detect and monitor this species, although it may be less suitable for monitoring *cis*-$[Pt(H_2O)_2(NH_3)_2]^{2+}$ (**3**), which gives a very broad peak under the conditions used.

Ultraviolet (UV) detection is convenient when exceptional sensitivity is not required, as the platinum(II) complexes all absorb strongly between 250 and 320 nm. For monitoring the platinum compounds in ultrafiltered plasma, it is useful to use 305 nm for detection, as many of the organic components in plasma do not absorb strongly at this wavelength *(45)*. Greater sensitivity may be obtained by the use of inductively coupled plasma-mass spectrometry (ICP-MS) techniques, *(60,63)*, and this also detects only species containing platinum, allowing platinum compounds to be monitored in the presence of complex mixtures of organic compounds.

7.2. NMR Spectroscopy

NMR spectroscopy offers significant advantages over other methods used for the determination of platinum compounds in biological media because it allows the possibility of the detection of species without the need for chemical separations. The application of NMR spectroscopy for studying the biospeciation of platinum drugs has been reviewed recently *(64,65)*. Several NMR nuclei can be used for studies of the aqueous solution of platinum drugs (Table 4) and spin-1/2 nuclei are the most useful because the sharper lines are more readily detected. The suitability of a given nucleus for direct NMR studies is roughly indicated by its receptivity, a quantity that takes into account both the natural abundance and inherent sensitivity to detection (determined by the gyromagnetic ratio, γ). The sensitivity increases at approx $B_o^{3/2}$ (where Bo is the magnetic field strength) and so the lowest detection limits (down to approx 5 μM) are achieved for ^{1}H at high magnetic field strengths (e.g., 600- or, 750-MHz spectrometers). ^{195}Pt is considerably less sensitive but has the advantage that changes in the metal coordination sphere can be monitored directly from the ^{195}Pt chemical shift, which is sensitive to the nature of the coordinated ligands. ^{14}N has a relatively high receptivity, but it is a quadrupolar nucleus, and quadrupolar relaxation, which dominates when the environment of ^{14}N has a low symmetry, can lead to very broad lines that are hard to detect.

On the other hand, one advantage of short relaxation times is that rapid pulsing can be employed, and a large number of transients can be acquired in a short time. ^{14}N NMR has been used to follow reactions of cisplatin in blood plasma at millimolar drug concentrations and to detect ammine release *(66)*. The spin-1/2 ^{15}N nucleus is usually preferred, and ^{15}N NMR studies have been used extensively to study the aqueous solution chemistry of cisplatin (see below). Increasingly ^{1}H NMR is being used for the inverse detection of other spin-1/2 nuclei to which it is coupled (especially ^{13}C and ^{15}N). By the use of inverse detection methods the sensitivity of ^{15}N detection can be improved by a factor of 306 ($|\gamma H/\gamma \mathrm{N}|^{5/2}$) such that signals can be detected at concentrations as low as 5 μM. These methods can be used to study ^{15}N-cisplatin and analogs that have measurable spin-spin couplings to ^{1}H (i.e., ammine, primary and secondary amines, not tertiary amines). Apart from the high sensitivity, a further advantage of inverse detection is that only those protons that are directly attached to ^{15}N are detected. Thus by the use of ^{1}H-{^{15}N} NMR methods, it is

Table 4
Properties of Some of the NMR Nuclei Useful in the Study of Platinum Anticancer Complexes

Nucleus	*Nuclear spin (I)*	*Abundance (%)*	*Relative receptivity*	*Frequency (MHz)*	*Approximate detection limit*
^{1}H	1/2	99.98	5682	600	5 μ*M*
^{13}C	1/2	1.11	1	150.87	10 m*M*[a]
^{195}Pt	1/2	33.8	19.1	128.46	5 m*M*
^{14}N	1	99.63	5.7	43.32	1 m*M*
^{15}N	1/2	0.37	0.02	60.81	50 m*M*[b]

[a] 10μ*M* with ^{1}H-{^{13}C} inverse detection.
[b] 1 m*M* with ^{15}N-{^{1}H} DEPT and 10 μ*M* with ^{1}H-{^{15}N} inverse detection.

now possible to follow the aqueous solution chemistry of cisplatin in body fluids or cell culture media, at concentrations close to those of physiological relevance.

7.2.1. ^{1}H NMR

^{1}H NMR studies are useful for studies of the interactions of cisplatin with biomolecules and with the components of biofluids, cell culture media, and cells. For example, ^{1}H NMR studies of cisplatin incubated with Dulbecco's cell culture medium showed that the ^{1}H singlet for the S-methyl of the L-methionine in the medium disappeared and a new peak characteristic of Pt-bound L-Met appeared *(67)*. A ^{1}H NMR study of urine samples from patients treated with carboplatin (7) demonstrated that by use of one-dimensional (1D) and 2D (COSY) methods it was possible to identify peaks for the intact drug and the free ligand CBCDA in the urine without the need for pre-concentration *(68)*. A major difficulty of ^{1}H NMR studies in biofluids has been the problem of "dynamic range", i.e., the detection of submillimolar metabolites in the presence of 55 M $^{1}H_2O$, but this has been largely overcome on modern spectrometers that allow the use of pulse sequences incorporating pulsed field gradients for solvent suppression (e.g., WATERGATE) *(69)*. ^{1}H-{^{15}N} NMR studies are now more useful than simple ^{1}H NMR studies of cisplatin in body fluids or cell culture media because they allow detection of only the drug metabolites without interference of the thousands of overlapping background resonances, which are completely filtered out (see below).

Direct ^{1}H NMR studies have been used to follow the reactions of *cis*- and *trans*-$[PtCl_2(NH_3)_2]$ inside intact red blood cells *(70)*. In this study, suppression of the $^{1}H_2O$ signal was aided by suspending the cells in D_2O-saline, and the use of a ^{1}H spin-echo pulse sequence allowed detection of only the mobile low molecular metabolites inside the cell. ^1H NMR signals from proteins and other high molecular weight metabolites were eliminated as a consequence of their short spin-spin (T_2) relaxation times. On addition of *trans*-[$PtCl_2(NH_3)_2$] to a suspension of red cells, there was a gradual decrease in the intensity of the ^1H resonances for free glutathione (GSH), and new peaks were observed that were assignable to coordinated GSH protons in *trans*-[$PtCl(SG)(NH_3)_2$], *trans*-[$Pt(SG)_2(NH_3)_2$], and possibly the S-bridged complex *trans*-[{$(NH_3)_2$ PtCl}$_2$SG]$^+$. For *cis*-[$PtCl_2(NH_3)_2$], although there was a gradual decrease in the intensity of the GSH ^1H spin-echo NMR resonances, no new peaks were resolved. This was interpreted as formation of high molecular weight Pt/GSH and mixed GS-Pt-S(hemoglobin) polymers inside the cell *(70)*.

7.2.2. ^{195}Pt NMR

^{195}Pt NMR would often be the method of choice for studying the solution chemistry of platinum complexes and its applications to the study of platinum drugs have been reviewed *(64,71)*. ^{195}Pt has a very large chemical shift range (approx 15,000 ppm), and ligand substitutions usually produce predictable chemical shift changes, Pt(II) is readily distinguished from Pt(IV) (chemical shifts are at the high field and low-field ends of the range, respectively), and there are usually ^{195}Pt chemical shift differences between geometrical isomers and diastereomers. The major limitation is the sensitivity of detection. Although ^{195}Pt NMR detection limits of 500 μ*M* have been quoted in the literature *(35)*, in the experience of the authors, drug concentrations of at least 5 m*M* are more realistic to obtain spectra within reasonable time limits (e.g., a few hours) and allow identification and quantification of cisplatin metabolites. The receptivity can be improved by a factor of three by isotopic enrichment of ^{195}Pt to >95%, but this is expensive. For ^{195}Pt, the advantage of increased sensitivity achievable at high magnetic field strengths is offset by the increase in linewidths as a consequence of efficient chemical shift anisotropy (CSA) relaxation, which can be the dominant relaxation mechanism for platinum complexes at high magnetic field strength. (CSA relaxation is proportional to B_o^2.) Similarly, ^{195}Pt satellites in ^{1}H (and ^{15}N) spectra of Pt(II) complexes are often broadened beyond detection at high magnetic fields (e.g., >7 T), due to CSA relaxation of ^{195}Pt, which precludes use of ^{1}H-{^{195}Pt} inverse detection methods to increase the sensitivity of detection. CSA relaxation is proportional also to the correlation time for molecular tumbling (τ_c) so that ^{195}Pt signals are usually very broad for Pt bound to macromolecules. A further source of broadening of ^{195}Pt resonances of platinum ammine/amine complexes is the quadrupolar effects of ^{14}N ligands. ^{195}Pt-^{14}N couplings in ^{195}Pt NMR spectra are usually better resolved at higher temperatures because the quadrupolar relaxation rate of ^{14}N decreases (decrease in correlation time). For best results, good temperature control of the sample is required because of the strong temperature dependence of ^{195}Pt NMR resonances (up to 1 ppm/K).

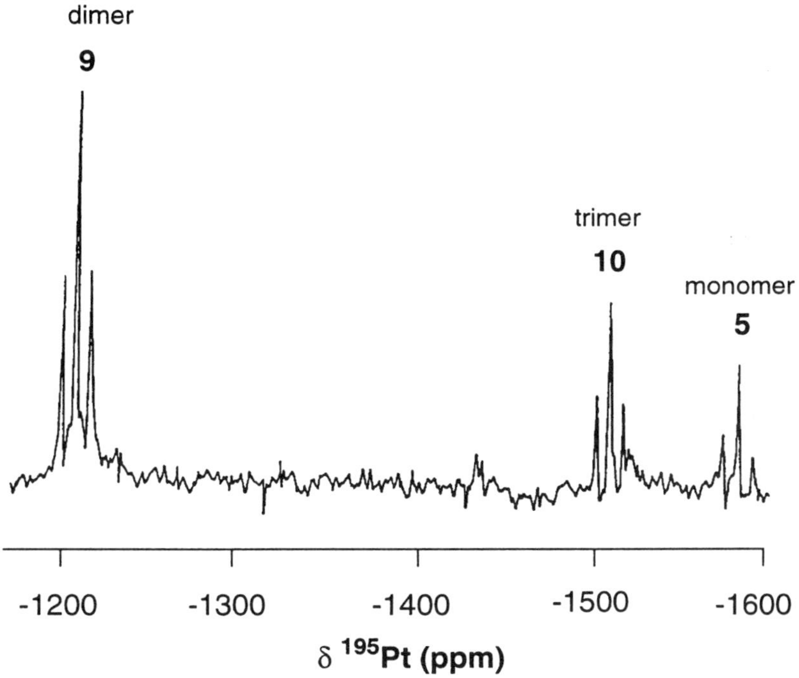

Fig. 3. The 38.7-MHz ^{195}Pt NMR spectrum of the hydroxo complex *cis*-$[Pt(OH)(H_2O)(^{15}NH_3)_2]^+$ (**5**) (at an initial concentration of 0.05 *M*) and the hydroxo-bridged dimer (**9**) and -trimer (**10**) at pD 6.4. (Adapted from ref. *72*.)

A useful application of ^{195}Pt NMR is in following the hydrolysis reactions of cisplatin and in particular the formation of hydroxo-bridged oligomers, as each hydrolysis product has a different chemical shift. If ^{15}N-labeled complexes are used, changes in $^1J(^{195}Pt\text{-}^{15}N)$ may also be observed. In an early (1978) study Rosenberg *(72)* used ^{195}Pt NMR to follow the rate of formation of hydroxo-bridged dimer (**9**) and trimer (**10**) from the monomer *cis*-$[Pt(OH)(H_2O)(NH_3)_2]$ (**5**) at pH 6.4 and an initial concentration of 50 m*M*. A spectrum showing the monomer, hydroxo-bridged dimer and trimer is shown in Figure 3. The chemical shift of the dimer is considerably downfield of the other two species, and this has been attributed *(40)* to ring strain at the metal center. The ^{195}Pt NMR chemical shifts of a range of cisplatin hydrolysis products and products of its reaction with buffer components are listed in Table 5.

7.2.3. ^{15}N NMR

^{15}N NMR is particularly useful in the study of the aqueous solution chemistry of cisplatin (and other platinum ammine/amine compounds) because ^{15}N-labeled compounds are readily prepared and both the ^{15}N chemical shift and

Table 5
^{15}N and ^{195}Pt Chemical Shifts and $^{1}J(^{15}N\text{-}^{195}Pt)$ Coupling Constants for Cisplatin and Carboplatin, the Hydrolysis Products of Cisplatin and Products of its Reaction with Buffer Components (in H_2O)

Compound	$\delta^{15}N^{a,b}$	$^{1}J(^{15}N\text{-}^{195}Pt)^{a}$	$\delta^{195}Pt^{c}$	*Ref.*
cis-[$PtCl_2(NH_3)_2$] (**1**)	−68.1 (Cl)	326		*4*
		312	−2168	*87*
cis-[$PtCl(H_2O)(NH_3)_2]^+$ (**2**)	−66.8 (Cl), −90.0 (O)			*27*
	−65.8 (Cl), −88.8 (O)	343 (Cl), 369 (O)	−1841	*19*
	−64.6 (Cl), −83.7 (O)	342 (Cl), 361 (O)	−1841	*40*
cis-[$Pt(H_2O)_2(NH_3)_2](X)_2$ (**3**)				
X = NO_3^-	−87.2 (O)	390		*70*
	−84.7 (O)	390	−1593	*40*
X = ClO_4^-	−85.8 (O)	391	−1584	*18*
cis-[$PtCl(OH)NH_3)_2$] (**4**)	−67.9 (Cl), −81.1 (O)			*70*
	−67.9 (Cl), −78.5 (O)	347 (Cl), 288 (O)	−1826	*19*
	−66.5 (Cl), −78.5 (O)	347 (Cl), 288 (O)	−1826	*40*
cis-[$Pt(OH)_2(NH_3)_2$] (**6**)	−79.9 (O)			*27*
	−76.9 (O)	293	−1572	*40*
cis-[$Pt(NH_3)_2$(CBDCA-*O,O'*)] (**7**)	−81.3 (O)	361		*4*
		360	−1723	*87*
[{$Pt(NH_3)_2(\mu\text{-}OH)\}_2]^{2+}$ (**9**)	−81.7 (O)	342		87
	−81.6 (O)	342	−1162	*40*
[{$Pt(NH_3)_2(\mu\text{-}OH)\}_3]^{3+}$ (**10**)	−79.1 (O)	339	−1499	*87*
	−78.0 (O)	342	−1520	*40*
[{$Pt(NH_3)_2(H_2O)\}_2(\mu\text{-}OH)]^{3+}$ (**12**)	−83.1 (OH_2)	397 (OH_2)	−1547	*18*
	−81.8 (OH)	339 (OH)		

$[\{Pt(NH_3)_2(OH)\}_2(\mu\text{-}OH)]^+$	−74.0 (OH) (terminal)	298	−1516	*18*
	−82.2 (OH) (bridging)	334		
$[Pt(NH_3)_2(\mu\text{-}Cl)(\mu\text{-}OH)]^{2+}$ (**13**)	−62.2 (Cl)	352	−1722	*19*
	−84.3 (O)	321		
$[Pt(NH_3)_2(\mu\text{-}OH)(\mu\text{-}O_2CCH_3)]^{2+}$ (**14**)	−77.4 (OH)	351	−1548	*18*
	−83.0 (OAc)	377		
cis-$[Pt(O_2CCH_3)(H_2O)(NH_3)_2]^+$	−87.2 (OH_2)	394	−1585	*18*
	−81.7 (OAc)	348		
cis-$[Pt(ONO_2)(H_2O)(NH_3)_2]^+$	−85.5 (OH_2)	403	−1598	*18*
	−85.5 (ONO_2)	378		
cis-$[Pt(OSO_3)(H_2O)(NH_3)_2]^+$	−85.1 (OH_2)	396	−1550	*18*
	−86.8 (OSO_3)	378		
cis-$[Pt(OPO_3H_2)(H_2O)(NH_3)_2]^+$	−85.5 (OH_2)	393	−1502	*18*
	−86.5 (OPO_3H_2)	377		
$[Pt(NH_3)_2(\mu\text{-}OH)(\mu\text{-}PO_4H)]^+$ (**15**)	−79.3 (OH)	342	−1481	*18*
	−83.4 (OPO_3H)	366		
cis-$[Pt(N,O\text{-}TrisH_{-1})(NH_3)_2]^+$ (**17**)	−65.3 (N)	d	−2304	*26*
	−81.4 (O)	d		
cis-$[Pt(N_1,N_4\text{-}HEPESH_{-1})(NH_3)_2]^+$ (**19**)	−60.4 (N)	d	−2606	*26*
	−62.7 (N)	d		

[a] Values in parentheses refer to the donor atom of the *trans* ligand.
[b] Referenced to 1.5 *M* NH_4Cl in 1 *M* HCl (refs. 4, 27), 2.4 *M* NH_4Cl in 1 *M* HCl (ref. 87), $^{15}NH_4^+$ signal from $^{15}NH_4{}^{15}NO_3$ (refs. 18, 19, 26, and 40).
[c] Referenced to $Na_2[PtCl_6]$.
[d] Not resolved.

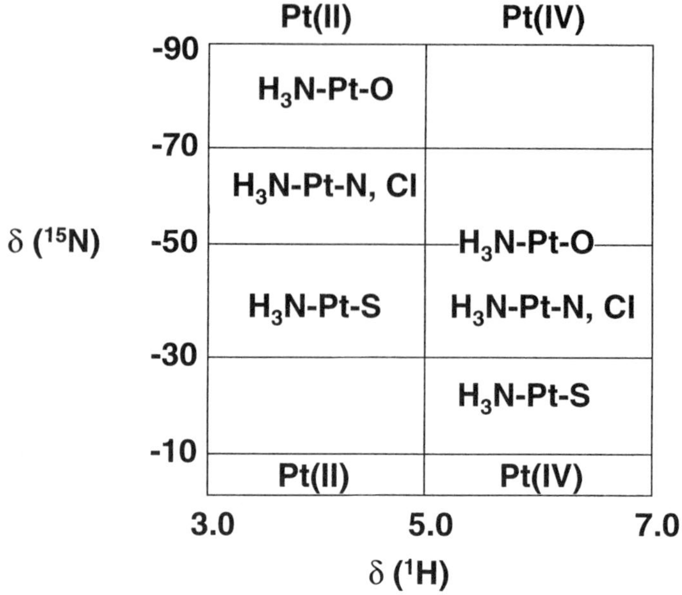

Fig. 4. Variation in ^{1}H and ^{15}N chemical shifts with the *trans* ligand in Pt-NH_3 complexes. A similar trend is obtained for Pt-NH_2 species, but the shifts are offset in both dimensions, e.g., for ethylenediamine the ^{1}H and ^{15}N peaks are shifted to higher frequency by about 2 and 40 ppm, respectively.

the $^1J(^{15}N-^{195}Pt)$ coupling constant are diagnostic of the ligand *trans* to the Pt-NH_3 group *(73)*. Typical ^{15}N shift ranges are shown in Figure 4. ^{15}N has been used extensively *(18,19,26)* to characterize the reaction products of ^{15}N-labeled cisplatin and its hydrolysis products with components of buffer solutions (e.g., phosphate, acetate, Tris, and HEPES), and the ^{15}N shifts and $^1J(^{195}Pt-^{15}N)$ coupling constants of these species are listed in Table 5.

The low receptivity of ^{15}N limits its usefulness for directly detected ^{15}N NMR studies of cisplatin, for example, in physiological fluids. The sensitivity of detection can be improved to some extent by isotopic enrichment of the 0.37% natural abundance, and further sensitivity enhancement (by a maximum of 9.8 (γH/γN)) can be achieved by polarization transfer from ^{1}H (e.g.,^{15}N-{^{1}H} INEPT and DEPT pulse sequences). These sequences have the additional advantage of allowing more rapid pulsing as the repetition time of the pulse sequence is governed by the ^{1}H rather than the longer ^{15}N spin-lattice relaxation time (T_1). For example, ^{15}N-{^{1}H} DEPT NMR methods have allowed detection of rapidly changing intermediates in the reaction of ^{15}N-cisplatin with GSH and also ammine release following reaction with intracellular components of intact red blood cells at concentrations as low as 1 m*M* *(70)*. However, inverse-detection ($^{1}H-\{^{15}N\}$) methods have now superseded these $^{15}N-\{^{1}H\}$ polarization transfer techniques, due to the far greater enhancement in the sensitivity of detection.

7.2.4. Inverse ^{1}H-{^{15}N} NMR

Over the past few years, inverse (^{1}H-detected) ^{15}N NMR methods have been applied to a wide range of studies of platinum anticancer drugs (reviewed in refs. *64* and *65*). These methods exploit the large one-bond $^{1}J(^{15}N-^{1}H)$ couplings (approx 73 Hz for $^{15}NH_3$) that are resolved for ^{15}N-cisplatin and related platinum ammine/amine complexes, to selectively detect these resonances. It is necessary to work in H_2O (as opposed to D_2O) since the NH protons usually exchange with D within minutes. The Pt-^{15}NH protons can be detected selectively by the use of heteronuclear single (or multiple) quantum coherence (HSQC and HMQC) pulse sequences. By acquiring only the first increment in a 2D experiment, a 1D ^{1}H spectrum containing only resonances from Pt-^{15}NH species is obtained; resonances for CH and OH (including water) are eliminated (Fig. 5). This is of particular value in studies in body fluids or cell culture media, in which it is possible to follow the speciation of the platinum complexes without interference from the thousands of other overlapping ^{1}H resonances, which are completely filtered out. If ^{15}N decoupling is employed during acquisition (e.g., the GARP method), then each distinct type of Pt-NH resonance appears as a singlet, sometimes together with the broadened ^{195}Pt satellites. By the use of pulse sequences incorporating pulsed field gradients (e.g., the HSQC sequence of Stonehouse et al. *(74)*, the $^{1}H_2O$ peak is eliminated without the need for additional solvent suppression techniques.

The combined detection of ^{1}H and ^{15}N in 2D inverse NMR experiments is especially powerful since the ^{15}N NMR chemical shifts [and $^{1}J(^{15}N-^{195}Pt)$ coupling constant where resolved] are diagnostic of the *trans* ligand (see above). [^{1}H, ^{15}N] NMR spectroscopy is of particular value in following the pathways of reactions of platinum ammine/amine complexes. It has the advantage that all Pt-NH species are detected simultaneously, without the need for trapping out reaction intermediates or chromatographic separation of products. It takes as little as 5–10 min to acquire a 2D [^{1}H,^{15}N] spectra, at millimolar concentrations, and pathways can be followed by observing time-dependent changes in the volumes of the ^{1}H,^{15}N resonances. These methods have recently proved particularly valuable in following the pathways of DNA platination reactions *(75–78)*. In studies of the platination of 10- and 14-mer oligonucleotides by ^{15}N-cisplatin (0.5–1 m*M*) it has been possible to determine the lifetime of the cisplatin aqua-chloro intermediate (**2**) and observe the formation of monofunctional adducts and closure to bifunctional adducts, in a single experiment *(75,76)*. The aqua-chloro intermediate **2** is readily monitored in these experiments, even though usually present at concentrations <10 μ*M*.

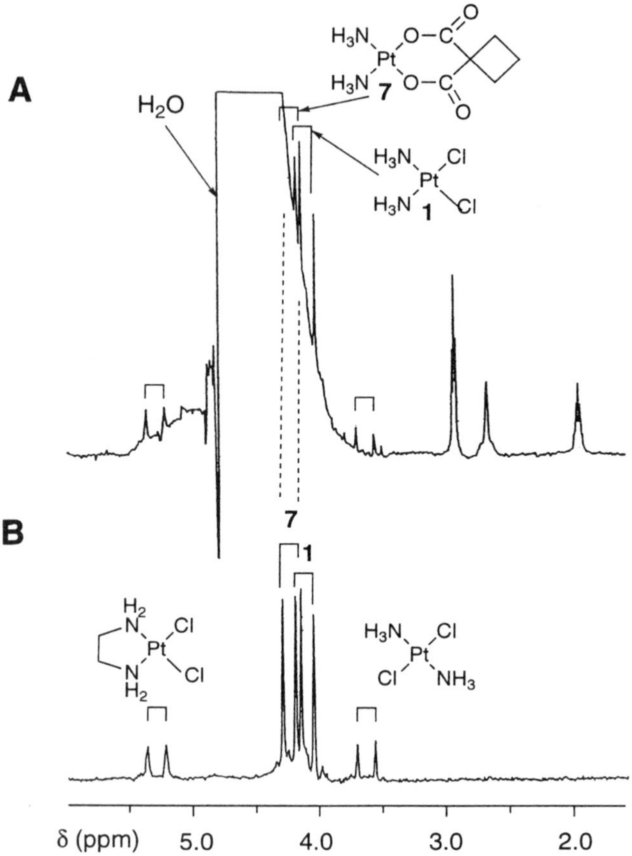

Fig. 5. ^{1}H NMR spectrum (**A**) of ^{15}N-labeled cisplatin (**1**), transplatin, carboplatin (**7**), and [Pt(en)Cl_2] in 95% H_2O-5% D_2O and (**B**) the ^{1}H-{^{15}N} spectrum. In **B**, only protons coupled to ^{15}N are selected, and these appear as doublets due to ^{15}N coupling [$^1J(^{15}N\text{-}^1H)$ approx 73 Hz]. Resonances for CH (i.e., the en- and carboplatin CH_2 protons) and OH (i.e., the ^1H_2O peak) are eliminated. If ^{15}N decoupling is used each different type of Pt-NH_3 environment appears as a singlet (along with broadened ^{195}Pt satellites). In this example, 0.5 *M* $(NH_4)_2SO_4$ was used as a relaxation agent to improve water suppression, but similar suppression could also be achieved using pulsed field gradients (see ref. *64*).

As discussed above (Section 3), by observation of ^{1}H and ^{15}N NMR chemical shifts as a function of pH, the first reliable pK_a values of both the cisplatin hydrolysis products (**2**) and (**3**) were determined by [^{1}H, ^{15}N] NMR spectroscopy *(27)* (Fig. 1). The pK_a values of aqua ligands of *cis*- and *trans*-[PtCl_2(NH_3)(cyclohexamine)] *(79)* and [Pt(dien)Cl]$^+$ *(80)* have been determined recently by [^{1}H, ^{15}N] NMR methods.

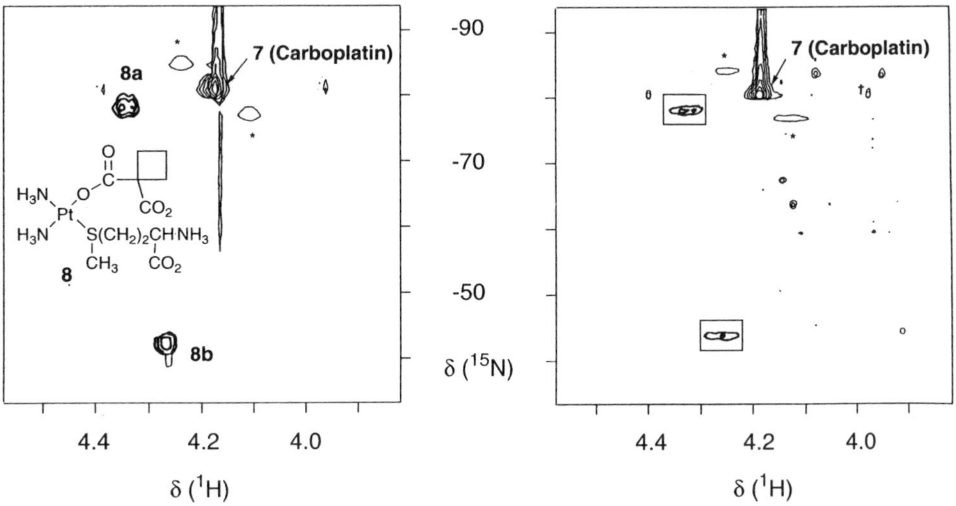

Fig. 6. [^{1}H, ^{15}N] HMQC NMR spectra of a solution containing ^{15}N-labeled carboplatin (**7**) and L-methionine in a 1:1 molar ratio 3.5 h after mixing (left) and of urine collected from mice treated with ^{15}N-carboplatin (right). The marked similarity of shifts for the boxed peaks in the spectrum of urine to those for the model complex shown on the left strongly suggests that a complex similar to the ring-opened complex **8** is excreted in urine. (Adapted from ref. *81*.)

[^{1}H, ^{15}N] NMR methods offer enormous potential for characterizing the metabolites of platinum drugs in intact body fluids, as it is possible to detect metabolites in animal urine after the administration of ^{15}N-labeled Pt complexes *(81)*. ^{15}N-editing removes background interference from other substances in urine so that detection limits are very low (10 μ*M*). For example, the spectra of urine of mice treated with ^{15}N-carboplatin have ^{1}H, ^{15}N peaks characteristic of a complex with NH_3 *trans* to O and S, which may be related to the ring opened complex [Pt(NH_3)$_2$(CBDCA-*O*)(L-Met-*S*)], which has similar shifts *(81) (Fig. 6)*.

The combination of [^{1}H,^{15}N] NMR with chromatography should be a powerful new technique for the identification of novel Pt metabolities.

8. CONCLUSIONS

The chemistry of cisplatin in aqueous solution plays an important role in the antitumor activity, metabolism, and toxicity of this and related platinum-based drugs. The popular model for the mechanism of action has assumed that cisplatin is activated by the lower intracellular chloride concentrations, which shift the equilibrium (Scheme 1) to favor the more reactive aquated species. Recent data available in the literature for equilibrium constants for the first and second hydrolysis steps of cisplatin (K_1 and K_2) *(25,31–33)*, together with reliable pK_a values for the hydrolysis product **2** and **3** *(27)* and a higher level of intracellular chloride than previously assumed *(30)*, allow calculation of revised estimates of the relative amounts of cisplatin and aquated species likely to be present under physiological conditions. However, the ready reactions of aquated platinum(II) complexes with phosphate suggest that this model is likely to be oversimplified.

In addition to phosphate, cisplatin hydrolysis products react readily with many substances commonly used in buffer solutions, (e.g., acetate, Tris, and HEPES), and there is no buffer that can be safely considered to be unreactive toward cisplatin and its hydrolysis products under physiological conditions. Caution is also needed if pH is controlled by addition of acids and bases due to the possible formation of hydroxo-bridged oligomers in solutions containing appreciable proportions of both aqua and hydroxo complexes.

Reversed-phase HPLC is a useful technique for monitoring cisplatin hydrolysis products and metabolites in body fluids, but insufficient care is often taken to exclude components from the mobile phase that can bind to platinum aqua complexes (e.g., phosphate, acetic, formic, and trifluoroacetic acids, acetonitrile). A mobile phase that does not contain any components that will bind to platinum(II) under the elution conditions has recently been proposed *(45)*.

NMR spectroscopy is a powerful tool for studying the biospeciation of platinum drugs, allowing the detection of species without the need for chemical separations. ^{195}Pt and ^{15}N NMR have been used extensively to characterize cisplatin hydrolysis products and reaction products with components of buffer solutions. Until recently, the relatively low receptivity of these isotopes has limited the usefulness of directly detected NMR studies of cisplatin in physiological fluids. However, by the use of inverse ^{1}H-{^{15}N} NMR methods, it is now possible to follow the aqueous solution chemistry of cisplatin in body fluids, at concentrations close to those of physiological relevance.

REFERENCES

1. Cleare, M. J. and Hoeschele, J. D. (1973) Studies on the antitumor activity of group VIII transition metal complexes. Part I. Platinum (II) complexes. *Bioinorg Chem.* **2,** 187–210.
2. Bancroft, D. P., Lepre, C. A., and Lippard, S. J. (1990) ^{195}Pt NMR kinetic and mechanistic studies of *cis*- and *trans*-diamminedichloroplatinum(II)binding to DNA. *J. Am. Chem. Soc.* **112,** 6860–6871.
3. Miller, S. E. and House, D. A. (1991) The hydrolysis products of *cis*-diammine-dichloroplatinum(II). 5. The anation kinetics of *cis*-Pt(X)$(NH_3)_2(OH_2)$+ (X = Cl, OH) with glycine, monohydrogen malonate and chloride. *Inorg. Chim. Acta* **187**, 125–132.
4. Frey, U., Ranford, J. D., and Sadler, P. J. (1993) Ring-opening reactions of the anticancer drug carboplatin: NMR characterisation of *cis*-[Pt$(NH_3)_2$(CBDCA-*O*)(5′GMP-N7)] in solution. *Inorg. Chem.* **32,** 1333–1340.

5. Barnham, K. J., Djuran, M. I., Murdoch, P. del S., Ranford, J. D., and Sadler, P. J. (1996) Ring-opened adducts of the anticancer drug carboplatin with sulfur amino acids. *Inorg. Chem.* **35,** 1065–1072.
6. Lempers, E. L. M. and Reedijk, J. (1991) Interactions of platinum ammine compounds with sulfur-containing biomolecules and DNA fragments. *Adv. Inorg. Chem.* **37**, 175–217.
7. Barnham, K. J., Djuran, M. I., Murdoch, P. del S., Ranford, J. D., and Sadler, P. J. (1995) L-Methionine increases the reaction of 5′-guanosine monophosphate with the anticancer drug cisplatin: mixed-ligand adducts and reversible methionine binding. *J. Chem. Soc. Dalton Trans.* 3721–3726.
8. Heudi, O., Cailleux, A., and Allain, P. (1998) Kinetic studies of the reactivity between cisplatin and its monoaquo species with L-methionine. *J. Inorg. Biochem.* **71**, 61–69.
9. van Boom, S. S. G. E. and Reedijk, J. (1993) Unprecedented migration of $[Pt(dien)]^{2+}$ (dien =1,5,-diamino-3-azapentane) from sulfur to guanosine-N^7 in S-guanosyl-L-methionine. *J. Chem. Soc. Chem. Commun.* 1397–1398.
10. Appleton, T. G., Hall, J. R., and Ralph, S. F. (1985) Reactions of platinum(II) aqua complexes. 3. Multinuclear (^{15}N, ^{195}Pt, ^{13}C and ^{1}H) NMR study of the reactions of aqua and hydroxo complexes with glycine and (methylimino)diacetic acid. *Inorg. Chem.* **24,** 673–677.
11. Faggiani, R., Lippert, B., Lock, C. J. L., and Rosenberg, B. (1977) Hydroxo-bridged platinum (II) complexes. 1. Di-μ-hydroxo-bis-[diammineplatinum(II)] nitrate, $[(NH_3)_2Pt(OH)_2Pt(NH_3)_2](NO_3)_2$. *J. Am. Chem. Soc.* **99,** 777–781.
12. Lippert, B., Lock, C. J. L., Rosenberg, B., and Zvagulis, M. (1978) Hydroxo-bridged platinum(II) complexes. 4. Crystal structure and vibrational spectra of di-μ-hydroxo-bis-[diammineplatinum(II)] carbonate dihydrate, $[(NH_3)_2Pt(OH)_2Pt(NH_3)_2](CO_3).2H_2O$. *Inorg. Chem.* **17,** 2971–2975.
13. Faggiani, R., Lippert, B., Lock, C. J. L., and Rosenberg, B. (1977) Hydroxo-bridged platinum(II) complexes. 2. Crystallographic characterization and vibrational spectra of *cyclo*-tri-μ-hydroxo-tris-[*cis*-diammineplatinum(II)] nitrate. *Inorg. Chem.* **16,** 1192–1196.
14. Gill, D. S. and Rosenberg, B. (1982) Synthesis, kinetics and mechanism of formation of polynuclear hydroxo-bridged complexes of (*trans*-1,2-diamino-cyclohexane)platinum(II)] trisulfate. *J. Am. Chem. Soc.* **104,** 4598–4604.
15. Macquet, J. P., Gros, S., and Beauchamp, A. L. (1985) Preparation and crystal structure of the hydroxo-bridged complex bis{cyclo-tri-μ-hydroxo-tris[*trans*-1,2-diaminocyclohexane) platinum(II)]trisulfate. *J. Inorg. Biochem.* **25,** 197–206.
16. Rochon, F. D., Morneau, A., and Melanson, R. (1988) Crystal structure of a hydroxo-bridged platinum(II) tetramer, *cyclo*-tetrakis(μ-hydroxo)tetrakis-(ethylenediamine)platinum(II) tetranitrate. *Inorg. Chem.* **27,** 10–13.
17. Rochon, F. D., Melanson, R., and Morneau, A. (1992) ^{195}Pt and ^{1}H NMR study of the products of hydrolysis of $Pt(L)X_2$, where L is an ethylenediamine derivative, and the crystal structure of $[Pt($*N,N*-dimethylenediamine$)(\mu\text{-}OH)]2(NO_3)_2$. *Magn. Reson. Chem.* **30,** 697–706.
18. Appleton, T. G., Berry, R. D., Davis, C. A., Hall, J. R., and Kimlin, H. A. (1984) Reactions of platinum(II) aqua complexes. 1. Multinuclear (^{195}Pt, ^{15}N, and ^{31}P) NMR study of reactions between the *cis*-diamminediaquaplatinum(II) cation and the oxygen-donor ligands hydroxide, perchlorate, nitrate, sulfate, phosphate, and acetate. *Inorg. Chem.* **23,** 3514–3521.
19. Appleton, T. G., Hall, J. R., Ralph, S. F., and Thompson, C. S. M. (1989) NMR study of acid-base equilibria and other reactions of ammineplatinum complexes with aqua and hydroxo ligands. *Inorg. Chem.* **28,,** 1989–1993.
20. Appleton, T. G., Mathieson, M., Byriel, K. A., and Kennard, C. H. L. (1998) Crystal structure of (μ-acetato-*O,O*')(μ-hydroxo)bis(diammine)platinum (II) nitrate. *Z. Krist.* **213**, 247–248.
21. Appleton, T. G., Hall, J. R., and Ralph, S. F. (1986) ^{15}N and ^{195}Pt NMR study of the effect of chain length, *n*, on the reactions of amino acids $^{+}NH_3(CH_2)nCO_2$- (n=1,2,3) with platinum(II)ammine complexes. *Aust. J. Chem.* **39,** 1347–1362.
22. Appleton, T. G., Hall, J. R., and McMahon, I. J. (1986) Multinuclear NMR study of reac-

tions of methylphosphonic acid, $CH_3PO_3H_2$ and aminoalkyl-phosphonic acids $NH_2(CH_2)nPO_3H_2$ (n=1,3) with the *cis*-diamminediaqua-platinum(II) cation and *cis*-diamminedihydroxoplatinum(II). *Inorg. Chem.* **25,** 720–725.

23. Orton, D. M., Gretton, V. A., and Green, M. (1993) Acidity constants for *cis*-diaquadi-ammineplatinum(II), the aquated form of cisplatin. *Inorg. Chim. Acta* **204,** 265–266.
24. Andersson, A., Hedenmalm, H., Elfsson, B., and Ehrsson, H. (1994) Determination of the acid dissociation constant for *cis*-diammineaqua-chloroplatinum(II) ion—a hydrolysis product of cisplatin. *J. Pharm. Sci.* **83,** 859–862.
25. Miller, S. E. and House, D. A. (1990) The hydrolysis products of *cis*-dichloro-diammine-platinum(II) 3. Hydrolysis kinetics at physiological pH. *Inorg. Chim. Acta* **173,** 53–60.
26. Prenzler, P. D. and McFadyen, W. D. (1997) Reactions of cisplatin and the *cis*-diamminedi-aqua platinum(II) cation with Tris and HEPES. *J. Inorg. Biochem.* **68,** 279–282.
27. Berners-Price, S. J., Frenkiel, T. A., Frey, U., Ranford, J. D., and Sadler, P. J. (1992) Hydrolysis products of cisplatin: pK_a determinations *via* [^{1}H,^{15}N] NMR Spectroscopy. *J. Chem. Soc. Chem. Commun.* 789–791.
28. Martin, R. B. (1983) Hydrolytic equilibria and N*7* versus N*1* binding in purine nucleosides of cis-diamminedichloroplatinum(II). *Am. Chem. Soc. Symp. Ser* **208,** 231–244.
29. Jensen, K. A. (1939) The acid strengths of the stereoisomeric diaquo-diammineplato ions. *Z. Anorg. Allgem. Chem* **242,** 87–91.
30. Jennerwein, M. and Andrews, P. A. (1995) Effect of intracellular chloride concentration on the cellular pharmacodynamics of *cis*-diammine-dichloroplatinum(II). *Drug Metab. and Dispos.* **23,** 178–184.
31. Miller, S. E. and House, D. A. (1989) The hydrolysis products of *cis*-diammine-dichloro-platinum(II), 1. The kinetics of formation and anation of the *cis*-diammine(aqua)chloroplat-inum(II) cation in acidic aqueous solution. *Inorg. Chim. Acta* **161,** 131–137.
32. Miller, S. E. and House, D. A. (1989) The hydrolysis products of *cis*-dichlorodiammine-platinum(II) 2. The kinetics of formation and anation of the *cis*-diamminedi(aqua)plat-inum(II) cation. *Inorg. Chim. Acta* **166,** 189–197.
33. Miller, S. E., Gerard, K. J., and House, D. A. (1991) The hydrolysis products of *cis*-di-amminedichloroplatinum(II) 6. A kinetic comparison of the *cis*- and *trans*-isomers and other *cis*-di(amine)di(chloro)platinum(II) compounds. *Inorg. Chim. Acta.* **190,** 135–144.
34. Hindmarsh, K., House, D. A., and Turnbull, M. M. (1997) The hydrolysis products of *cis*-diamminedichloroplatinum(II) 9. Chloride and bromide anation kinetics for some $[Pt(II)(N)_2(OH_2)_2]^{2+}$ complexes and the structures of $[Pt(IV)Br_4(N)_2]$ ((N_2) = en,tn). *Inorg. Chim. Acta* **257,** 11–18.
35. Briere, K. M., Goel, R., Shirazi, F. H., Stewart, D. J., and Smith, I. C. P. (1996) The integrity of cisplatin in aqueous and plasma ultrafiltrate media studied by ^{195}Pt and ^{15}N nuclear magnetic resonance. *Cancer Chemother. Pharmacol.* **37,** 518–524.
36. Basolo, F., Bailar, J. C., and Tarr, B. R. (1950) The stereochemistry of complex inorganic compounds. X. The stereoisomers of dichlorobis(ethylenediamine)-platinum(IV)chloride. *J. Am. Chem. Soc.* **72,** 2433–2438.
37. Glass, G. E., Scwabacher, W. B., and Tobias, R. S. (1968) Oxygen-17 nuclear magnetic resonance studies of the hydration of organometallic cations. *Inorg. Chem.* **7,** 2471–2478.
38. Appleton, T. G. and Hall, J. R. (1970) Complexes with six-membered chelate rings. I. Preparation of platinum(II) and palladium(II) complexes of trimethylene-diamine and some methyl-substituted derivatives. *Inorg. Chem.* **9,** 1800–1806.
39. Dhara, S. C. (1970) A rapid method for the synthesis of *cis*-$[Pt(NH_3)_2Cl_2]$. *Ind. J. Chem.* **8,** 193–194.
40. Boreham, C. J., Broomhead, J. A., and Fairlie, D. P. (1981) A ^{195}Pt and ^{15}N NMR study of the anticancer drug, *cis*-diamminedichloroplatinum(II) and its hydrolysis and oligomerization products. *Aust. J. Chem.* **34,** 659–664.
41. O'Halloran, T. V., Lippard, S. J., Richmond, T. J., and Klug, A. (1987) Multiple heavy-atom

reagents for molecular X-ray structure determination. Application to the nucleosome core particle. *J. Mol. Biol.* **194,** 705–712.

42. Lippert, B., Lock, C. J. L., Rosenberg, B., and Zvagulis, M. (1977) *cis*-Dinitratodiammineplatinum(II), *cis*-$Pt(NH_3)_2(NO_3)_2$. *Inorg. Chem.* **16,** 1525–1529.
43. Rochon, F. D. and Melanson, R. (1987) Molecular and crystal structure of a platinum(II) complex with aquo and sulfate ligands: aquo(*N,N*'-dimethyl-ethylenedeiamine)(sulfato)platinum(II) hydrate. *Inorg. Chem.* **26,** 989–992.
44. Harrison, R. C., McAuliffe, C. A., and Zaki, A. M. (1980) An efficient route for the preparation of highly soluble platinum(II) antitumour agents. *Inorg. Chim. Acta* **46,** L15-L16.
45. El-Khateeb, M., Appleton, T. G., Charles, B. G., and Gahan, L. R. (1999) Development of HPLC conditions for valid determination of hydrolysis products of cisplatin. *J Pharm. Sci.* **88,** 319–326.
46. Gonnet, F., Lemaire, D., Kozelka, J., and Chottard, J.-C. (1993) Isolation of *cis*-$[PtCl(NH_3)_2(H_2O)](ClO_4)$, the monohydrated form of the anti-tumour drug cisplatin, using cation-exchange high performance liquid chromatography. *J. Chromatogr.* **648,** 279–282.
47. Hacker, M. P., Khokhar, A. R., Krakoff, I. H., Brown, D. F., and McCormack, J. (1986) Water-soluble N-substituted iminodiactetate(1,2-diamino-cyclohexane)platinum(II) complexes as potential antitumor agents. *J. Cancer. Res.* **46,** 6250–6254.
48. Hoeschele, J. D., Farrell, N., Turner, W. R., and Rithner, C. D. (1988) Synthesis and characterisation of diastereomeric (substituted iminodiacetate)(1,2-diaminocyclohexane)platinum(II) complexes. *Inorg. Chem.* **27,** 4106–4113.
49. Gandolfi, O., Apfelbaum, H. C., and Blum, J. (1987) Aminomalonate(1,2-diamino-cyclohexane)platinum(II): a competitive antitumour compound with a new class of neutral, chemically stable, water soluble, functionalized platinum(II) complexes. *Inorg. Chim. Acta* **135,** 27–31.
50. Gibson, D., Rosenfeld, A., Apfelbaum, H., and Blum, J. (1990) Multinuclear (^{195}Pt, ^{15}N, ^{13}C) NMR studies of the reactions between *cis*-diammine-diaquaplatinum(II) complexes and aminomalonate. *Inorg. Chem.* **29,** 5125–5129.
51. Appleton, T. G., Hall, J. R., Neale, D. W., and Thompson, C. S. M. (1990) Reactions of the *cis*-diamminediaquaplatinum(II) cation with with 2-amino-malonic acid and its homologues, aspartic and glutamic acids. Rearrangement of metastable complexes with carboxylate-bound ligands to N,O chelates and formation of di- and tri-nuclear complexes. *Inorg. Chem.* **29,** 3985–3990.
52. Talebian, A. H., Bensely, D., Ghiorghis, A., Hammer, C. F., Schein, P. S., and Green, D. (1991) Asparto(1,2-cyclohexanediamine)platinum(II) complexes: synthesis and characterisation; effects of minor impurities on antitumour activity. *Inorg. Chim. Acta* **179,** 281–287.
53. Shooter, K. V., Howse, R., Merrifield, R. K., and Robins, A. B. (1972) Interaction of platinum(II) compounds with bacteriophages. *Chem. Biol. Interact.* **5,** 289–307.
54. Wood, F. E., Hunt, C. T., and Balch, A. L. (1982) ^{195}Pt and ^{31}P nuclear magnetic resonance studies of the binding of the *cis*-$Pt(NH_3)_2^{2+}$ moiety to phosphate in aqueous solution. *Inorg. Chim. Acta* **67,** L19-L20.
55. Bose, R. N., Goswani, N., and Moghaddas, S. (1990) Phosphato complexes of platinum(II): phosphorus-31 NMR and kinetics of formation and isomerization studies. *Inorg. Chem.* **29,** 3461–3467.
56. Appleton, T. G., Berry, R. D., and Hall, J. R. (1982) `Platinum phosphate blues'. A comparison with `amide blues.' *Inorg. Chim. Acta* **64,** L229-L233.
57. Andersson, A., Fagerberg, J., Lewensohn, R., and Ehrsson, H. (1996) Pharmacokinetics of cisplatin and its monohydrated complex in humans. *J. Pharm. Sci.* **85,** 824–827.
58. Wenclawiak, B. W. and Wollmann, M. (1996) Separation of platinum(II) anti-tumour drugs by micellar electrokinetic capillary chromatography. *J. Chromatogr. A* **724,** 317–326.
59. Shearan, P., Alvarez, J. M. F., Zayed, N., and Smyth, M. R. (1990) High performance liquid chromatography separation of cisplatin and its hydrolysis products on alumina and application to studies of their interaction with cysteine. *Biomed. Chromatogr.* **4,** 78–82.

60. DeWaal, W. A. J., Maessen, F. J. M. J., and Kraak, J. C. (1987) Analysis of platinum species originating from *cis*-diamminedichloroplatinum(II) cisplatin in human and rat plasma by high-performance liquid chromatography with on-line inductively coupled plasma atomic emission spectrometric detection. *J. Chromatogr.* **407,** 253–272.
61. Heudi, O., Caillieux, A., and Allain, P. (1997) Interactions between cisplatin derivatives and mobile phase during chromatographic separation. *Chromatographia* **44,** 19–24.
62. Daley-Yates, P. T. and O'Brien, D. C. H. (1984) Cisplatin metabolites in plasma. A study of their pharmacokinetics and importance in the nephrotoxic and antitumour activity of cisplatin. *Biochem. Pharmacol.* **33,** 3063–3067.
63. Zhao, Z., Tepperman, K., Dorsey, J. G., and Elder, R. C. (1993) Determination of cisplatin and some possible metabolites by ion-pairing chromatography with inductively coupled plasma mass spectroscopic determination. *J. Chromatogr. Biomed. Applic.* **615,** 83–89.
64. Berners-Price, S. J. and Sadler, P. J. (1996) Coordination chemistry of metallodrugs—insights into biological speciation from NMR spectroscopy. *Coord. Chem. Rev.* **151,** 1–40.
65. Barnham, K. J., Berners-Price, S. J., Guo, Z., Murdoch, P. del S., and Sadler, P. J. (1996) NMR spectroscopy of platinum drugs: from DNA to body fluids, in *Platinum and Other Metal Coordination Compounds in Cancer Chemotherapy 2* (Pinedo, H. M. and J. H. Schmogale, eds.), Plenum, New York, pp. 1–16.
66. Norman, R. E. and Sadler, P. J. (1988) ^{14}N NMR studies of amine release from anticancer drugs: models and human blood plasma. *Inorg. Chem.* **27,** 3583–3587.
67. Bell, J. D., Norman, R. E., and Sadler, P. J. (1987) Coordination chemistry in biological media: reactions of antitumour Pt(II) and Au(III) complexes with cell culture media. *J. Inorg. Biochem.* **31,** 241–246.
68. Ranford, J. D., Sadler, P. J., Balmanno, K., and Newell, D. R. (1991) ^{1}H NMR studies of human urine: urinary elimination of the anticancer drug carboplatin. *Magn. Reson. Chem.* **29,** S125–129.
69. Piotto, M., Saudek, V., and Sklenar, V. (1992) Gradient-tailored excitation for single-quantum NMR spectroscopy of aqueous solutions. *J. Biomol. NMR* **2,** 661–665.
70. Berners-Price, S. J. and Kuchel, P. W. (1990) The reaction of *cis*- and *trans*-$[PtCl_2(NH_3)_2]$ with reduced glutathione inside human red blood cells studied by ^{1}H and ^{15}N-{^{1}H} DEPT NMR. *J. Inorg. Biochem.* **38,** 327–345.
71. Macdonald, F. and Sadler, P. J. (1986) ^{195}Pt NMR spectroscopy: applications to the study of anticancer drugs, in *Biochemical Mechanisms of Platinum Antitumour Drugs* (McBrien, D. C. H. and T. F. Slater, eds.), IRL , Oxford, pp. 361–381.
72. Rosenberg, B. (1978) Platinum complex-DNA interactions and anticancer activity. *Biochimie* **60,** 859–867.
73. Appleton, T. G., Hall, J. R., and Ralph, S. F. (1985) ^{15}N and ^{195}Pt NMR spectra of platinum ammine complexes: *trans* and *cis*-influence series based on ^{195}Pt-^{15}N coupling constants and ^{15}N chemical shifts. *Inorg. Chem.* **24,** 4685–4693.
74. Stonehouse, J., Shaw, G. L., Keeler, J., and Laue, E. D. (1994) Minimizing sensitivity losses in gradient-selected ^{15}N-^{1}H HSQC spectra of proteins. *J. Magn. Reson. Series A* **107,** 174–184.
75. Barnham, K. J., Berners-Price, S. J., Frenkiel, T. A., and Sadler, P. J. (1995) Platination pathways for reactions of cisplatin with GG single-stranded and double-stranded decanucleotides. *Angew. Chem. Int. Ed.* **34,** 1874–1877.
76. Berners-Price, S. J., Barnham, K. J., Frey, U., and Sadler, P. J. (1996) Kinetic analysis of the stepwise platination of single- and double-stranded GG oligonucleotides with cisplatin and *cis*-$[PtCl(H_2O)(NH_3)_2]^+$. *Chem. Eur. J.* **2,** 1283–1291.
77. Reeder, F., Guo, Z., Murdoch, P. del S., Corazza, A., Hambley, T. W., Berners-Price, S. J., Chottard, J.-C., and Sadler, P. J. (1997) Platination of a GG single- and double-stranded 14-mer oligonucleotide with diaqua cisplatin followed by NMR and HPLC. Influence of the platinium ligands and base sequence on 5′-G versus 3'-G platination selectivity . *Eur. J. Biochem.* **249,** 370–382.

78. Davies, M. S., Berners-Price, S. J., and Hambley, T. W. (1998) Rates of platination of double stranded AG and GA containing oligonucleotides: insights into why cisplatin binds to AG but not GA Sequences in DNA. *J. Am. Chem. Soc.* **120,** 11380–11390.
79. Barton, S. J., Barnham, K. J., Habtemariam, A., Sue, R. E., and Sadler, P. J. (1998) pK_a values of aqua ligands of platinum(II) anticancer complexes: [^{1}H,^{15}N] and ^{195}Pt NMR studies of *cis*- and *trans*-[$PtCl_2(NH_3)$(cyclohexamine)]. *Inorg. Chim. Acta* **273,** 8–13.
80. Guo, Z., Chen, Y., Zang, E., and Sadler, P. J. (1997) [^{1}H,^{15}N] nuclear magnetic resonance studies of $[Pt(dien)Cl]^+$ (dien = diethylenetriamine): hydrolysis and reactions with nucleotides. *J. Chem. Soc. Dalton Trans.* 4107–4111.
81. Barnham, K. J., Frey, U., Murdoch, P. del S., Ranford, J. D., and Sadler, P. J. (1994) [Pt(CBDCA-*O*)$(NH_3)_2$(L-methionine-*S*)]: ring-opened adduct of the anticancer drug carboplatin ("paraplatin"). Detection of a similar complex in urine by NMR spectroscopy. *J. Am. Chem. Soc.* **116,** 11175–11176.
82. Grinberg, A. A., Stetsenko, A. I., Mitkinova, N. D., and Tikhonova, L. S. (1971) Acid properties of aqua complexes of platinum(II). *Russ. J. Inorg. Chem.* **16,** 137. (*Zh. Neorg. Khim.* **116** 1264–1266).
83. LeRoy, A. F., Lutz, R. J., Dedrick, R. L., Litterst, C. L., and Gaurino, A. M. (1979) Pharmacokinetic study of *cis*-dichlorodiammineplatinum(II) (DDP) in the beagle dog: thermodynamic and kinetic behaviour of DDP in the biologic milieu. *Cancer Treat. Rep.* **63,** 59–71.
84. Howe-Grant, M. E. and Lippard, S. J. (1980) Aqueous platinum(II) chemistry: binding to biological molecules. *Metal Ions Biol. Syst.* **11,** 63–125.
85. Lee, K. W. and Martin, D. S. Jr. (1976) *cis*Dichlorodiammineplatinum(II) aquation equilibria and isotopic exchange of chloride ions with free chloride and tetrachloroplatinate(II). *Inorg. Chim. Acta* **17,** 105–110.
86. Lim, M. C. and Martin, R. B. (1976) The nature of *cis* amine Pd(II) and antitumour *cis* amine Pt(II) complexes in aqueous solutions. *J. Inorg. Nucl. Chem.* **38,** 1911–1914.
87. Ismail, I. M. and Sadler, P. J. (1983) ^{195}Pt and ^{15}N NMR studies of antitumor complexes. *Am. Chem. Soc. Symp. Ser.* **209,** 171–190.

2 Chemistry and Structural Biology of 1,2-Interstrand Adducts of Cisplatin

Viktor Brabec

CONTENTS

1. FREQUENCY

Shortly after the discovery of the cytostatic activity of cis-diamminedichloroplatinum(II) (cisplatin) *(1)* it was suggested that the mechanism of antitumor activity of cisplatin involves its binding to DNA (for review, see refs. *2–4*). In addition, it was suggested that the mechanism of antitumor activity of cisplatin might be analogous to the biologic activity of bifunctional alkylating agents (such as nitrogen mustard), which also exhibit cytostatic effects *(5)*. As the cytostatic effect of di-alkylating agents was generally accepted to be associated with their DNA interstrand crosslinking efficiency, the first hypotheses on the mechanism underlying the cytotoxicity of cisplatin in tumor cells were derived from its ability to form interstrand crosslinks in DNA *(6)*. On the basis of this analogy, cisplatin was sometimes incorrectly called an "alkylating agent."

Cisplatin is typically administered intravenously. Extracellular and extranuclear fluids contain relatively high concentrations of chlorides, in which cisplatin exists in stable, i.e., nonreactive, dichloro form. Cisplatin is activated as

From: *Platinum-Based Drugs in Cancer Therapy*
Edited by: L. R. Kelland and N. Farrell © Humana Press Inc., Totowa, NJ

it crosses cellular membranes. During this process, the concentration of chloride drops from approx 0.15 *M* to approx 4 m*M*, producing the kinetically more reactive monoaqua and diaqua species *(7)*.

When a solution of freshly dissolved cisplatin is added to linear. high-molecular-mass DNA, the drug loses one chloride ligand and preferentially forms on DNA a monofunctional adduct at guanine residues [at the N(7) atom]. The next step involves hydrolysis of the second chloride ion and closure of monofunctional adducts to bifunctional lesions. A typical experiment, in which DNA adducts of cisplatin were analyzed after a 16-h reaction in a cell-free medium at $r_b = 0.002$ (r_b is the number of platinum atoms fixed per nucleotide) showed that the major adducts are 1,2-intrastrand crosslinks between purine residues (approx 90%). The minor adducts were interstrand crosslinks, 1,3-intrastrand adducts, and monofunctional adducts. Recent results showed that interstrand crosslinks represented 5–10% of the bound cisplatin *(8–10)*. However, it was shown more recently *(11)* that in negatively supercoiled DNA of the plasmid pSP73 the frequency of interstrand crosslinks was noticeably higher than in the corresponding relaxed or linearized forms and increased with growing negative supercoiling. For instance, at low levels of platination of the naturally supercoiled plasmid DNA (r_b approx 10^{-4}), the frequency of interstrand crosslinks was approx 30% of all platinum adducts, i.e., considerably higher than in linear DNA.

Contradictory data have been published on DNA interstrand crosslinking by cisplatin in different cell lines treated with this drug. Whereas numerous studies have reported the correlation between interstrand crosslinking and the cytotoxicity of cisplatin *(12–15)*, others have not *(16,17)*.

2. SEQUENCE PREFERENCE

The mechanism by which interstrand crosslinks formed by cisplatin in DNA elicit their biologic responses remains unclear. To shed light on this question, these interstrand lesions have been intensively analyzed, although to a lesser extent than the more frequent DNA intrastrand adducts formed by cisplatin between neighboring base residues.

An important step in this analysis is to identify the sites in DNA at which cisplatin forms interstrand adducts. Initial studies employing in particular chromatographic analysis of DNA modified by cisplatin in cell-free media, which was subsequently hydrolyzed to monomeric nucleosides or various products containing cisplatin, revealed that DNA interstrand crosslinks of cisplatin occurred predominantly between N(7) atoms of guanine residues in opposite strands *(18,19)*. This conclusion was further corroborated by the observation that in the reaction of the synthetic double-helical polydeoxyribonucleotide complex poly(dG-dC)·poly(dG-dC) (in which in each guanine strand alternates regularly with cytosine) with cispiatin, interstrand crosslinks were only formed between guanine residues in neighboring base pairs *(20)*. This result, however, did not allow us to distinguish whether the crosslink was preferentially oriented in the 3′→3′ or 5′→5′ direction, i.e., in the 5′-CG or 5′-GC sequences. The distance between the leaving (reactive) groups in cisplatin is approx 0.3 nm, so that two neighboring guanine residues on the opposite strands, either in 5′-CG or 5′-GC sequences, are the most likely sites on DNA for interstrand crosslinking by cisplatin *(21)*. Manipulation of three-dimensional molecular models inferred that the 5′-CG sequence should be more capable of matching the interstrand crosslinking by cisplatin *(19,22)*. This finding was surprising since the distance between two N(7) atoms of guanine residues in the 5′-CG sequence is larger (0.9 nm) than in the 5′-GC sequence (0.7 nm) *(23)*.

A convincing conclusion about the bases preferentially involved in the interstrand crosslinks formed by cisplatin under physiologic conditions (in a cell-free medium) was obtained with the aid of transcriptional footprinting of the platinum adducts on DNA. Recent work has shown that the in vitro RNA synthesis by bacterial RNA polymerases on DNA templates containing several types of bifunctional adducts of platinum complexes can be prematurely terminated at the site or in the proximity of adducts *(10,24)*. The resulting RNA transcripts are separated using high-resolution sequencing gels, and quantification of blocked transcripts is performed by conventional autoradiography or by a phosphorimaging technique. Importantly, monofunctional DNA adducts of cisplatin and several other platinum(II) complexes {for instance, those of chlorodiethylenetriamineplatinum(II) chloride, $[PtCl(NH_3)_3]Cl$, or the trans isomer of cisplatin (transplatin)} are incapable of terminating RNA synthesis *(10,24)*. This assay was applied to a restriction fragment (212 base pairs) modified by cisplatin, which contained only interstrand adducts. This was achieved by treatment of the cisplatin-modified fragment with sodium cyanide at slightly alkaline pH. It was shown that at pH 8.3 and 37°C treatment with NaCN could remove approx 90% of intrastrand crosslinks and monofunctional adducts formed by cisplatin in double-helical DNA, whereas interstrand crosslinks were more stable under these conditions. (Only approx 15% of all interstrand adducts were removed.) Transcriptional footprinting using this template revealed that cisplatin-interstrand crosslinks were formed in linear DNA between two guanine residues, preferentially in the 5′-GC sequence. This finding was further confirmed by assays employing dimethyl sulphate and formic acid as chemical probes of platinum binding to N(7) atoms of adenine and guanine residues in DNA.

Interstrand crosslinks of cisplatin can be formed in negatively supercoiled DNA with a higher frequency than in linear DNA *(11) (see above)*. However, the topology of DNA does not affect only the amount of interstrand crosslinks. Transcriptional footprinting of interstrand crosslinks formed by cisplatin in nega-

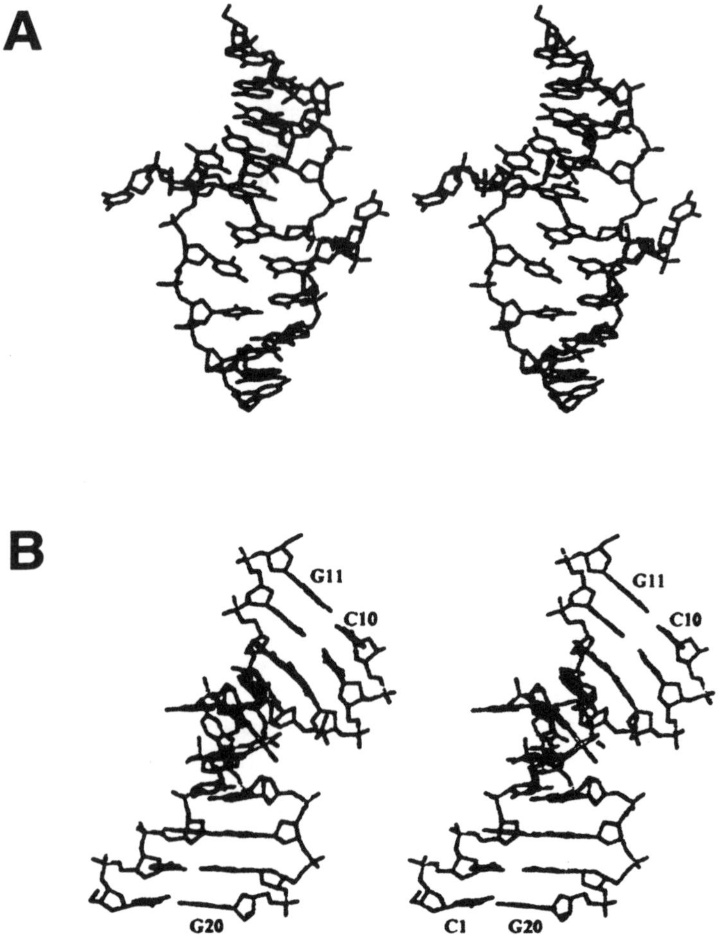

Fig. 1. Structure of *cis*-$(NH_3)_2Pt:[d(C_1C_2T_3C_4G^*{}_5C_6T_7C_8T_9C_{10})\cdot d(G_{11}A_{12}G_{13}A_{14}G^*{}_{15}C_{16}G_{17}A_{18}G_{19}G_{20})]$, where G_5^* and G_{15}^* are guanine residues on opposite strands of DNA crosslinked by cisplatin at the N7 position. Stereoviews of the atomic model. (A) View showing the minor groove and the bound platinum residue. (B) View after a 90° rotation around a vertical axis. Reproduced with permission from *ref. 32.*

tively supercoiled DNA revealed that these lesions were formed at both 5′-GC and 5′-CG sequences, which was in contrast to linear DNA *(11)*. Thus, DNA topology also controls sequence preferences of cisplatin to form this type of DNA adduct.

Interestingly, interstrand crosslinks between guanine and cytosine residues were formed by cisplatin in the synthetic polydeoxyribonucleotide complex poly(dG)·poly(dC). In this double-helical DNA, one strand contains only guanine residues, whereas the other strand contains cytosine residues *(25)*. This type of interstrand crosslink was also formed in a short oligodeoxyribonucleotide duplex (20 base pairs) at its central sequence 5′-TCGT/5′-ACGA (Vrana et al., unpublished results). However, this interstrand adduct of cisplatin was formed only very slowly ($t_{1/2}$>48 h at 37°C), which was consistent with the inability to detect crosslinks of this type in natural linear DNA randomly modified by cisplatin at 37°C *(22)*.

3. STRUCTURE

In B-DNA the distance between the N(7) atoms of the opposite guanine residues in the 5′-GC sequence [i.e., between the sites at which cisplatin preferentially forms interstrand crosslinks *(see above)*] are separated by 0.7 nm. On the other hand, the crosslinking reaction by cisplatin requires a distance of DNA binding sites of about 0.3 nm *(26,27)*. It is therefore evident that DNA interstrand crosslinking by cisplatin requires a distortion of the canonical B-DNA conformation.

A double-stranded oligodeoxyribonucleotide (22 base pairs) containing a single interstrand crosslink of cisplatin within the central sequence 5′-TGCT/5′-AGCA was analyzed by using gel electrophoresis, chemical probes of DNA conformation, and molecular modeling *(28)*. The electrophoretic mobility of multimers obtained by ligation of crosslinked oligonucleotide duplexes was anomalously slow. It was concluded that the interstrand adducts at GC sites bent DNA more than the 1,2-G,G intrastrand adduct. Chemical probing by hydroxylamine showed that cytosine residues complementary to the platinated guanines were largely exposed to the solvent, whereas the flanking adenines and thymines were not reactive with diethyl pyrocarbonate and osmium tetroxide, respectively. These results indicated that the distortion induced by the crosslink formation was localized at the platinated GC/CG base pairs and no local denaturation took place in the vicinity of the platination site. These conclusions were corroborated by molecular mechanics modeling, which yielded two different lowest energy structures. Both structures were similar to B-DNA on the 3′ and 5′ sites of the adduct and exhibited a lack of stacking interactions of the cytosine residues complementary to platinated guanines. The two structures differed by the magnitude of bending at the platinated site toward the major groove; the bending angles were 24° and 57°, respectively. The bending angle of the latter model corresponded well with the angle determined from the gel electrophoresis experiment.

Another study *(29)* was performed by using gel electrophoresis of ligated oligodeoxyribonucleotides that differed in the central platinated sequences (5′-TGCT/5′-AGCT, 5′-AGCT/5′-AGCT, and 5′-CGCT/5′-AGCG). The results of this study were interpreted to mean that the interstrand crosslink formed by cisplatin in the GC/GC sequences induced bending of the duplex axis at the platinated site by approximately 45° and unwinding by 79°, the distortion being independent of the flanking base residues. It should be noted, however, that the unwinding was not compatible with the simple model based on the N(7)-Pt-N(7) bond localized in the major groove, which would rather lead to overwinding of the DNA double helix at the platination site *(30)*.

A novel solution structure of the cisplatin-induced interstrand crosslink of DNA was proposed on the basis of ^{1}H nuclear magnetic resonance measurements (NMR) in two laboratories nearly simultaneously *(30,31)*. The experiments were carried out with short duplexes, deoxyribonucleotide decamers [(5′-CATAG*CTATG)$_2$ *(30)* or 5′-CCTCG*CTCTC/5′-GAGAG*CGAGG *(31)*], which were treated with an aqueous solution of cisplatin to obtain a single interstrand crosslink between two central opposite guanine residues (denoted in the sequences by asterisks). Even though the central sequences of the two duplexes were different, the general features of the solution structures were in a good agreement.

The NMR data were used to assign the imino and nonexchangeable protons. Several irregularities in the crosslinked base pairs and their immediate neighbor pairs indicated that the structure of the central region of the duplex had features not present in B-DNA. Evidence was obtained that the crosslinked deoxyriboguanosine residues were not paired with hydrogen bonds to the complementary deoxyribocytidines, which were located outside the duplex and not stacked with other aromatic rings. All other base residues were paired. Furthermore, the spectra indicated an unusual glycosidic angle for the crosslinked deoxyriboguanosines and a close proximity between the platinated guanine and the flanking neighbor base pair.

Solution structures were calculated and refined by molecular dynamics and energy minimization *(30)*. The refined structures corresponded closely to the features derived from the NMR spectra. The two crosslinked guanines adopted a head-to-tail arrangement and were stacked with flanking neighbor base pairs. An entirely unforseen feature was that the *cis*-diammineplatinum(II) bridge resided in the minor groove, and not in the major groove as reported earlier *(28)*. Also surprising was the finding that the double helix was locally reversed to a left-handed, Z-DNA-like form. The change of the helix sense and the extrusion of deoxyribocytidine residues (complementary to the platinated deoxyriboguanosine residues) from the duplex resulted in the helix unwinding by approximately 80° [precisely by 87°, as determined by Huang et al. *(30)*, or 76°, as determined by Paquet et al. *(31)*] relative to B-DNA. This angle is in a good agreement with the value deduced from electrophoretic measurements *(29)*. It was demonstrated by an electrophoretic retardation technique that the helix axis was bent at the crosslinked site toward the minor groove *(30)*. The bending angle determined by Huang et al. *(30)* (20°) was smaller than that reported by Paquet et al. *(31)* or determined by electrophoresis measurements *(29)* (40° and 45°, respectively).

The crosslinking reaction of cisplatin requires that the N(7) atoms of guanines in opposite strands be brought closer to a distance that is less than half that in B-DNA. Both spin relaxation measurements and molecular dynamic calculations demonstrated that in solution at room temperature the glycosidic angle in B-DNA could vary within ± 28°. It has been suggested that such restricted diffusion around the glycosidic angle induces large coupled motions of the backbone and deoxyribose conformation that can bring the bases closer *(31)*.

Quite recently, the crystal structure of a double-stranded DNA decamer containing a single interstrand crosslink of cisplatin formed between opposite guanine residues in the 5′-GC sequence was solved (Figure 1) *(32)*. 47° for double-helix bending towards the minor groove and 70° for unwinding were found. The major conformational distortions were located at the level of the adduct and did not extend over the flanking nucleotide residues. The platinum residue protruded in the minor groove of the DNA duplex and the N7 atoms of the crosslinked guanine residues localized initially in the major groove of B-DNA mooved in the minor groove. The minor groove was enlarged to >1.0 nm and the planar character of the platinum coordination remained preserved. The structure also exhibited a network of ordered water molecules forming a cage which surrounded the platinum atom and the crosslinked guanine residues.

4. ISOMERIZATION

A local distortion of the canonical conformation of DNA due to the formation of interstrand crosslinks by cisplatin can occur because the DNA conformation is dynamic. Double-helical DNA exists in solution in various transient and distorted conformations, which differ in the extent of, for instance, base pair opening, the duplex unwinding, and the bending of the duplex axis *(32a,b)*. In addition, accessibility of the binding sites, conformation of the duplex (its geometry), nucleotide sequence, electrostatic potential, flexibility, and the formation of transient reactive species can affect the DNA binding mode of cisplatin, but each to a different extent. Interestingly, the reactivity of the monofunctional adduct of cisplatin (which is formed in the first step of bidentate binding of cisplatin to DNA) to close to bifunctional adducts in double-helical DNA was sequence dependent *(33)*. The half-times of closure of the monofunctional adduct of cisplatin at guanine residues were 14 and 3 h if this adduct was formed in the sequence 5′-TGCT and 5′-AGCT, respectively. In both cases, only the interstrand crosslinks were formed. This is particularly interesting for the sequence 5′-AGCT, since the monofunctional adduct at the guanine residue reacted preferentially with the guanine residue in the opposite strand and not with the neighboring adenine residue on the 5′ site of the same strand to form one of the major adducts of cisplatin, 1,2-AG-intrastrand crosslink. In addition, it was shown using an assay based on the DNA cleavage by exonuclease III that in a double-helical DNA fragment (49 base pairs) randomly modified by cisplatin the drug formed in the sequence 5′-CGCGGG an unexpected interstrand crosslink, rather than the expected intrastrand adduct at a GG site *(34)*. These results have indicated that in some sequences of double-helical DNA, in which cisplatin could form both a 1,2-intrastrand adduct between purine residues and an interstrand adduct between opposite guanine residues in the neighboring base pairs, cisplatin preferentially forms the interstrand crosslink.

Another example of the higher stability of an interstrand adduct in comparison with the 1,2-intrastrand adduct of cisplatin is the isomerization of a 1,2-G,G-intrastrand crosslink in double-helical DNA into a more stable interstrand crosslink. This isomerization was observed in several DNA duplexes. It was shown recently *(35)* that the adjacent guanine bases in the 1,2-intrastrand crosslink formed by cisplatin in double-helical DNA were rolled toward one another by 49° and that one possible consequence of this roll is the strain induced in the Pt-N(7) bonds, which may labilize the platinum-guanine linkages. NMR analysis of the short oligodeoxyribonucleotide duplex (8 base pairs) whose upper strand, CCTG*G*TCC, contained a single intrastrand adduct of cisplatin at the central GG sequence (designated in the sequence by asterisks) clearly revealed transformation of intrastrand to interstrand adduct, which was promoted by the presence of the nucleophilic chloride ion in the medium *(36)*. The new crosslink was formed between 5′G* and the 5′ terminal guanine residue of the complementary strand; (Fig. 2).

In the initially formed 1,2-intrastrand crosslinked structure, N(7) of the 5′ terminal guanine residue of the complementary strand was 0.12 nm away from the platinum atom, but there was probably enough flexibility at the end of the duplex to facilitate the intramolecular isomerization. The finding that 1,2-intrastrand adducts of cisplatin can isomerize to interstrand crosslinks was reinforced by investigation of the palindromic dodecamer 5′-d(GACCATATG*G*TC) containing a 1,2-intrastrand crosslink between guanine residues (designated in the sequence by asterisks). Using NMR analysis *(37)*, it was observed that during incubation of this platinated oligonucleotide various reactions took place and one resulted in the formation of the crosslinks between guanine residues belonging to two duplexes. Another example of this transformation was its induction by irradiation with 300–350 nm of light. Short restriction fragments (123 or 82 base pairs) were modified by cisplatin, irradiated with 300–350 nm of light, and analyzed by gel electrophoresis under denaturing conditions *(38)*. This analysis revealed a considerably increased amount of interstrand

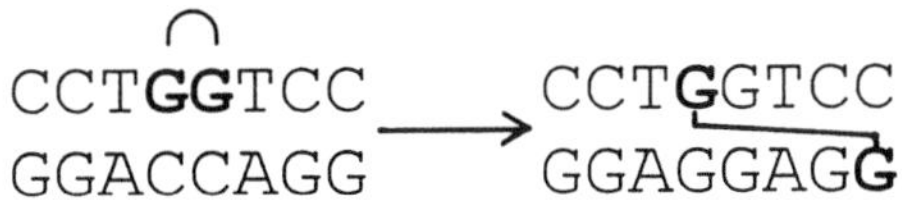

Fig. 2. Example of the isomerization of a 1,2-GG-intrastrand adduct of cisplatin into an interstrand cross-link *(36)*.

crosslinks in comparison with control, nonirradiated platinated samples. Similarly, irradiation of a short oligodeoxyribonucleotide duplex (15 base pairs) containing a single 1,2-GG-intrastrand crosslink of cisplatin in the center resulted in interstrand crosslinked DNA. It was suggested *(38)* that, starting with a 1,2-GG-intrastrand adduct in double-helical DNA, irradiation with 300 nm of light resulted in photodissociation of one of the purine ligands, producing a reactive intermediate in which the vacant site was filled with a more labile ligand, presumably a water molecule. This labile ligand could be displaced by a nucleobase in the opposite DNA strand, producing a DNA interstrand crosslink. Another likely pathway would involve photosubstitution of one of the ammine ligands of cisplatin, a possibility supported by the observation that DNA containing a $[Pt(NH_3)_3]^{2+}$ adduct also formed interstrand crosslinks upon irradiation.

It was also shown recently *(39)* that in short oligodeoxyribonucleotide duplexes (10 and 20 base pairs) containing a central sequence AGCGA/TCGCT the interstrand crosslink formed by cisplatin between guanine residues in the opposite strands in the 5′-GC sequence was labile at 37°C and rearranged into an intrastrand crosslink (Fig. 3). Importantly, this isomerization took place considerably less readily in the longer duplex. ($t_{1/2}$ values were 29 h and 5 d for the isomerization in the short and long oligonucleotide duplexes, respectively.) We extended these studies to the oligonucleotide duplex, containing a single interstrand crosslink of cisplatin formed in the same central sequence, incorporated by ligation approximately into the center of a linearized plasmid DNA (2464 base pairs). We found (Brabec et al., unpublished results) that the interstrand crosslink was stable at 37°C for at least 2 weeks without any sign of decrease of the amount of interstrand crosslinked molecules. In addition, we prepared a sample of linearized plasmid DNA (2464 base pairs) that was randomly modified by cisplatin so that approximately 50% of the DNA molecules contained one interstrand crosslink. This sample was incubated for 2 weeks at 37°C, but the amount of interstrand crosslinked molecules, detected using gel electrophoresis under denaturing conditions, remained unchanged. Thus, the rearrangement of interstrand crosslinks into intrastrand adducts in DNA modified by cisplatin is specific only for some short oligonucleotide duplexes and should not be generalized to natural, high-molecular-mass DNA. The effect of isomerization observed

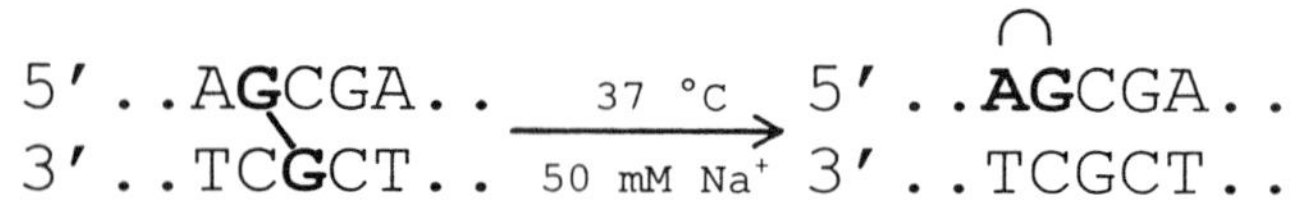

Fig. 3. Rearrangement of the interstrand crosslink of cisplatin into intrastrand adduct in short oligonucleotide duplexes *(39)*.

in very short oligonucleotide duplexes was consistent with the labile Pt-N(7)(guanine) coordination bond involved in the interstrand crosslink of cisplatin. If this bond was ruptured in the case of an interstrand crosslinked short duplex, a monofunctional adduct was formed, which might considerably decrease the melting temperature of the short duplex, particularly if the base residue on the 5′ side of the guanine monoadduct was a pyrimidine base *(40–42)*. In this way the strands in a very short duplex separate, and the interstrand crosslink could not be reformed. Then it was not surprising that the transient monofunctional adduct closed into the intrastrand crosslink if the neighboring base on the 5′ side of the platinated gunanine was adenine or guanine. Thus, the isomerization of interstrand crosslinks of cisplatin into intrastrand crosslinks appears to be not only specific for very short oligonucleotide duplexes but probably also sequence dependent.

In the past, the stability of the cisplatin intrastrand and interstrand adducts was not systematically studied. It is well known that the Pt-N(7)(guanine) bond can be reverted by stronger nucleophilic ligands such as CN^- *(24, 43–45)*, but it is still not entirely clear how stable this bond is in individual types of cisplatin adducts. In this chapter *(see above)* we have summarized several examples of the metastability of both intrastrand and interstrand crosslinks, although understanding the detailed mechanisms involved in the processes by which the Pt-N(7)(guanine) bond is ruptured requires further studies.

The findings on the instability of DNA adducts of cisplatin and their isomerization observed in vitro may have biologic implications. It has been suggested *(36)* that the same reactions, which involve rupture of the Pt-N(7)(guanine) bond, can be promoted in vivo by other nucleophilic biologic ligands, such as sulphhydryl or amine groups of proteins. In addition, if the Pt-N(7)(guanine) bond is broken at one place and reformed at another place, it might also be hypothesized that the platinum atom can "migrate" on the DNA duplex. It can also be speculated that the rate of isomerization of DNA adducts of cisplatin could be affected by DNA conformation or topology, which can be locally changed during genetic processes involved in the mechanisms underlying the antitumor activity of the drug. Thus, the frequency of the individual types of the cisplatin adducts could be locally and transiently altered in DNA in the cell nucleus during some phase (or phases) of the cell cycle and could be different from that found in DNA randomly modified in cell-free media.

5. RECOGNITION BY SPECIFIC PROTEINS

Studies on the mechanisms underlying antitumor activity of cisplatin often employ inactive compounds such as, e.g., the *trans* isomer of cisplatin (transplatin). In this approach, one searches for differences between active and inactive compounds, which may be responsible for their different pharmacologic effects. DNA serves as a template for polymerases that copy the genetic code and transcribe it into messenger RNA. Important results were obtained when the effect of cisplatin and transplatin on replication of chromosomal DNA was examined by using African green monkey CV-1 cells infected by simian virus 40 *(46)*.The results of these studies indicated that: (1) equal numbers of cisplatin and transplatin lesions per nucleotide residue produced the same degree of inhibition of DNA replication; (2) the cellular uptake of cisplatin and transplatin was equal; (3) a time-course analysis of platinum binding to DNA in CV-1 cells treated with the two platinum isomers revealed that cisplatin adducts continuously accumulated on the DNA, whereas transplatin adducts did not. On the basis of these results, it has been suggested that the DNA adducts formed by the two isomers in cells might be differentially processed and that cellular components, presumably cellular proteins, must exist that interact with specific platinum lesions on DNA.

Gel mobility shift assays revealed the presence of proteins in mammalian cellular extracts that bind specifically to DNA modified by antitumor cisplatin and its direct analogs, but not by inactive transplatin or monofunctional chlorodiethylenetriamineplatinum(II) chloride *(47–50)*. One class of the proteins, which bind selectively to DNA modified by cisplatin, was identified as proteins containing a high mobility group (HMG) domain, HMG1 and HMG2 proteins *(51–53)*. These proteins belong to architectural chromatin proteins that play some kind of structural role in the formation of functional higher order protein/DNA or protein/protein complexes *(54)*. Other bacterial and mammalian proteins were also identified that bind selectively to cisplatin adducts (reviewed recently in ref. 55), but in most studies the recognition of platinated DNA by HMG-domain proteins was investigated.

Unfortunately, the initial studies were only aimed at recognition by these proteins of 1,2- and 1,3-intrastrand crosslinks and monofunctional adducts, and no attention was paid to interstrand crosslinks of cisplatin. These studies were performed with oligodeoxyribonucleotide probes containing defined and unique platinum adducts. It was found *(48,53)* that HMG-domain proteins bound selectively to the 1,2-GG or AG adducts of cisplatin, but not to the 1,3-intrastrand crosslinks and monofunctional adducts. At the same time, HMG-domain proteins were reported not to bind to 1,3-intrastrand crosslink and monofunctional adducts of transplatin *(48,53)*.

Later we extended these studies to DNA interstrand crosslinks produced by cisplatin or transplatin by using oligodeoxyribonucleotide probes containing only one type of interstrand crosslink (the cisplatin crosslink between opposite guanine residues in the 5′-GC sequence or transplatin crosslink between guanine and complementary cytosine, i.e., the crosslinks located at the sites where interstrand adducts of these platinum compounds are formed preferentially) *(56)*. It was found that mammalian HMG1 protein bound to the interstrand crosslink of cisplatin with a similar affinity as to the 1,2-GG-intrastrand crosslink. On the other hand, no binding of the HMG1 protein to the probe containing transplatin interstrand crosslink was noted.

Another protein that has been tested for its specific recognition of DNA interstrand adducts of cisplatin and transplatin was an enzyme with deoxyribonuclease activity, T4 endonuclease Vll. This bacteriophage T4-encoded protein cleaves branched DNA structures, most notably four-way junctions, and is regarded as a repair enzyme *(57,58)*. Again, DNA recognition properties of this protein were characterized initially only with respect to 1,2-GG or AG intrastrand crosslinks of cisplatin and the 1,3-GNG crosslink of both cisplatin and transplatin *(58)*. It was discovered that T4 endonuclease Vll recognized 1,2-intrastrand crosslinks of cisplatin, whereas 1,3-intrastrand crosslinks of both isomers were recognized much less efficiently. In later studies *(56)*, we used oligodeoxyribonucleotide duplexes (22 base pairs) containing a single, site-specific interstrand crosslink of cisplatin or transplatin to investigate whether DNA interstrand crosslinked by either platinum isomer was a substrate for cleavage by T4 endonuclease VII. It was shown that the DNA duplex containing a single interstrand crosslink of cisplatin was precisely cleaved in both strands by this DNA-debranching enzyme with an efficiency similar to that observed with DNA containing a single 1,2-GG-intrastrand adduct or a four-way junction. In contrast, the duplex containing the interstrand crosslink of clinically ineffective transplatin was cleaved considerably less efficiently, a property shared by HMG-domain proteins. Thus, T4 endonuclease VII recognized interstrand crosslinks of cisplatin and transplatin like HMG1 protein. The cleavage of branched DNA structures is highly specific in that the enzyme leaves two or three nucleotides to the 3′ side of the point of strand exchange *(57)*. Interestingly, both strands of the duplex containing an interstrand crosslink of cisplatin were cleaved at approximately the same rate, and the sites of cleavage by T4 endonuclease VII were positioned symmetrically to the crosslink, two nucleotides on the 3′ side of the platinated guanine residues in both strands *(56)*. This result was in favor of a symmetric distortion induced in both strands of DNA by the interstrand crosslink of cisplatin. Such symmetry of conformational distortions is apparent from the experiments describing equal chemical reactivity of both opposite cytosine residues in the 5′-GC sequence in which the interstrand crosslink of cisplatin was formed and has been confirmed by the structural model of this lesion based on NMR analysis *(28,30,31)*. The results describing cleavage of interstrand crosslinked DNA by T4 endonuclease VII, in conjunction with the fact that this enzyme interacts with four-way junction DNA, suggest that T4 endonuclease VII recognizes DNA that is distorted in a particular way, such as DNA that contains mutually inclined DNA helical segments.

It has been suggested *(52,53,58–60)* that distortions such as bending and/or unwinding at the site of platination induced in DNA by platinum complexes are important for the recognition and affinity of the platinum-damaged DNA binding proteins. The data so far available show no clear correlation between the magnitude of bending and/or unwinding induced in DNA by the individual types of the platinum adducts and the resulting fixation of HMG1 or T4 endonuclease VII (Table 1).

On the other hand, these data strongly support the view that the platinum-damaged DNA binding proteins utilize kinked, unwound, platinated DNA as a basis for recognition and binding. The 1,2-intrastrand adduct of cisplatin bends DNA toward the major groove *(35,61,62–73)* whereas the interstrand crosslink of this drug bends DNA toward the minor groove *(30–32)*. The recognition of both these lesions by HMG1 and T4 endonuclease VII implies that the DNA bending at the platinated site is recognized by HMG-domain proteins or T4 endonuclease VII independently of whether it is directed toward the major or minor groove. An important feature of the interstrand crosslink of cisplatin is that the crosslinked guanine residues are moved into the minor grove where the cis-diammineplatinum(II) bridge is then located *(30–32)*. The observation that HMG-domain proteins readily bind to the DNA interstrand crosslinks of cisplatin also implies that the presence of the *cis*-diammineplatinum(II) bridge in the minor groove represents no marked sterical hindrance for the binding of these proteins to DNA. This is an interesting observation since generally HMG-domain proteins bind to their recognition sequences in the minor groove.

The 1,3-GNG-intrastrand adduct of cisplatin is not recognized by HMG1 or T4 endonuclease VII even though the bending and unwinding induced in DNA by this adduct are rather similar to those induced by the 1,2-GG-intrastrand adduct (which is recognized when formed in double-helical DNA) (Table 1). This suggests that there are another factors controlling recognition of platinum adducts by the DNA binding proteins. At present the factors that hinder the binding of these proteins to the platinum adducts capable of bending and unwinding of DNA are unknown. Some data on local conformation of DNA around the individual types of platinum adducts (Table 1) are consistent with the hypothesis that the recognition of DNA bending and/or unwinding induced by these lesions might be obscured, if the formation of the platinum-induced DNA lesion is accompanied by a local denaturation and/or by a lowered rigidity of the duplex around the adduct. This hypothesis is supported by the fact that the HMG-domain proteins have a considerably lower affinity for cisplatin adducts in flexible, single-stranded DNA than for the same lesions in the rigid, double-helical DNA *(74)* and that considerably decreased levels of binding are

Table 1
Conformational Distortions Induced in DNA by Platinum Adducts and Their Recognition by HMG1 Protein and T4 Endonuclease VII

DNA adduct type[a]	*Bending angle (deg)*	*Unwinding angle (deg)*	*Denaturation, flexibility*	*Recognition*	
				HMG1	*T4endoVII*
Cisplatin 1,2-intra	32–34,[b,c] 58,[d] 78[e]	13,[f] 21,[d] 25[e]	(−)[c,f–i]	(+)[j,k]	(+)[l]
Cisplatin 1,3-intra	35[c]	23[f]	(+)[m–o]	(−)[j,k]	ND
Cisplatin inter	20,[p] 40,[q] 45,[r] 47[s]	70,[s] 76,[q] 79,[r] 87[p]	(−)[r]	(+)[t]	(+)[t]
Transplatin 1,3-intra	hinge joint[f]	6–13[f]	(+)[m]	(−)[j]	(−)[l]
Transplatin inter	26[u]	12[u]	(+)[u]	(−)[t]	(~)[t]

[a]cisplatin 1,2-intra = 1,2-intrastrand crosslink of cisplatin; cisplatin 1,3-intra = 1,3 intrastrand crosslink of cisplatin; cisplatin inter = interstrand crosslink of cisplatin; transplatin 1,3 intra = 1,3-intrastrand crosslink of transplatin; transplatin inter = interstrand crosslink of transplatin.
[b]Rice et al., 1988 (*61*).
[c]Bellon and Lippard, 1990 (*62*).
[d]Yang et al., 1995 (*63*).
[e]Gelasco and Lippard, 1998 (*35*).
[f]Bellon et al., 1991 (*64*).
[g]Brabec et al., 1990 (*65*).
[h]den Hartog et al., 1985 (*66*).
[i]Sherman and Lippard, 1987 (*67*).
[j]Pil and Lippard, 1992 (*53*).
[k]Huang et al., 1994 (*68*).
[l]Murchie and Lilley, 1993 (*58*).
[m]Anin and Leng, 1989 (*69*).
[n]Marrot and Leng, 1989 (*70*).
[o]van Garderen and van Houte, 1994 (*71*).
[p]Huang et al., 1995 (*30*).
[q]Paquet et al., 1996 (*31*).
[r]Malinge et al., 1994 (*29*).
[s]Coste et al., 1999 (*32*).
[t]Kašpárková and Brabec, 1995 (*56*).
[u]Brabec et al., 1993 (*72*).

observed when a cisplatin-damaged double-helical DNA substrate contains a single-strand break in the phosphodiester backbone *(75)*. It was suggested *(56)* that the formation of the complex between the DNA binding protein and platinated DNA might require contacts or linkages of the specific groups in both interacting biomacromolecules. It cannot be excluded that these contacts or linkages could be difficult to constitute if the specific groups in DNA were contained in denatured base pairs or in more flexible segments of DNA. Such groups may have more freedom to adopt various geometries in comparison with the same groups in rigid DNA segments. In other words, the reduced rigidity of the DNA duplex around the platinated site could decrease the probability that the groups in DNA capable of specific contacts with the DNA binding protein occur in positions favorable for these specific interactions. Further studies are warranted to reveal all factors involved in the recognition of DNA adducts of platinum compounds by DNA binding proteins.

The cisplatin-damaged DNA binding proteins apparently occur in nature for other purposes than for specific recognition of platinum adducts in DNA, since platinum compounds do not belong to natural components of our environment. The capability of cisplatin-damaged DNA to bind DNA binding proteins, which may have a fundamental relevance to the antitumor activity of cisplatin and its simple antitumor analogs, is probably a coincidence when the formation of some platinum adducts in double-helical DNA adopts a structure that mimics the recognition signal for these proteins.

6. REPAIR

The mechanism by which DNA binding proteins might mediate cisplatin cytotoxicity has not yet been elucidated, although several models have been proposed *(76)*. For example, specific binding of HMG-domain proteins to cisplatin-modified DNA could shield the adducts from nucleotide excision repair, which is one of the many cellular defense mechanisms involved in elimination of the toxic effects of cisplatin *(77–79)*. This type of repair includes removal of the damaged base by hydrolyzing phosphodiester bonds on both sides of the lesion. It was found *(80)* using a reconstituted system containing highly purified nucleotide excision repair factors that 1,2- and 1,3-intrastrand crosslinks were efficiently repaired. Importantly, this repair of the 1,2-, but not 1,3-intrastrand crosslink was blocked upon addition of an HMG-domain protein. This is consistent with the observation that HMG-domain proteins bind to 1,2- and not 1,3-intrastrand crosslinks and also with the "shielding" model *(see above)*.

An in vitro excision repair of a site-specific cisplatin interstrand crosslink was also studied *(80)* using mammalian cell-free extracts containing HMG-domain proteins at the levels that were not sufficient to block excision repair of the 1,2-intrastrand adducts. Repair of the interstrand crosslink formed by cisplatin between opposite guanine residues in the 5′-GC sequence was not detected. Similarly, in cell strains derived from patients with Fanconi's anemia nucleotide excision repair of cisplatin-interstrand crosslinks was not observed *(81,82)*, although nucleotide excision repair can readily occur in these cells. Fanconi's anemia cells were described as being extremely sensitive to crosslinking agents so that their noticeably high sensitivity to cisplatin was explained by the inability of these cells to repair cisplatin interstrand crosslinks *(83)*. On the other hand, repair of these lesions was detected with the aid of a repair synthesis assay, which measured the amount of new DNA synthesized after the damage removal in whole cell extracts *(84)*. In this way, however, the repair could also result from a mechanism different from that of nucleotide excision.

The pathways for the repair of DNA interstrand crosslinks of cisplatin and other genotoxic agents in mammalian cells are poorly defined. DNA interstrand crosslinks pose a special challenge to repair enzymes because they involve both strands of DNA and therefore cannot be repaired using the information in the complementary strand for resynthesis. So far most of the studies have been performed using bacterial cells. Based on the genetic and biochemical evidence from bacterial systems, it is thought that interstrand crosslinks are eliminated from DNA by the combined actions of excision repair and recombination systems. Recently, the activities of various human cell extracts and purified human excinuclease on a duplex containing a site-specific interstrand crosslink of psoralen have been tested *(85)*. It was found that, in contrast to monoadducts, which were removed by dual incisions bracketing the lesion, the interstrand crosslink also caused dual incisions, but both were 5′ to the crosslink in one of the two strands. The result of this dual incision was a 22- to 28-nucleotide-long gap immediately 5′ to the crosslink. This gap was suggested to act as a recombinogenic signal to initiate interstrand crosslink removal. On the other hand, there is also a recombination-independent pathway capable of repairing nitrogen mustard interstrand crosslinks, but not psoralen interstrand crosslink *(86)*. It has been suggested that not all interstrand crosslinks are repaired comparably, which might have an influence on the relative ability of each one to be repaired and contribute to the cytotoxicity. Further work is required to find a mechanism effective in the repair of interstrand crosslinks of cisplatin.

7. COMPARISON WITH CLINICALLY INEFFECTIVE TRANSPLATIN

Cisplatin and transplatin exhibit distinctly different antitumor activities in spite of their very similar chemistry. An argument for substantiating the view that DNA interstrand crosslinks of cisplatin are unlikely candidates of antitumor effects of this drug was also based on the observations that clinically ineffective transplatin does not form a considerably lower amount of interstrand

Table 2
Characteristics of Interstrand Crosslinks Formed in DNA by Cisplatin and Transplatin in Cell-Free Media

	Cisplatin	*Transplatin*
Quantity after 48 h[a]	~6% in linearized plasmid DNA[b,c]	~12% in linearized plasmid DNA[b]
Rate of the interstrand cross-linking[a]	$t_{1/2} = 4$ h[b,c]	$t_{1/2} > 11$ h[b]
Bases preferentially involved in the interstrand cross-links	5′-**G**C-[d] \ -C**G**-5′	-**G**-[b] | -**C**-
Bending at the site of platination	20–47° towards minor groove[e]	26° towards major groove[f]
Unwinding of the duplex at the site of platination	70–87° [e]	12° [f]
Some characteristics of the helix distortion	Pt in the minor groove, in the platinated sequence Z-DNA-like form and G not H-bonded with complementary C, which are extrahelical, cross-strand base-base stacking[e]	Nondenaturational, distortion extending over approx. 4 bp around the crosslink, platinated guanosine in *syn* conformation, duplex locally flexible[f]
Recognition by DNA binding proteins,[e,g]	Yes	No

[a]Estimated in linearized plasmid (2464 base pairs) in 10 m*M* $NaClO_4$ at 37°C.
[b]Brabec and Leng, 1993 (*10*).
[c]Vrána et al., 1996 (*11*).
[d]Lemaire et al., 1991 (*24*).
[e]See Table 1 and Sections 3 and 5 of the present article.
[f]Brabec et al., 1993 (*72*).
[g]Recognition by HMG1 and T4 endonuclease VII proteins.

crosslinks in DNA than cisplatin. The acceptance of this argument would, however, require us to admit that, for instance, the structural or conformational properties of the interstrand crosslinks formed by cisplatin and transplatin in DNA are identical. Here we summarize the data on cisplatin and transplatin interstrand crosslinks formed in DNA in cell-free media (Table 2) with the goal of showing how these lesions are structurally different.

The data in Table 2 show that there are considerable differences not only in the base residues preferentially involved in the interstrand crosslinks of cisplatin and its *trans* isomer, but also in the rate of their formation and conformational alterations induced by the two interstrand adducts. Also importantly, the interstrand crosslinks of cisplatin are recognized by DNA binding proteins (HMG-domain proteins and T4 endonuclease VII), whereas those of transplatin are not *(see above)*. Taken together, it cannot be excluded that the different clinical effectiveness of cisplatin and its *trans* isomer may also be associated with the differences in their DNA interstrand crosslinks.

8. FINAL REMARKS

The interstrand crosslink was the first bifunctional adduct of cisplatin detected in vitro and in vivo more than 25 years ago, and it was initially considered the main lesion associated with the antitumor effect of cisplatin. However, later much more attention was paid to the more frequent intrastrand crosslinks formed by cisplatin between neighboring purine residues, but the relative antitumor efficacy of intrastrand and interstrand crosslinks still remains unknown. In the following text we present several examples consistent with the hypothesis and supporting the view that interstrand crosslinks of cisplatin, although they are not the major adducts, play an important role in the mechanisms underlying the antitumor activity of cisplatin, or that at least the possibility of a contribution of interstrand crosslinks to these mechanisms cannot be ruled out.

1. Interstrand crosslinks of cisplatin strongly inhibit DNA transcription elongation by prokaryotic and eukaryotic RNA polymerases *(87)*.
2. Increased gene-specific DNA repair efficiency of interstrand but not intrastrand crosslinks of cisplatin is associated with resistance of cells to the drug *(88–91)*.
3. Interferon-α significantly increases the sensitivity to cisplatin of glioblastoma cells strongly resistant to the cytotoxic effect of this drug. Importantly, interferon-α alone is not cytotoxic in this cell line, but increases considerably the magnitude of cisplatin-induced DNA interstrand crosslinks *(92)*.
4. Antitumor fludarabine nucleoside and arabinosyl-2-fluoroadenine (efficient DNA replication inhibitors) and topoisomerase I inhibitors synergistically enhance cisplatin-induced cytotoxicity in vitro, and the synergism parallels the inhibition of removal of cellular cisplatin-induced DNA interstrand crosslinks *(93–95)*.

In general, interstrand crosslinks formed by various compounds of biologic significance are more inhibitory to DNA replication and transcription because of the damage sustained by both complementary strands, and the resultant severe blockages imposed on DNA-dependent polymerases. In addition, interstrand crosslinks are more difficult to repair, probably requiring both nucleotide excision and recombinational repair, and thus leading to greater cytotoxicity than that expected for monoadducts or intrastrand lesions (which can be repaired solely by nucleotide excision). The fact that interstrand crosslinks of cisplatin are more difficult to repair also suggests that cytotoxic effects of these lesions could rely less on the recognition by and binding of DNA binding proteins, as they probably have to in the case of 1,2-intrastrand crosslinks. In addition, the importance of DNA interstrand crosslinks of cisplatin is reinforced since some regulatory sequences associated with proliferation are known to contain a high number of GC sequences at which cisplatin just preferentially forms interstrand crosslinks.

Exploring new structural classes of platinum antitumor drugs resulted in the discovery of dinuclear *bis*(platinum) complexes with equivalent coordination spheres, represented by the general formula $[PtCl(NH_3)_2]_2(H_2N\text{-}R\text{-}NH_2)]^{2+}$. (R is a linear alkane chain.) To date, the properties of *trans*-$[PtCl(NH_3)_2]_2(H_2N\text{-}R\text{-}NH_2]^{2+}$ and [*cis*-$[PtCl(NH_3)_2]_2(H_2N\text{-}R\text{-}NH_2]^{2+}$ have been reported, including their high activity in vitro and in vivo in both murine and human tumor cell lines resistant to cisplatin *(96–98)*. Importantly, these novel platinum drugs, structurally different from cisplatin, exhibit a spectrum of antitumor activity different from that of cisplatin, and also the major DNA adducts formed by these dinuclear platinum compounds are interstrand crosslinks *(99)*. Moreover, these interstrand adducts are formed at sites that differ from those preferentially involved in the interstrand crosslinking by cisplatin, and conformational distortions induced in DNA by the interstrand crosslinks of dinuclear platinum compounds are markedly distinct from those induced by interstrand and intrastrand crosslinks of cisplatin *(99)*.

Furthermore, in contrast to ineffective transplatin, platinum(II) complexes of the types *trans*-$[PtCl_2L_2]$ and *trans*-$[PtCl_2(NH_3)L]$ (L = planar N-donor) exhibit greatly enhanced cytotoxicity, including activity in cisplatin-resistant tumor cells *(100)*. Interestingly, formal substitution of an NH_3 ligand in transplatin by a planar base, such as quinoline, considerably enhances the interstrand crosslinking efficiency of these transplatin derivatives *(100,101)*. The interstrand adduct formed by both *trans*-$[PtCl_2(NH_3)$(quinoline)] was identified as a 1,2-GG-interstrand crosslink in the sequence 5′-GC, thus being formally equivalent to that of cisplatin rather than transplatin (Neplechová, Kašpárková, Brabec, Bierbach and Farrell, submitted for publication). This result is unique and represents the first demonstration of alteration of a DNA binding site of an inactive drug into a DNA adduct characteristic of an active drug by simple chemical modification of the drug structure. The most intriguing finding proved to be the fact that DNA randomly platinated by *trans*-$[PtCl_2(NH_3)$(quinoline)] is recognized by cisplatin-specific antibodies that exhibit a strict requirement for 1,2-intrastrand crosslinked DNA *(101)*. Thus, one or several unique adducts of the drug produce changes in DNA conformation that efficiently mimic the most frequently formed cisplatin-DNA adduct.

Understanding the formation of DNA interstrand crosslinks of different platinum antitumor compounds is a challenge, not only from the mechanistic view, but also from the therapeutic one. Comprehension of the physiologic roles of

DNA interstrand crosslinks of antitumor platinum compounds in functions of tumor cells requires integration of inorganic chemistry, molecular and cell biology and pharmacology. A coordinated effort in the research of interstrand crosslinks induced by genotoxic agents is under way to resolve the remaining problems of their structures, cellular processing, and biologic significance.

ACKNOWLEDGMENTS

We thank the Grant Agency of the Academy of Sciences of the Czech Republic (grant no. A5004702) and the Grant Agency of the Czech Republic (grant no. 305/99/0695) for support. V.B. is grateful for an International Research Scholar's award from the Howard Hughes Medical Institute. This research is part of the European COST program (project D8/0009/97). This work is funded in part through the US-Czech International Cooperation Program of the NSF.

REFERENCES

1. Rosenberg, B., Van Camp, L., Trosko, J. E. and Mansour, V. H. (1969) Platinum compounds: a new class of potent antitumor agents. *Nature* **222,** 385–386.
2. Kleinwächter, V. (1978) Interaction of platinum(II) coordination complexes with deoxyribonucleic acid . *Studia biophys.* **73,** 1–17.
3. Roberts, J. J. and Thomson, A. J. (1979) Mechanism of action of antitumor platinum compounds. *Prog. Nucleic Acid Res. Mol. Biol.* **22,** 71–134.
4. Drobník, J. (1983) Antitumor activity of platinum complexes. *Cancer Chemother. Pharmacol.* **10,** *145–149.*
5. Drobník, J. and Horáček, P. (1973) Specific biological activity of platinum complexes. Contribution to the theory of molecular mechanism. *Chem. Biol. Interact.* **7,** 223–229.
6. Pascoe, J. M. and Roberts, J. J. (1974) Interactions between mammalian cell DNA and inorganic platinum compounds. I. DNA interstrand crosslinking and cytotoxic properties of platinum(II) compounds. *Biochem. Pharmacol.* **23,** 1345–1357.
7. Johnson, N. P., Hoeschele, J. D., and Rahn, R. O. (1980) Kinetic analysis of the in vitro binding of radioactive *cis-* and *trans-*dichlorodiammineplatinum(II) to DNA *Chem. Biol. Interact.* **30,** 151–169.
8. Hansson, J. and Wood, R. D. (1989) Repair synthesis by human cell extracts in DNA damaged by *cis-* and *trans-*diamminedichloroplatinum(II). *Nucleic Acids Res.* **17,** 8073–8092.
9. Jones, J. C., Zhen, W., Reed, E., Parker, R. J., Sancar, A., and Bohr, V. A. (1991) Gene-specific formation and repair of cisplatin intrastrand adducts and interstrand crosslinks in Chinese hamster ovary cells. *J. Biol. Chem.* **266,** 7101–7107.
10. Brabec, V. and Leng, M. (1993) DNA interstrand crosslinks of *trans-*diamminedichloroplatinum(II) are preferentially formed between guanine and complementary cytosine residues. *Proc. Natl. Acad. Sci. USA* **90,** 5345–5349.
11. Vrana, O., Boudný, V., and Brabec, V. (1996) Superhelical torsion controls DNA interstrand crosslinking by antitumor *cis-*diamminedichloroplatinum(II). *Nucleic Acids Res.* **24,** 3918–3925.
12. Zwelling, L. A., Anderson, T., and Kohn, K. W. (1979) DNA protein and DNA interstrand crosslinking by *cis-* and *trans-*platinum(II)diamminedichloride in L1210 mouse leukemia cells and relation to cytotoxicity. *Cancer Res.* **39,** 365–369.
13. Pera, M. F., Rawlings, C. J., and Roberts, J. J. (1981) The role of DNA repair in the recovery of human cells form cisplatin toxicity. *Chem. Biol. Interact.* **37,** 245–261.

14. Plooy, A. C.M., Van Dijk, M., and Lohman, P. H.M. (1984) Induction and repair of DNA crosslinks in Chinese hamster ovary cells treated with various platinum coordination compounds in relation to platinum binding to DNA cytotoxicity, mutagenicity, and antitumor activity. *Cancer Res.* **44,** 2043–2051.
15. Bedford, P., Walker, M. C., Sharma, H. L., Perera, A., M. A.liffe, C.A., Masters, J. R.W., and Hill, B. T. (1987) Factors influencing the sensitivity of two human bladder carcinoma cell lines to cis-diamminedichloroplatinum(II). *Chem.Biol. Interact.* **61,** 1–15.
16. Strandberg, M. C., Bresnick, E., and Eastman, A. (1982) The significance of DNA crosslinking to *cis*-diamminedichloroplatinum(II)-induced cytotoxicity in sensitive and resistant lines of murine leukemia L1210 cells. *Chem.Biol. Interact.* **39,** 169–180.
17. Pinto, A. L. and Lippard, S. J. (1984) Binding of the antitumor drug *cis*-diamminedichloroplatinum(II) (cisplatin) to DNA *Biochim. Biophys. Acta* **780,** 167–180.
18. Fichtinger-Schepman, A. M. J., Van der Veer, J. L., Den Hartog, J. H. J., Lohman, P. H. M., and Reedijk, J. (1985) Adducts ol the antitumor drug *cis*-diamminedichloroplatinum(II) with DNA formation, identification, and quantitation. *Biochemistry* **24,** 707–713.
19. Eastman, A. (1987) The formation, isolation and characterization of DNA adducts produced by anticancer platinum complexes. *Pharmacol. Ther.* **34,** 155–166.
20. Rahmouni, A. and Leng, M. (1987) Reaction of nucleic acids with *cis*-diamminedichloroplatinum(II): interstrand crosslinks. *Biochemistry* **26,** 7229–7234.
21. Síp, M. and Leng, M. (1993) DNA cis-platinum and intercalators: catalytic activity of the DNA double helix, in *Nucleic Acids and Molecular Biology* (Eckstein, F. and Lilley, D. M.J., eds.), Springer-Verlag, Berlin, pp. 1–15.
22. Eastman, A. (1985) Interstrand crosslinks and sequence specificity in the reaction of *cis*-dichloro(ethylenediamine)platinum(II) with DNA *Biochemistry* **24,** 5027–5032.
23. Castleman, H. and Erlanger, B. F. (1983) Stabilization of (dG-dC)n.(dG-dC)n in the Z conformation by a crosslinking reaction. *Nucleic Acids Res.* **11,** 8421–8429.
24. Lemaire, M. A., Schwartz, A., Rahmouni, A. R., and Leng, M. (1991) Interstrand crosslinks are preferentially formed at the d(GC) sites in the reaction between *cis*-diamminedichloroplatinum(II) and DNA *Proc. Natl Acad. Sci. USA* **88,** 1982–1985.
25. Harder, H. C. and Lee, C. C. (1983) Coordination of interstrand crosslinks between polydeoxyguanylic acid and polydeoxycytidylic acid by *cis*-diamminedichloroplatinum(II). *Cancer Res.* **43,** 4799–4804.
26. Sherman, S. E., Gibson, D., Wang, A. H.J. and Lippard, S. J. (1988) Crystal and molecular structure of *cis*-[Pt(NH_3)$_2${d(pGpG)}], the principal adduct formed by *cis*-diamminedichloroplatinum(II) with DNA *J. Am. Chem. Soc.* **110,** 7368–7380.
27. Lippert, B. (1989) Platinum nucleobase chemistry. *Prog. Inorg. Chem.* **37**, 1–97.
28. Sip, M., Schwartz, A., Vovelle, F., Ptak, M., and Leng, M. (1992) Distortions induced in DNA by *cis*-platinum interstrand adducts. *Biochemistry* **31,** 2508–2513.
29. Malinge, J. M., Perez, C., and Leng, M. (1994) Base sequence-independent distorsions induced by interstrand crosslinks in *cis*-diaminedichloroplatinum (II) modified DNA *Nucleic Acids Res.* **22,** 3834–3839.
30. Huang, H. F., Zhu, L. M., Reid, B. R., Drobny, G. P., and Hopkins, P. B. (1995) Solution structure of a cisplatin-induced DNA interstrand crosslink. *Science* **270,** 1842–1845.
31. Paquet, F., Perez, C., Leng, M., Lancelot, G., and Malinge, J. M. (1996) NMR solution structure of a DNA decamer containing an interstrand crosslink of the antitumor drug *cis*-diamminedichloroplatinum(II). *J. Biomol. Struct. Dyn.* **14,** 67–77.
32. Coste, F., Malinge, J.-M., Serre, L., Shepard, W., Roth, M., Leng, M. and Zelwer, Ch. (1999) Crystal structure of a double-stranded DNA containing a cisplatin interstrand crosslink at 1.63 Å resolution: hydration at the platinated site. *Nucleic Acids Res.* **27,** 1837–1846.
32a. Leroy, J. L., Charretier, E., Kochyian, M., and Guéron, M. (1988) Evidence from base-pair kinetics for two types of adenine tract structures in solution: their reaction to DNA curvature. *Biochemistry* **27,** 8894–8898.

32b. Ramstein, J. and Lavery, R. (1990) Base pair opening pathways in B-DNA. *J. Biomol. Struct. Dyn.* **7,** 915–933.
33. Payet, D., Gaucheron, F., Šíp, M., and Leng, M. (1993) Instability of the monofunctional adducts in *cis*-[Pt(NH_3)$_2$(N7-N-methyl-2-diazapyrenium)CI]$^{2+}$-modified-DNA: rates of crosslinking reactions in *cis*-platinum-modified DNA *Nucleic Acids Res.* **21,** 5846–5851.
34. Zou, Y., Vanhouten, B., and Farrelll, N. (1994) Sequence specificity of DNA DNA interstrand crosslink formation by cisplatin and dinuclear platinum complexes. *Biochemistry* **33,** *5404–5410.*
35. Gelasco, A. and Lippard, S. J. (1998) NMR solution structure of a DNA dodecamer duplex containing a *cis*-diammineplatinum(II) d(GpG) intrastrand crosslink, the major adduct of the anticancer drug cisplatin. *Biochemistry* **37,** 9230–9239.
36. Yang, D. Z., Vanboom, S. S. G. E., Reedijk, J., Vanboom, J. H., and Wang, A. H.J. (1995) Structure and isomerization of an intrastrand cisplatin-crosslinked octamer DNA duplex by NMR analysis. *Biochemistry* **34,** 12912–12920.
37. Yang, D. Z. and Wang, A. H. J. (1996) Structural studies of interactions between anticancer platinum drugs and DNA. *Prog. Biophys. Mol. Biol.* **66,** 81–111.
38. Kane, S. A. and Lippard, S. J. (1996) Photoreactivity of platinum(II) in cisplatin-modified DNA affords specific crosslinks to HMG domain proteins. *Biochemistry* **35,** 2180–2188.
39. Perez, C., Leng, M., and Malinge, J. M. (1997) Rearrangement of interstrand crosslinks into intrastrand crosslinks in *cis*-diamminedichloroplatinum(II)-modified DNA *Nucleic Acids Res.* **25,** 896–903.
40. Brabec, V., Reedijk, J., and Leng, M. (1992) Sequence-dependent distortions induced in DNA by monofunctional platinum(II) binding. *Biochemistry* **31,** 12397–12402.
41. Van Garderen, C. J., Van den Elst, H., Van Boom, J. H., Reedijk, J., and Van Houte, L. P.A. (1989) A double-stranded DNA fragment shows a significant decrease in double-helix stability after binding of monofunctional platinum amine compounds. *J. Am. Chem. Soc.* **111**, 4123–4125.
42. Brabec, V., Boudný, V. and Balcarová, Z. (1994) Monofunctional adducts of platinum(II) produce in DNA a sequence-dependent local denaturation. *Biochemisty* **32**, 1316–1322.
43. Lippard, S. J. and Hoeschele, J. D. (1979) Binding of *cis*-dichlorodiammineplatinum(II) and *trans*-dichlorodiammineplatinum(II) to the nucleosome core. *Proc. Natl Acad. Sci. USA* **76,** 6091–6095.
44. Tullius, T. D. and Lippard, S. J. (1981) *cis*-Diamminedichloroplatinum(II) binds in a unique manner to oligo(dG).oligo(dC) sequences in DNA—a new assay using exonuclease III. *J. Am. Chem. Soc.* **103,** 4620–4622.
45. Schwartz, A., Sip, M., and Leng, M. (1990) Sodium cyanide—a chemical probe of the conformation of DNA modified by the antitumor drug *cis*-diamminedichloroplatinum(II). *J. Am. Chem. Soc.* **112,** 3673–3674.
46. Ciccarelli, R. B., Solomon, M. J., Varshavsky, A., and Lippard, S. J. (1985) In vivo effects of *cis*-and *trans*-diamminedichloroplatinum(II) on SV 40 chromosomes: differential repair, DNA protein crosslinking, and inhibition of replication. *Biochemistry* **24,** 7533–7540.
47. Chu, G. and Chang, E. (1988) Xeroderma pigmentosum group E cells lack a nuclear factor that binds to damaged DNA *Science* **242,** 564–567.
48. Donahue, B. A., Augot, M., Bellon, S. F., Treiber, D. K., Toney, J.H., Lippard, S. J., and Essigmann, J. M. (1990) Characterization of a DNA damage-recognition protein from mammalian cells that binds specifically to intrastrand d(GpG) and d(ApG) DNA adducts of the anticancer drug cisplatin. *Biochemistry* **29,** 5872–5880.
49. Andrews, P. A. and Jones, J. A. (1991) Characterization of binding proteins from ovarian carcinoma and kidney tubule cells that are specific for cisplatin modified DNA *Cancer Commun.* **3,** 1–10.
50. Chao, C. C.-K., Huang, S. L., Lee, L .Y., and Lin-Chao, S. (1991) Identification of in-

ducible damage-recognition proteins that are overexpressed in HeLa cells resistant to *cis*-diamminedichloroplatinum(II). *Biochem. J.* **277,** 875–878.

51. Toney, J. H., Donahue, B. A., Kellett, P. J., Bruhn, S. L., Essigmann, J.M., and Lippard, S. J. (1989) Isolation of cDNAs encoding a human protein that binds selectively to DNA modified by the anticancer drug *cis*-diamminedichloroplatinum(II). *Proc. Natl Acad. Sci. USA.* **86,** 8328–8332.
52. Bruhn, S. L., Pil, P. M., Essigmann, J. M., Housman, D. E., and Lippard, S. J. (1992) Isolation and characterization of human cDNA clones encoding a high mobility group box protein that recognizes structural distortions to DNA caused by binding of the anticancer agent cisplatin. *Proc. Natl Acad. Sci. USA.* **89,** 2307–2311.
53. Pil, P. M. and Lippard, S. J. (1992) Specific binding of chromosomal protein HMG1 to DNA damaged by the anticancer drug cisplatin. *Science* **256,** 234–237.
54. Bustin, M. and Reeves, R. (1996) High-mobility-group chromosomal proteins: architectural components that facilitate chromatin function. *Prog. Nucleic Acid Res. Mol. Biol.* **54,** 35–100.
55. Zlatanova, J., Yaneva, J., and Leuba, S. H. (1998) Proteins that specifically recognize cisplatin-damaged DNA: a clue to anticancer activity of cisplatin. *FASEB J.* **12,** 791–799.
56. Kašpárková, J. and Brabec, V. (1995) Recognition of DNA interstrand crosslinks of *cis*-diamminedichloroplatinum(II) and its *trans* isomer by DNA binding proteins. *Biochemistry* **34,** 12379–12387.
57. Duckett, D. R., Murchie, A. I. H., Bhattacharyya, A., Clegg, R. M., Diekmann, S., Von Kitzing, E., and Lilley, D. M. J. (1992) The structure of DNA junctions, and their interactions with enzymes. *Eur. J. Biochem.* **207,** 285–295.
58. Murchie, A. I.H. and Lilley, D. M.J. (1993) T4 endonuclease VII cleaves DNA containing a cisplatin adduct. *J. Mol. Biol.* **233,** 77–82.
59. Bruhn, S. L., Housman, D. E., and Lippard, S. J. (1993) Isolation and characterization of cDNA clones encoding the *Drosophila* homolog of the HMG-box SSRP family that recognizes specific DNA structures. *Nucleic Acids Res.* **21,** 1643–1646.
60. Lilley, D. M.J. (1996) Cisplatin adducts in DNA: distortion and recognition. *J. Biol. Inorg. Chem.* **1,** 189–191.
61. Rice, J. A., Crothers, D. M., Pinto, A. L., and Lippard, S. J. (1988) The major adduct of the antitumor drug *cis*-diamminedichloroplatinum(II) with DNA bends the duplex by ~40° toward the major groove. *Proc. Natl Acad. Sci. USA.* **85,** 4158–4161.
62. Bellon, S. F. and Lippard, S. J. (1990) Bending studies of DNA site-specifically modified by cisplatin, *trans*-diamminedichloroplatinum(II) and *cis*-$[Pt(NH_3)_2(N3\text{-cytosine})Cl]^+$. *Biophys. Chem.* **35,** 179–188.
63. Yang, D. Z., Van Boom, S. S. G. E., Reedijk, J., Van Boom, J. H., and Wang, A. H. J. (1995) Structure and isomerization of an intrastrand cisplatin-crosslinked octamer DNA duplex by NMR analysis. *Biochemistry* **34,** 12912–12920.
64. Bellon, S. F., Coleman, J. H., and Lippard, S. J. (1991) DNA unwinding produced by site-specific intrastrand crosslinks of the antitumor drug *cis*-diamminedichloroplatinum(II). *Biochemistry* **30,** 8026–8035.
65. Brabec, V., Kleinwachter, V., Butour, J. L., and Johnson, N. P. (1990) Biophysical studies of the modification of DNA by antitumour platinum coordination complexes. *Biophys. Chem.* **35,** 129–1411.
66. Den Hartog, J. H. J., Altona, C., Van Boom, J. H., Van der Marel, G.A., Haasnoot, C. A.G., and Reedijk, J. (1985) *cis*-Diamminedichloroplatinum(II) induced distortion of a single and double stranded deoxydecanucleosidemonophosphates studied by nuclear magnetic resonance. *J. Biomol. Struct. Dyn.* **2,** 1137–1155.
67. Sherman, S. E. and Lippard, S. J. (1987) Structural aspects of platinum anticancer drug interactions with DNA *Chem. Rev.* **87,** 1153–1181.

68. Huang, J. C., Zamble, D. B., Reardon, J. T., Lippard, S. J., and Sancar, A. (1994) HMG-domain proteins specifically inhibit the repair of the major DNA adduct of the anticancer drug cisplatin by human excision nuclease. *Proc. Natl Acad. Sci. USA.* **91,** 10394–10398.
69. Anin, M. F. and Leng, M. (1990) Distortions induced in double-stranded oligonucleotides by the binding of *cis*-diamminedichloroplatinum(II) or *trans*-diamminedichloroplatinum(II) to the d(GTG) sequence. *Nucleic Acids Res.* **18,** *4395–4400.*
70. Marrot, L. and Leng, M. (1989) Chemical probes of the conformation of DNA modified by *cis*-diamminedichloroplatinum(II). *Biochemistry* **28,** 1454–1461.
71. Van Garderen, C. J. and Van Houte, L. P.A. (1994) The solution structure of a DNA duplex containing the *cis*-$Pt(NH_3)_2$[d(GTG)N7(G),N7(G)] adduct, as determined with high-field NMR and molecular mechanics/dynamics. *Eur. J. Biochem.* **225,** 1169–1179.
72. Brabec, V., Śíp, M. and Leng, M. (1993) DNA conformational distortion produced by site-specific interstrand crosslink of *trans*-diamminedichloroplatinum(II). *Biochemistry* **32,** 11676–11681.
73. Takahara, P. M., Frederick, C. A. and Lippard, S. J. (1996) Crystal structure of the anticancer drug cisplatin bound to duplex DNA *J. Am. Chem. Soc.* **118,** 12309–12321.
74. Marples, B., Adomat, H., Billings, F. C., Farrell, N. P., Koch, C. J., and Skov, K. A. (1994) Recognition of platinum-induced DNA damage by nuclear proteins: screening for mechanisms. *Anti-Cancer Drug Design* **9,** 389–399.
75. Turchi, J. J., Li, M., and Henkels, K. M. (1996) Cisplatin-DNA binding specificity of calf high-mobility group 1 protein. *Biochemistry* **35,** 2992–3000.
76. Whitehead, J. P. and Lippard, S. J. (1996) Proteins that bind to and mediate the biological activity of platinum drug-DNA adducts, in *Metal Ions in Biological Systems* (Siegel, A. and Siegel, H., eds.), Marcel Dekker, New York, pp. 687–726.
77. Chaney, S. G. and Sancar, A. (1996) DNA repair: enzymatic mechanisms and relevance to drug response. *J. Natl Cancer Inst.* **88,** 1346–1360.
78. Sancar, A. (1996) DNA excision repair. *Annu. Rev. Biochem.* **65,** 43–81.
79. Naegeli, H. (1997) *Mechanisms of DNA Damage Recognition in Mammalian Cells.* Springer-Verlag, New York.
80. Zamble, D. B., Mu, D., Reardon, J. T., Sancar, A., and Lippard, S. J. (1996) Repair of cisplatin-DNA adducts by the mammalian excision nuclease. *Biochemistry* **35,** 10004–10013.
81. Plooy, A. C.M., Van Dijk, M., Berends, F., and Lohman, P. H. M. (1985) Formation and repair of DNA interstrand crosslinks in relation to cytotoxicity and unscheduled DNA synthesis induced in control and mutant human cells treated with *cis*-diamminedichloroplatinum(II). *Cancer Res.* **45,** 4178–4184.
82. Dijt, F. J., Fichtinger-Schepman, A. M. J., Berends, F., and Reedijk, J. (1988) Formation and repair of cisplatin-induced adducts to DNA in cultured normal and repair-deficient human fibroblasts. *Cancer Res.* **48,** 6058–6062.
83. Fujiwara, Y., Tatsumi, M., and Sasaki, M. S. (1977) *J. Mol. Biol.* **113**, 635–649.
84. Calsou, P., Frit, P., and Salles, B. (1992) Repair synthesis by human cell extracts in cisplatin-damaged DNA is prefentially determined by minor adducts. *Nucleic Acids Res.* **20,** 6363–6368.
85. Bessho, T., Mu, D., and Sancar, A. (1997) Initiation of DNA interstrand crosslink repair in humans: the nucleotide excision repair system makes dual incisions 5′ to the crosslinked base and removes a 22- to 28-nucleotide-long damage-free strand. *Mol. Cell. Biol.* **17,** 6822–6830.
86. Berardini, M., Mackay, W., and Loechler, E. L. (1997) Evidence for a recombination-independent pathway for the repair of DNA interstrand crosslinks based on a site-specific study with nitrogen mustard. *Biochemistry* **36,** 3506–3513.
87. Corda, Y., Job, C., Anin, M. F., Leng, M., and Job, D. (1991) Transcription by eucaryotic and procaryotic RNA polymerases of DNA modified at a d(GG) or a d(AG) site by the antitumor drug *cis*-diamminedichioroplatinum(II). *Biochemistry* **30,** 222–230.

88. Zhen, W. P., Link, C. J., O'Connor, P. M., Reed, E., Parker, R., Howell, S. B., and Bohr, V. A. (1992) Increased gene-speciflic repair of cisplatin interstrand crosslinks in cisplatin-resistant human ovarian cancer cell lines. *Mol. Cell. Biol.* **12,** 3689–3698.
89. Larminat, F., Zhen, W., and Bohr, V. A. (1993) Gene-specific DNA repair of interstrand crosslinks induced by chemotherapeutic agents can be preferential. *J. Biol. Chem.* **268,** 2649–2654.
90. Johnson, S. W., Perez, R. P., Godwin, A. K., Yeung, A. T., Handel, L.M., Ozols, R. F., and Hamilton, T. C. (1994) Role of platinum-DNA adduct formation and removal in cisplatin resistance in human ovarian cancer cell lines. *Biochem. Pharmacol.* **47,** 689–697.
91. Larminat, F. and Bohr, V. A. (1994) Role of the human ERCC-1 gene in gene-specific repair of cisplatin-induced DNA damage. *Nucleic Acids Res.* **22,** 3005–3010.
92. Stanzione, S., Cimoli, G., Debernardis, D., Michelotti, A., Conte, P.F., Parodi, S., and Russo, P. (1995) Interferon-α or β potentiate platinum analogous in human glioblastoma cell lines. *Mutat. Res.* **348,** 131–135.
93. Yang, L. Y., Li, L., Keating, M. J., and Plunkett, W. (1995) Arabinosyl-2-fluoroadenine augments cisplatin cytotoxicity and inhibits cisplatin-DNA crosslink repair. *Mol. Pharmacol.* **47,** 1072–1079.
94. Li, L., Keating, M. J., Plunkett, W., and Yang, L. Y. (1997) Fludarabine-mediated repair inhibition of cisplatin-induced DNA lesions in human chronic myelogenous leukemia-blast crisis K562 cells: induction of synergistic cytotoxicity independent of reversal of apoptosis resistance. *Mol. Pharmacol.* **52,** *798–806.*
95. Li, L., Liu, X. M., Glassman, A. B., Keating, M. J., Stros, M., Plunkett, W., and Yang, L. Y. (1997) Fludarabine triphosphate inhibits nucleotide excision repair of cisplatin-induced DNA adducts in vitro. *Cancer Res.* **57,** 1487–1494.
96. Farrell, N., Qu, Y., Feng, L., and Van Houten, B. (1990) Comparison of chemical reactivity, cytotoxicity, interstrand crosslinking and DNA sequence specificity of bis(platinum) complexes containing monodentate or bidentate coordination spheres with their monomeric analogues. *Biochemistry* **29,** 9522–9531.
97. Hoeschele, J. D., Kraker, A. J., Qu, Y., Van Houten, B., and Farrell, N. (1990) Bis(platinum) complexes, chemistry, antitumor activity and DNA binding, in *Molecular Basis of Specificity in Nucleic Acid-Drug Interactions* (Pullman, B. and Jortner, J., eds.), Academic, Dordrecht, pp. 301–321.
98. Farrell, N. (1991) Structurally novel platinum antitumor compounds, in *Platinum and Other Metal Coordination Compounds in Cancer Chemotherapy* (Howell, S. B., ed.), Plenum, New York, pp. 81–91.
99. Zaludová, R., Zákovská, A., Kašpárková, J., Balcarová, Z., Kleinwächter, V., Vrána, O., Farrell, N., and Brabec, V. (1997) DNA interactions of bifunctional dinuclear platinum(II) antitumor agents. *Eur. J. Biochem.* **246,** *508–517.*
100. Zou, Y., Van Houten, B., and Farrell, N. (1993) Ligand effects in platinum binding to DNA A comparison of DNA binding properties for *cis*-and *trans*-[$PtCl_2(amine)_2$] (amine = NH_3, pyridine). *Biochemistry* **32,** 9632–9638.
101. A., Nováková, O., Balcarová, Z., Bierbach, U., Farrell, N., and Brabec, V. (1998) DNA interactions of antitumor *trans*-[$PtCl_2(NH_3)$(quinoline)]. *Eur. J. Biochem.* **254,** 547–557.

3 Transplatin-Modified Oligonucleotides as Potential Antitumor Drugs

Marc Leng, Annie Schwartz, and Marie-Josephe Giraud-Panis

CONTENTS

1. INTRODUCTION

The discovery by Rosenberg and co-workers *(1,2)* of the induction of filamentous growth in bacteria cells by platinum-amine complexes has been the starting point of much work devoted to the chemistry of these complexes, their binding to biomolecules (particularly to DNA), and their biologic activity. One major achievement is the successful use of *cis*-diamminedichloroplatinum(II) (cisplatin) in the treatment of several human cancers. Cisplatin triggers cell death by apoptosis, but the complete mechanism of action of the drug and the development of resistance have not yet been elucidated *(3–5)*. Cellular DNA is the target of cisplatin through covalent interaction *(6–8)*. The lesions formed in the reaction between DNA and cisplatin have been identified in vitro and in vivo (mainly intrastrand and interstrand crosslinks), as well as the distortions they induce in the DNA double helix *(9,10)*. Recently, several studies have demonstrated that proteins that bend DNA also interact specifically with cisplatin-modified DNA at d(GpG) and d(ApG) sites *(11–19)*. This gives strong support to the hypothesis that the major 1,2-intrastrand crosslinks between adjacent purine nucleotides play a key role, although one cannot discard the role of the interstrand crosslinks.

From: *Platinum-Based Drugs in Cancer Therapy*
Edited by: L. R. Kelland and N. Farrell © Humana Press Inc., Totowa, NJ

The systematic study of platinum complexes led to empirical pharmacologic structure-activity relationships *(7,8,20)*. The complexes must have the *cis* conformation since *trans*-diamminedichloroplatinum(II) (transplatin), the stereoisomer of cisplatin, is clinically inefficient. For steric reasons, transplatin cannot form intrastrand crosslinks between adjacent purine residues, which could explain its inefficiency. However, platinum(IV) complexes with *trans* geometry for the leaving groups have antitumor activity and are able to overcome the cisplatin resistance of cancer cells *(21,22)*. In transplatin, substitution of NH_3 ligands by heterocyclic amines *(23,24)* or iminoethers *(25, 26)* produces complexes with significant antitumor activity. Furthermore, the new family of bis(platinum(II)) complexes with bridging diamine ligands of composition *trans*-$\{[Pt(NH_3)_2]_2(\mu\text{-}NH_2(CH_2)_xNH_2\}Cl_2$ presents promising features for clinical activity *(27)*. All these results show that the difference in geometry between the two isomers cannot be the only explanation for the clinical inefficiency of transplatin and are in agreement with the conclusion of a recent review *(28)* on the properties of transplatin, pointing out that a simple answer cannot be given to the question: what makes transplantin different from its isomer?

Our purpose in this review is to describe another family of compounds that bind specifically and covalently to nucleic acids. The bound compounds can interfere with the cellular machinery at different levels, such as replication, transcription, or translation, and thus have a potential use in cancer therapy by specifically modulating gene expression, eventually leading to cell death. These compounds are transplatin derivatives in which the platinum residue is coordinated to four nitrogen ligands. They are prepared by reacting transplatin with oligonucleotides containing a GNG triplet (N being any nucleotide residue). The resulting (G1,G3)-intrastrand crosslinks are stable within single-stranded oligonucleotides under physiologic conditions. The pairing of the platinated oligonucleotides with their complementary sequences within DNA or RNA triggers the rearrangement of the 1,3-intrastrand crosslinks into interstrand crosslinks *(29,30)*.

We have divided this review into three main parts. In the first part, we recall some results on the reaction between DNA and transplatin (nature of the adducts, distortions of the double helix). In the second part, we describe in detail the promoted rearrangement of the (G1,G3)-intrastrand crosslinks into interstrand crosslinks by the formation of a double helix. In the third part, we discuss the potential use of the transplatin-modified oligonucleotides as antitumor drugs.

2. TRANSPLATIN-MODIFIED DOUBLE-STRANDED DNA

2.1. Nature of the Adducts

The chemical properties of transplatin and its covalent binding to DNA through a solvent-assisted pathway have been the subject of several reviews *(7,8,20,28,31)*. The first DNA binding step results in the formation of the monofunctional adducts *trans*-$[Pt(NH_3)_2(dG)Cl]^+$, which can react further to form bifunctional lesions. The nature of the adducts in the in vitro reaction was first identified by nuclear magnetic resonance (NMR) and atomic absorption after high-performance liquid chromatography (HPLC) separation of the enzymatic digestion of the transplatin-modified DNA *(32,33)*. The closure of the monofunctional adducts into bifunctional adducts is slow (being only 80% complete in 48 h). The crosslinks are between G and C (50%), G and G (40%), and G and A (10%), some of them corresponding to interstrand crosslinks. Quite different results were obtained in another study *(34)*, the kinetics of closure being followed by ^{195}Pt NMR. The monofunctional adduct closure is fast ($t_{1/2}$ = 3.1 h), with formation of 1,3- and longer range intrastrand crosslinks.

However, the very existence of intrastrand crosslinks has been questioned. T4 DNA polymerase, acting as a 3′→ 5′ exonuclease, is able to digest completely a platinated DNA restriction fragment whereas, in the same experimental conditions, model studies have shown that the enzyme is stopped by (G1,G3)- and (C1,G4)-intrastrand crosslinks *(35)*.

Another piece of evidence against the formation of intrastrand crosslinks is to be found in the RNA polymerase mapping experiments reported here. T7 and SP6 RNA polymerases were used previously to reveal adducts in cisplatin- and transplatin-modified DNAs *(36,37)*. We have repeated the mapping experiment on a DNA restriction fragment platinated at a low r_b (molar ratio bound platinum per nucleotide). After 24 h of reaction between transplatin and DNA, the fragments with and without interstrand crosslinks were separated by electrophoresis on agarose gel under denaturing conditions. (Those containing interstrand crosslinks had a slower migrating rate than those without interstrand crosslinks). The two kinds of fragments were transcribed and their products analyzed by gel electrophoresis. As shown in Fig. 1, the sample without any interstrand crosslink (lane labeled intra) is fully transcribed, whereas the sample containing interstrand crosslinks (lane inter) generates a population of RNA fragments of defined sizes. For comparison, the results obtained with cisplatin-modified DNA are shown. [The main stops correspond to intrastrand crosslinks at d(GG) and d(AG) sites.]

Several conclusions can be drawn from these mapping experiments and previously reported experiments *(37,38)*. First is that the formation of intrastrand crosslinks, if it occurs, is a rare event. Second is that the closure of monofunctional *trans*-$[Pt(NH_3)_2(dG)Cl]^+$ adducts leads essentially to interstrand crosslinks. To react with the complementary C residue, the monofunctional *trans*-$[Pt(NH_3)_2(dG)Cl]^+$adduct, initially in the anti conformation and paired with the C residue, has to rotate around its glycosidic bond, as schematically represented in Fig. 2. A third conclusion is that the rate of closure of the monofunctional adducts into interstrand crosslinks is slow ($t_{1/2}$ in the range 20–40 h). This is notably slower than the rate of closure of most of the cisplatin monofunctional adducts.

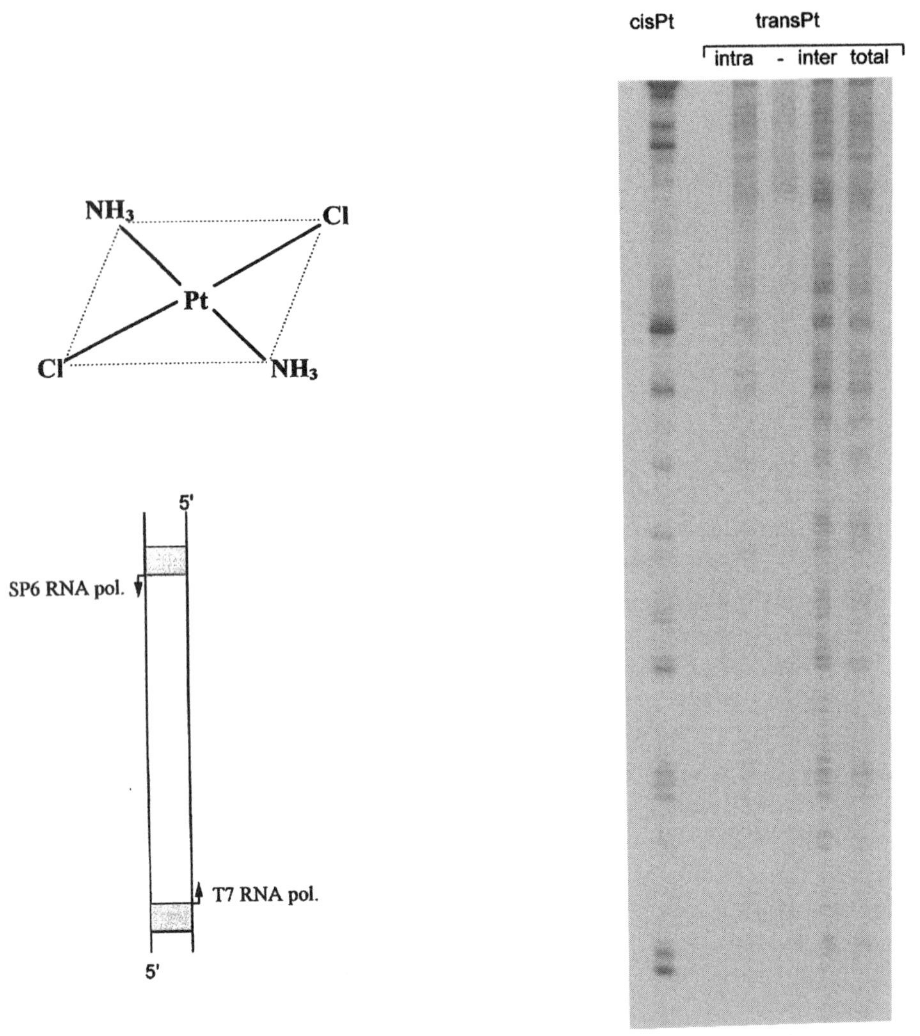

Fig. 1. Inhibition of RNA synthesis on transplatin- or cisplatin-modified DNA restriction fragments. The formula of transplatin is given on the top (left) of the figure. The mapping of the adducts was done on the platinated *(NdeI/HpaI)* restriction fragments with convergent T7 and SP6 promoters. Either strand can be used as a template for RNA synthesis in vitro *(bottom, left)*. Right: Autoradiogram of a 6% polyacrylamide/7 M urea sequence gel showing inhibition of RNA synthesis by T7 RNA polymerase on cisplatin- or transplatin-modified DNA at r_b = 0.005. Lanes intra and inter are for transplatin-modified DNAs, which do not contain or contain interstrand crosslinks.

In summary, in the reaction between transplatin and double-stranded DNA, monofunctional adducts are formed that slowly evolve into interstrand crosslinks and not into intrastrand crosslinks. It is likely that the discrepancy in

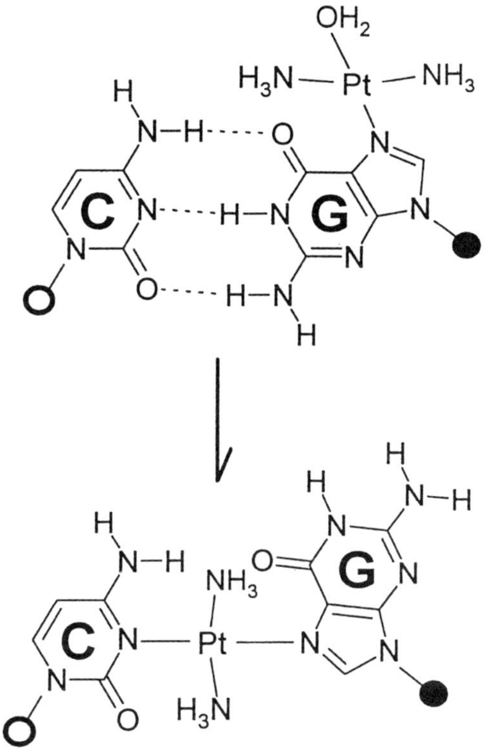

Fig. 2. Representation of the interstrand crosslink formed in the reaction between transplatin and double-stranded DNA. The monofunctional *trans*-[Pt$(NH_3)_2$(dG)Cl]$^+$ adduct, initially paired with the complementary C residue, rotates around the glycosidic bond from anti to syn conformation, which allows its reaction with the complementary C residue.

the literature on the nature of the adducts originates from a too high level of platination of the samples. A recent study *(39)* based on model systems has shown that the closure of the monofunctional *trans*-[Pt$(NH_3)_2$(dG)Cl]$^+$ adducts results in the formation of interstrand crosslinks between complementary G and C residues but eventually to other lesions (intrastrand and interstrand crosslinks) if other adducts are near the reacting species. An interstrand crosslink between G and A residues separated by 4–5 base pairs was even detected.

2.2. Distortion of the DNA Double Helix by the Interstrand Crosslinks

The conformational changes induced in the double helix by the transplatin interstrand crosslinks have been characterized by several techniques. Qualitative data at the nucleotide level were obtained by means of chemical probes such as diethyl pyrocarbonate, chloroacetaldehyde, and osmium tetroxide. The rates of reaction of these chemical compounds with nucleotide residues are strongly dependent on the structure of DNA. Moreover, subsequent to the specific modifications, the residues are sensitive to cleavage by piperidine, and hence the generated fragments can be resolved as a ladder of bands on a denaturing gel *(40,41)*. The local distortion due to the interstrand crosslink spreads over 4 base pairs without unpairing of the bases adjacent to the crosslink *(38)*.

From the comparative study *(38)* of the electrophoretic mobility of multimers of double-stranded oligonucleotides of various lengths (19–22 base pairs), containing or not a single interstrand crosslink, the extent of unwinding and bending of the double helix was calculated according to the procedure described for other platinated oligonucleotides *(42)*. The interstrand crosslink unwinds DNA by about 12° and bends its axis by about 26°. Molecular modeling calculations support the hypothesis that the platinated G residue is in the syn conformation and that the double helix is bent toward the DNA minor groove.

These findings are in agreement with a recent two-dimensional (2D) NMR study *(43)* of a double-stranded dodecamer containing a single interstrand crosslink, although the values of the bending and unwinding of the double helix are smaller (14° and approx 4°, respectively) than those deduced from the electrophoretic mobility experiments. They confirm that the platinated G residue is in the syn conformation and that the bases adjacent to the crosslink are paired. They show that the two NH_3 molecules of platinum residue are on either side of the plane of the crosslinked bases and push away the adjacent paired bases along the axis of the double helix (Fig. 3).

This model could explain the slow closure of the monofunctional adduct into an interstrand crosslink. Two events (rotation of the platinated G residue from the anti to syn conformation, vertical displacement of the adjacent base pairs) have to occur concomitantly in order to locate the platinum residue near the N3 of the cytosine residue. One expects the rate of the interstrand crosslinking reaction to be sensitive to local conformational modifications of the DNA double helix. This can be achieved by several ways. An extreme way is to replace the monofunctional *trans*-$[Pt(NH_3)_2(dG)Cl]^+$ adduct by the monofunctional *trans*-$[Pt(NH_3)_2(dC)Cl]^+$ adduct. It is likely that the monofunctional *trans*-$[Pt(NH_3)_2(dC)Cl]^+$ adduct is inserted into the double helix and is no longer paired with the complementary G residue. The unpairing of the (G.*trans*-$[Pt(NH_3)_2(dC)Cl]^+$) base pair facilitates the anti-syn rotation of the G residue. Indeed, the closure of monofunctional *trans*-$[Pt(NH_3)_2(dC)Cl]^+$ adduct into an interstrand crosslink is relatively fast ($t_{1/2}$ = 2–3 h) *(44)*. For both *trans*-$[Pt(NH_3)_2(dG)Cl]^+$ and *trans*-$[Pt(NH_3)_2(dC)Cl]^+$ adducts, the formation of an aqua species is assumed. However, one cannot exclude a direct reaction of the chloro species, especially if the monofunctional *trans*-$[Pt(NH_3)_2(dC)Cl]^+$ adduct is inserted into the DNA.

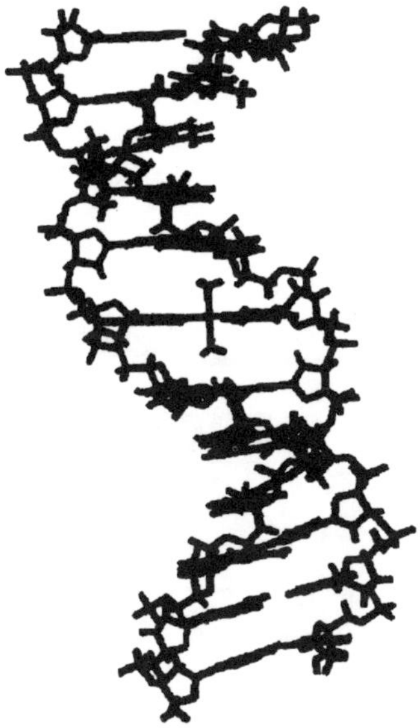

Fig. 3. Transplatin interstrand crosslink. View derived from 2D NMR data of the double-stranded oligonucleotide d(CTCTCG*AGTCTC).d(GAGACTC*GAGAG) containing a single transplatin interstrand crosslink (the platinated residues are indicated by *.)

Another way of modifying DNA locally is to change the chemical nature of the nonleaving groups of the platinum residues. Compared with transplatin, *trans*-[$PtCl_2(NH_3)$(quinoline)] forms more interstrand crosslinks and the reaction is faster ($t_{1/2}$ = 5 h) *(45)*, whereas [$PtCl_2${HN=C(OMe)Me}$_2$] and *trans*-[$PtCl_2${HN=C(OEt)Me}$_2$] *(46–48)* form fewer interstrand crosslinks and the reaction is slower.

2.3. Comparison Between Cisplatin and Transplatin Interstrand Crosslinks

In the reaction between DNA and cisplatin, interstrand crosslinks are preferentially formed between the two G residues at the d(GpC).d(GpC) sites *(36,49)*. The distortions induced in the DNA duplexes by the interstrand crosslinks have been characterized by several techniques *(50,51)*. The two C residues complementary to the crosslinked G residues are largely exposed to the solvent, and the conformational changes occur only at the level of the adducts. The double helix is unwound (79°), and its axis is bent (45°). 2D NMR studies *(52,53)* of two DNA duplexes containing a single interstrand crosslink but differing in their sequences confirm the previous conclusions but also reveal unexpected results. The two C residues complementary to the crosslinked G residues are no longer paired and are extruded from the double helix. This extrusion allows a rotation

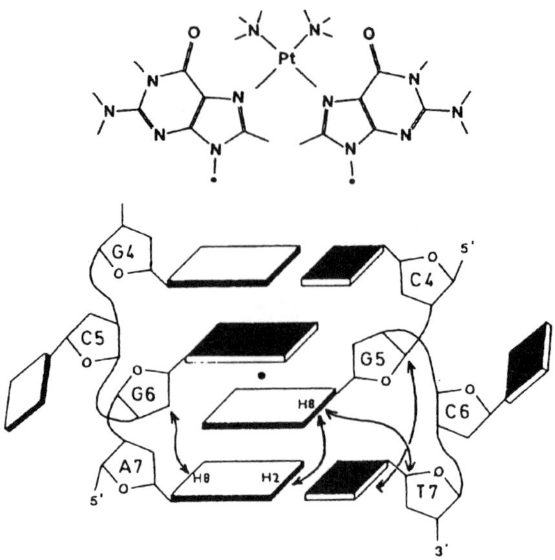

Fig. 4. Cisplatin interstrand crosslink. Top: Cisplatin crosslinked to the two G residues as in the interstrand crosslink. Bottom: Schematic representation, deduced from 2D NMR data, of the relative location of the nucleotides surrounding the crosslinked G*(5) and G*(6) on the opposite strands of the duplex d(CCTCG*CTCTC).d(GAGAG*CGAGG) containing a single interstrand crosslink. The double arrows indicate unusual NOE cross-peaks. (Reproduced with permission from ref. *53).*

of 180° of the platinated G residues, which brings the crosslinked N7 into the minor groove of the double helix. (In B-DNA, the N7 of the G residues are in the major groove.) The reorganization of the duplex leads to a permutation of the relative positions of the two crosslinked G with their sugars pointing in a direction opposite to that of the sugars of the same strand (Fig. 4). At the level of the crosslink, the phosphodiester backbone forms a kind of chicane, the double helix is unwound, and its axis is bent toward the minor groove.

One of the two platinated duplexes studied by NMR has been crystallized. The crystals are of very good quality, and the electron density map at 1.7 Å is directly interpretable at the atomic level *(54)*. The global distortions of the crystallographic and NMR models are qualitatively in good agreement. In addition, the crystallographic model shows that the conformational rearrangement of the platinated duplex originates essentially from changes in the values of the three backbone angles P-—O5′ , P-—O3′, and C5′-—C4′ belonging to the crosslinked residues. The exposure of the complementary C residues arises mainly from a change of about 80° of the C3′-—O3′ angle value. The other residues are in a B-like form. The model also shows a network of ordered water molecules surrounding the crosslink (Fig. 5). Two water molecules are located

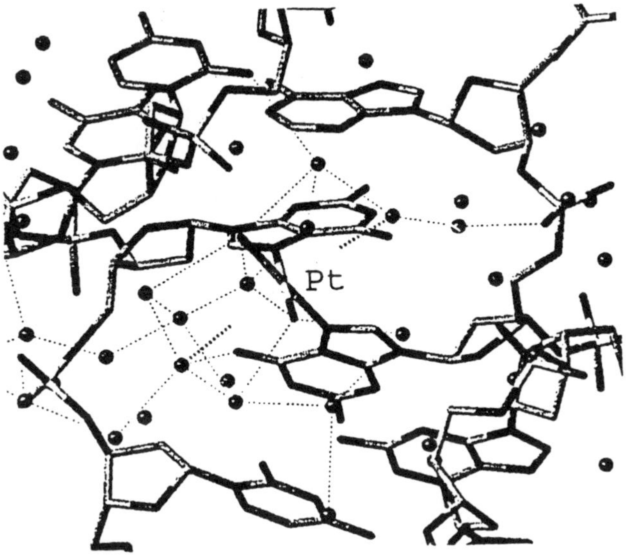

Fig. 5. Representation of the water molecules (•) surrounding the cisplatin interstrand crosslink derived from the X-ray structure of the platinated oligonucleotide d(CCTCG*CTCTC).d(GAGAG*CGAGG).

on either side of the square plane of the platinum residue at about 3.6 Å from the platinum along its quaternary axis. These two water molecules, seven other water molecules, the two NH_3 groups of platinum, and the O6 of the crosslinked G residues form a well-defined cage embeding the platinum residue. The cage is linked by other water molecules to the phosphate groups of the crosslinked G residues and participates in the widening of the minor groove (from 4–6 Å in B-DNA to more than 10 Å in the platinated DNA).

These ordered water molecules could explain, at least in part, the relative instability of the interstrand crosslinks. The bonds between platinum and the N7 of G residues are spontaneously cleaved with essentially one cleavage per crosslinked duplex in either of both DNA strands ($t_{1/2}$ for the cleavage reaction is about 29 h) *(55)*. The cleavage generates monofunctional adducts, which can further react and form intrastrand and interstrand crosslinks. The highly distorted conformation allows the formation of intrastrand crosslinks, whereas they are not formed during the closure of *cis*-$[Pt(NH_3)_2(dG)Cl]^+$ within the same double-stranded oligonucleotide in a B-like form. It is proposed that the instability of the interstrand crosslinks is due to a destabilization of the G-Pt bond by one of the two water molecules in apical position with respect to the square plane of the platinum.

The rate of closure of the monofunctional adduct into an interstrand crosslink depends on the sequence of the oligonucleotides, but it can be almost as fast as the closure of the monofunctional adduct into an intrastrand crosslink at the d(GpG) site. The successive steps of the interstrand crosslinking reaction are not yet known, but it is tempting to speculate that the water molecules play a major role as driving forces during the dramatic conformational changes of the double helix. More generally, the results on the ordered water molecules around the interstrand crosslinks show that it is important to know more about the hydration of DNA for the understanding of the reaction of platination and the plasticity of DNA.

3. TRANSPLATIN-MODIFIED-SINGLE-STRANDED DNA

3.1. Nature of the Adducts

The adducts formed in the reaction between transplatin and single-stranded DNA differ notably from those formed with double-stranded DNA. Although the G residues are the preferred sites, several other sites are available. [Cisplatin and transplatin bind to the four mononucleotides but with different affinity, GMP > AMP > CMP > > UMP *(56)*.] Moreover, the flexibility of single-stranded DNA makes possible contacts between residues located far away along the chain. The closure of the monofunctional adducts leads to the formation of intrastrand crosslinks between two Gs (60%), between G and A (35%), and between G and C (5%) *(32,33)*. Preferential transplatin binding to G residues within single-stranded oligonucleotides is obtained by carrying out the reaction of platination at acidic pH (the p*K*s of AMP and CMP are 3.7 and 4.2, respectively) *(37,57)*. However, unexpected platination can happen with C-rich oligonucleotides. At acidic pH, the C-rich oligonucleotides adopt the i-form. It is a four-stranded structure built by head-to-tail intercalation of two duplexes with C^+.C base pairs *(58)*. With oligonucleotides containing the right stretches of C residues, the i-DNA can be formed by the assembly of four oligonucleotides, of two folded oligonucleotides or by the folding of a single oligonucleotide. This structure, first observed with the oligonucleotide d(TCC-CCC), is also adopted by less regular sequences such as d(5mCCTTTACC), d(5mCCTTTCCTTTACCTTTCC), and sequences containing G residues *(59,60)*. The reactivity of the nucleotide residues in the loops of i-DNA has not yet been studied in detail.

4. REARRANGEMENT OF THE TRANSPLATIN (G1,G3)-INTRASTRAND CROSSLINKS

4.1. Rearrangement Within Single-Stranded DNA

It is generally accepted that the transplatin crosslinks, once formed, are stable. However, two examples have shown that rearrangement of the 1,3-*trans*-$\{Pt(NH_3)_2[GNG]\}$-intrastrand crosslink, N being any nucleotide residue [abbreviated (G1,G3)-intrastrand crosslinks] can occur as schematically represented in Fig. 6.

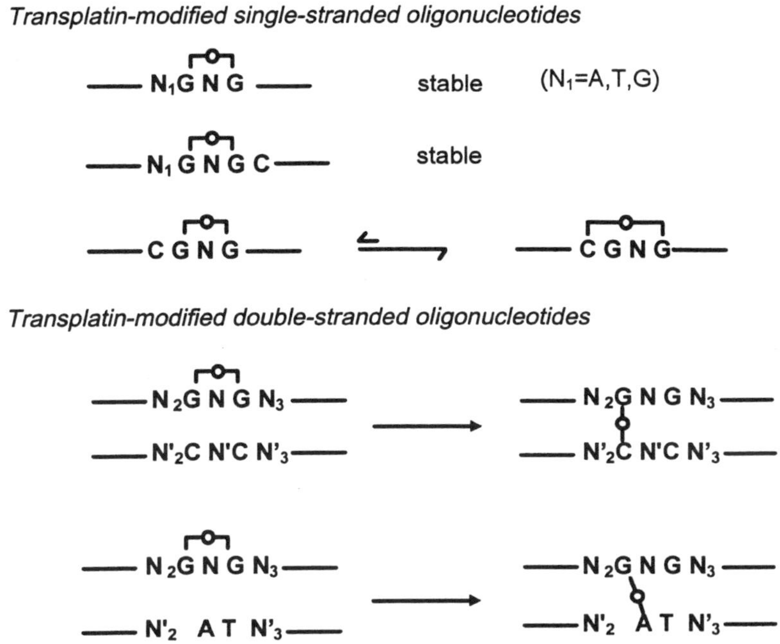

Fig. 6. Rearrangement of the transplatin (G1,G3)-intrastrand crosslink within single-stranded or double-stranded oligonucleotides. N'_1, N'_2, and N'_3 are nucleotide residues complementary to the residues N_1, N_2 and N_3, respectively .

First, we will consider the case dealing with the (G1,G3)-intrastrand crosslink within a single-stranded oligonucleotide *(57,61)*. As long as the 5′-residue adjacent to the crosslink is not a C, the crosslink is stable. If it is a C, the metal migrates from the 5′ G to the 5′ C residue, and an equilibrium between the two isomers, (G1,G3)- and (C1,G4)-intrastrand crosslinks, is attained. The rate of the reaction depends on temperature ($t_{1/2}$ approx 38 h at 37°C) but not on the nature of the salt (NaCl or $NaClO_4$). This independence of the salt nature is not in favor of an intermediate step involving an aqua species during the linkage isomerization reaction.

4.2. Rearrangement Within Double-Stranded DNA

The pairing of the single-stranded oligonucleotides containing a 1,3-*trans*-{$Pt(NH_3)_2$[GNG]}-intrastrand crosslink with their complementary strands has two consequences: on the one hand, the rearrangement of the (G1,G3)-intrastrand crosslink into the (C1,G4)-intrastrand crosslink is blocked; on the other hand, the (G1,G3)-intrastrand crosslink rearranges into an interstrand crosslink whatever the nature of the nucleotide residue adjacent to the intrastrand crosslink on its 5′ side (Fig. 6). This linkage isomerization reaction is triggered by the formation of the double helix *(29, 30)*.

Initially, platinated DNA.DNA duplexes were studied. The interstrand crosslink was formed between the 5′ G of the former intrastrand crosslink and its complementary C. It is identical to the interstrand crosslink in the reaction between transplatin and double-stranded DNA. However, the rate of the interstrand crosslinking reaction ($t_{1/2}$ in the range 3–12 h) is faster than that corresponding to the closure of the monofunctional *trans*-$[Pt(NH_3)_2(dG)Cl]^+$ adduct within double-stranded DNA and is not slowed down in the presence of NaCl. Thus, one can exclude the cleavage of the Pt-3′ G bond with formation of a monofunctional adduct during the rearrangement of the intrastrand crosslink. A direct nucleophilic attack of the Pt-3′ G bond by the C complementary to the 5′ G is proposed.

Although the NMR or crystal structure of a duplex containing a single (G1,G3)-intrastrand crosslink has still to be determined, molecular mechanics modeling indicates that the C residue has the appropriate location and orientation to attack the Pt-3′ G bond. Molecular modeling *(62)* is also in agreement with the bending (45°) and the unwinding (26°) of the double helix, as deduced from gel electrophoresis experiments, and, with the accessibility of 4–5 base pairs (the three base pairs at the level of to the adduct and the 5′ base pair adjacent to the adduct) to chemical probes *(63)*.

4.3. Kinetics of the Rearrangement

A study of various kinds of platinated duplexes has been undertaken to prove the unusual mechanism of the linkage isomerization reaction and also to determine whether the rate of the reaction could be increased to be compatible with biologic applications *(30,35,64,65)*.

At the level of the (G1,G3)-intrastrand crosslink, the sugars, the phosphate groups, and the intervening base between the two crosslinked G do not interfere directly in the reaction. The replacement of either the intervening nucleoside by a propylene link, or the phosphate groups by uncharged methylphosphonate groups, or the deoxyribose by a 2′-O-Me-ribose has a minor effect on the rate of the rearrangement. On the other hand, cleavage of the phosphodiester backbone between the crosslinked G greatly decreases the rate, which shows the importance of the strains imposed by the platinated macrocycle. Some strains are also imposed by the double helix since the rate of the reaction is very slow when the (G1,G3)-intrastrand crosslink is located at the 3′- or 5′-end of the platinated oligonucleotide.

In addition to the strains, assumed to be not very different whatever the shape (A-like or B-like), the double helix interferes with the relative positions of the attacking C residue and the platinum residue. About a 20-fold decrease of the rate occurs when the deoxystrand complementary to the platinated strand is replaced by a ribo strand.

A dramatic increase of the rate is obtained by replacing the triplet CN′ C complementary to the intrastrand crosslink by the doublet 5′-TA or 5′-UA. The interstrand crosslink is formed between the N7 of the 5′ G and the N1 of the A. The rearrangement is complete in a few minutes in the hybrids between the platinated 2′-O-Me-ribo strand and the RNA strand. No rearrangement occurs if 5′-TA or 5′-UA is replaced by 5′-AT or 5′-UA, which stresses the importance of the location of the attacking base.

In summary, the binding of an oligonucleotide containing a (G1,G3)-intrastrand crosslink to its complementary sequence triggers the rearrangement of the intrastrand crosslink into an interstrand crosslink. The rearrangement can be done in a few minutes at 37°C, even in the presence of NaCl, by the right choice of the targeted sequence. This reaction allows specific and irreversible linkage of a platinated oligonucleotide to its target.

5. OLIGONUCLEOTIDES AND MODULATION OF GENE EXPRESSION

It is well established that oligonucleotides can form duplexes with single-stranded RNA and DNA through Watson-Crick hybridization or triplexes with double-stranded RNA or DNA through Hoogsteen and reverse Hoogsteen hybridization. Many studies have recently been undertaken to demonstrate that in vivo oligonucleotides bind to their complementary sequences in mRNA or DNA and subsequently act on the cell machinery [the so-called antisense and antigene strategies *(66–68)*]. In principle, these strategies should make it possible to target one given gene and thus to affect selectively "sick" cells *(69–71)*.

Our purpose is to present briefly the potential interest of oligonucleotides containing a (G1,G3)-intrastrand crosslink in the context of the antisense and antigene strategies. We will limit ourselves to the binding of these platinated oligonucleotides to single-stranded nucleic acids. The rearrangement of the (G1,G3)-intrastrand crosslinks does not seem to be promoted in triplexes. Although it is possible to link oligonucleotides containing a monofunctional *trans*-$[Pt(NH_3)_2(dG)Cl]^+$ or *trans*-$[Pt(NH_3)_2(dC)Cl]^+$ adduct specifically and irreversibly to their complementary sequences within single-stranded or double-stranded DNA *(72,73)*, this will not be discussed here.

5.1. Accessibility of the Target to Oligonucleotides

Assuming that the oligonucleotides have reached the cytoplasm or the nucleus, they have first to bind their targets and then exert their activity. The target must be accessible to the oligonucleotides. Concerning mRNA, even if it is a single-stranded molecule, it folds on itself in a complex way with formation of several stem-loops with further interactions between these stem-loops. In eukaryotic cells, the site of synthesis of mRNA is in the nucleus, whereas the translation of mRNA into protein occurs in the cytoplasm. During all the steps from synthesis up to translation, mRNA undergoes several transformations and interacts with proteins. The prediction of the accessibility of the target is still approximate, but improvements are done in the determination of the 3D structure of RNA and of the regions interacting with proteins *(74,75)*.

In the nucleus, DNA is in a compact B-form, interacting with histones and other proteins. Binding sites for oligonucleotides become available when the double helix is transiently open during transcription and replication. Another potential binding site is the single-stranded 3′-end of the G-rich strand of telomeric DNA. In fact, the state of this 3′-end is still under debate. In vitro, G-rich oligonucleotides form tetraplexes by association of four oligonucleotides or, of two folded oligonucleotides, or by folding of one oligonucleotide with Hoogsteen pairing between four G (the so-called G-quartet) *(76)*. Whatever its structure in vivo, during DNA replication the telomeric 3′-end becomes accessible to the ribonucleoprotein telomerase, a telomere-specific reverse transcriptase, which restores the integrity of DNA *(77)*.

5.2. Inhibition of Cell Machinery by Oligonucleotides

The mechanism of action of the oligonucleotides depends on the target. We consider first the case of mRNA.

Once bound to RNA, the oligonucleotides lead to inhibition of translation or RNA metabolism by two general mechanisms, which are either degradation of the targeted mRNA through an RNase H-mediated cleavage or steric blocking of the cellular machinery *(71)*.

RNase H presents two major advantages *(78)*. It is an ubiquitous protein, and, after RNase H-mediated cleavage of the mRNA, the oligonucleotide is available to bind to another RNA molecule. However, this mechanism presents two drawbacks. RNase H is less active but still active on hybrids containing mismatches, leading to a possible loss in the specificity of the oligonucleotides. Activation of RNase H implies the use of oligodeoxyribonucleotides, which are highly sensitive to the action of nucleases present in the cells. There are ways to minimize these drawbacks such as chemical modifications of the phosphate groups (for example, phosphorothioate and phosphorodithioate) or of the bases (for example, C-5 propynyl pyridine instead of C) *(79, 80)*.

Steric blocking has been less exploited *(81,82)*. Although some experiments are very promising, such as the restoration of correct splicing of thalassemic human β-globin mRNA in mammalian cells *(83)*, the steric blocking presents a major constraint. The oligonucleotide-RNA hybrids have to be stable enough to avoid dissociation by the cellular machinery. When directed to the coding region, antisense oligonucleotides are dissociated from their target by translating ribosomes *(82)*. A major advantage of the steric blocking is that chemically modified oligonucleotides can be used; these make them resistant to nucleases, increase their affinity for their targets, and stabilize the corresponding hybrids. However, the so-called second generation of oligonucleotides as peptide nucleic acids *(84)* and N3′→P5′ phosphoramidate oligonucleotides *(85,86)*, which fulfil these conditions, are still displaced by translating ribosomes *(87)*.

When the target is DNA, the oligonucleotides act by steric blocking and as previously, the cellular machinery can displace the oligonucleotides *(88)*.

To avoid the displacement, a possibility is to crosslink the oligonucleotides to the targets. This has been achieved by tethering a photocrosslinking or a chemical crosslinking (generally an alkylating electrophile) reagent to the oligonucleotides *(89)*. Irradiation of the samples is not easy to do in vivo, and the chemical reactions are often nonspecific and slow. The use of the oligonucleotides containing an (G1,G3)-intrastrand crosslink presents several advantages for irreversible and specific crosslinkage of the oligonucleotides to their targets.

5.3. Efficacy of the Platinated Oligonucleotides

Up to now, the efficacy of the oligonucleotides containing a (G1,G3)-intrastrand crosslink has been assayed by targeting mRNA.

The specificity of the crosslinking reaction has been shown by mixing capped Ha-ras mRNA (820 residues) with a complementary platinated oligo-2′-O-Me-nucleotide (17-mer), named Ras1(Pt) *(30)*. After incubation of the mixture, the location of the oligonucleotide was revealed by primer extension with AMV reverse transcriptase. The polymerization reaction was stopped at the level of the oligonucleotide, and no other stops were detected. This demonstrates that the platinated oligonucleotide is crosslinked at the expected location and is not displaced by the enzyme.

The specificity of the crosslinked reaction was further tested by looking at the efficiency of the crosslinked oligonucleotides in inhibiting protein synthesis in a cell-free system *(30)*. Capped Ha-ras mRNA and the platinated oligonucleotide Ras1(Pt) were mixed, and after 10 min incubation, amino acids and rabbit reticulocyte lysate were added. The products of the reaction were analyzed by gel electrophoresis. As shown in Fig. 7, the platinated oligonucleotide is able to inhibit Ha-ras mRNA translation completely.

The specificity and efficacy of the platinated oligonucleotides have also been confirmed by in vitro translation of vesicular stomatitis virus mRNA. In the absence of oligonucleotide, the three major viral proteins are synthesized, whereas in the presence of the appropriate platinated oligonucleotide, only the synthesis of one of the three proteins *(87)* is inhibited.

The specific and irreversible binding of the platinated oligonucleotides to their targets occurs in complex medium, as shown by the binding of Ras1(Pt) to Ha-ras mRNA in HBL100ras 1 cells *(30)*. It is known that the selective de-

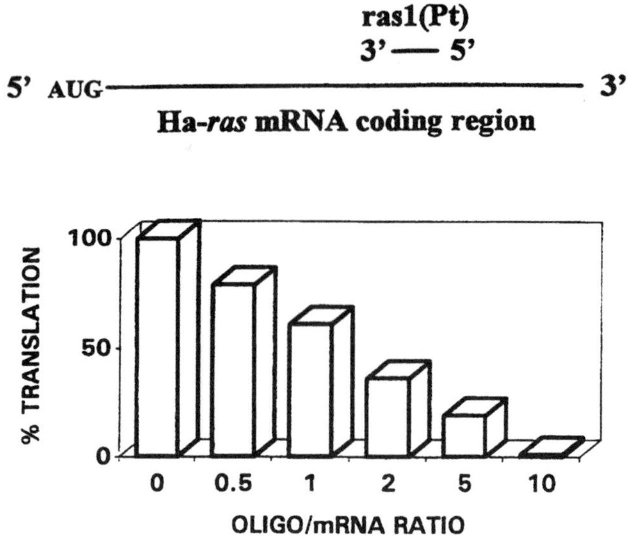

Fig. 7. In vitro inhibition of capped Ha-ras mRNA translation by the oligo-2′-O-methylnucleotide Ras1(Pt) containing a single (G1,G3)-intrastrand crosslink.

pletion of Ha-ras proteins in HBL100ras 1 cells leads to inhibition of cell division. It has been verified that the treatment of these cells by the platinated oligonucleotide Ras1(Pt) induces a dose-dependent inhibition of cell proliferation in the range 0–4 μM.

6. SUMMARY AND PERSPECTIVES

In their reaction with DNA, both cisplatin and transplatin form monofunctional adducts at approximately the same rate. The cisplatin monofunctional adducts close into intrastrand crosslinks, essentially at the d(GpG) and then d(ApG) sites, whereas the transplatin adducts close mainly into interstrand crosslinks at complementary (G.C) base pairs. The rate of closure is faster by at least one order of magnitude for cisplatin than for transplatin monofunctional adducts. Transplatin interstrand crosslinks are found at most but not all of the (G.C) base pairs. This suggests that transplatin, contrary to cisplatin, does not react preferentially at $d(G)_n$ sequences and/or that the closure of transplatin monofunctional adducts depends strongly on the nature of the base pairs flanking the adducts. The long lifetime of transplatin monofunctional adducts and their strong reactivity with sulfur-containing nucleophiles, could explain at least in part, the clinical inefficiency of transplatin *(32,39)*. This is supported by the facts that transplatin monofunctional adducts react with glutathione much faster than cisplatin monofunctional adducts *(32,34)* and that depletion of glutathione increases the sensitivity of ovarian carcinoma cells to transplatin but not to cisplatin *(90,91)*.

Do these results mean that a platinum complex has to form bifunctional lesions to be an antitumor drug? This is generally accepted because platinum complexes that bind monofunctionally to DNA, such as $[Pt(NH_3)_3Cl]^+$ and chlorodiethylenetriammineplatinum(II) chloride, are inactive. However, some platinum complexes do not seem to obey this rule.

Trisubstituted complexes of general formula *cis*-$[Pt(NH_3)_2(Am)Cl]^{n+}$ where Am is an heterocyclic amine such as pyridine, pyrimidine, ellipticine, etc., react with DNA and form monofunctional adducts. Some of these trisubstituted platinum(II) complexes are active against a number of murine and human cell lines *(92)*. Whether this activity is related essentially to the monofunctional *cis*-$[Pt(NH_3)_2(Am)(G)]^{n+1}$ adducts and/or to the transformation of these monofunctional adducts into the monofunctional *cis*-$[Pt(NH_3)_2(dG)(H_2O)]^{2+}$ adducts, and eventually into bifunctional crosslinks, is still under study *(64)*.

Another fascinating field concerns the antitumor activity exhibited by transplatin derivatives in which the NH_3 groups are substituted by iminoether. The transplatin-iminoether complexes react preferentially with G residues in double-stranded DNA and form monofunctional adducts *(46–48)*. These monofunctional adducts evolve slowly into interstrand crosslinks, even more slowly than transplatin monofunctional adducts. Moreover, the former are more resistant to the action of thiourea than the latter, probably for steric reasons. It is tempting to speculate that bifunctional lesions are not involved in the antitumor activity of the transplatin-iminoether complexes, unlike cisplatin. In cells, the long-lived transplatin-iminoether monofunctional adducts are expected to be hardly reactive with small sulfur-containing compounds for steric reasons. Nevertheless, they are good candidates for crosslinking proteins that interact with DNA along its major groove, eventually distort it, and, have a relatively long dwelltime. The DNA-protein crosslinks could be responsible for the cytotoxicity of the transplatin-iminoether complexes. Such a scheme has been already proposed for some cisplatin derivatives *(93)*. The *trans* configuration seems more favorable for a crosslinking reaction with proteins than the *cis* configuration. Experiments are in progress to test this hypothesis.

The studies on single-stranded nucleic acids containing a transplatin (G1,G3)-intrastrand crosslink lead us to consider these platinated oligonucleotides as new derivatives with distinct structure-activity relationships. The platinum residue is coordinated to four nitrogen ligands. The platinated oligonucleotides are prepared by reacting transplatin with the appropriate single-stranded oligonucleotides. The resulting (G1,G3)-intrastrand crosslinks are inert under normal conditions. However, the pairing of the platinated oligonucleotides with their complementary sequences within nucleic acids triggers the rearrangement of the (G1,G3)-intrastrand crosslinks into interstrand crosslinks. Conditions have been established in which the rate of the crosslinking reaction is relatively fast (*$t_{1/2}$* in the range of a few minutes). The specificity of the reaction has been proved in cell-free and cell systems. The crosslinked oligonucleotides are able to stop the cell machinery at different levels and to inhibit cell growth. The platinated oligonucleotides can regulate gene expression and thus can be considered potential antitumor drugs.

Several problems are encountered when the platinated oligonucleotides are tested in cells. The targeted sequence must be accessible to the oligonucleotide, long enough to form a stable double-helix, and contain preferentially a 5′-TA or 5′-UA doublet. It should not be a C-rich sequence. In addition to the GNG triplet, the presence of several G in the oligonucleotides decreases the yield of the platination reaction at the GNG triplet. Furthermore, relatively large quantities of the platinated oligonucleotides are necessary for in vivo assays. It is clear that the automated solid-phase synthesis of site-specifically platinated oligonucleotides *(94,95)* will be highly useful in this field. A major hurdle in the antisense and antigene approaches is the poor passage of the oligonucleotides through biologic barriers and thus their low concentrations in the appropriate intracellular compartments. Physical association to various compounds including cationic lipids improve the cellular uptake of the oligonucleotides *(96,97)*. It should be mentioned that several control experiments have to be done to prove that the oligonucleotides are effective as antisense or antigene agents.

Since the pioneering work of Zamecnick and Stephenson *(98)* on the inhibition of Rous sarcoma virus replication by oligonucleotides, numerous studies have been devoted to the development of oligonucleotides as therapeutic drugs. An ever increasing body of information strengthens the potential of oligonucleotides for modulating gene expression. There are already promising results showing that the oligonucleotides are effective against viral and cancer targets both in vivo and in vitro, and human clinical trials are in progress. Surprisingly, several therapeutic oligonucleotides display greater potency in animal than in cell culture. All these studies have greatly contributed to our knowledge of oligonucleotides (and nucleic acids) and their behavior in cell-free and cell systems, as well as to the larger use of oligonucleotides in biotechnology. Although many problems remain to be solved, this new class of drug offers an attractive possibility for various diseases.

ACKNOWLEDGMENTS

We are deeply indebted for many helpful discussions to Pr. B. Lippert (Dortmund, Germany), Dr. J. Arpalahti (Turku, Finland), and our collaborators Drs. C. Janke, J.-M. Malinge, and R. Rahmouni. This work was supported in part by la Ligue Contre le Cancer and the European Community (COST D8 and BMH4-CT97–2485).

REFERENCES

1. Rosenberg, B., van Camp, L. and Krigas, T. (1965) Inhibition of cell division in *E. coli* by electrolysis products from a platinum electrode. *Nature* **205,** 698–699.
2. Rosenberg, B., Van Camp, L., Grimley, E. B., and Thomson, A. J. (1967) The inhibition of growth or cell division in *Escherichia coli* by different ionic species of platinum(IV) complexes. *J. Biol. Chem.* **242,** 1347–1352.
3. Barry, M. A., Behnke, C. A., and Eastman, A. (1990) Activation of programmed cell death (apoptosis) by cisplatin, other anticancer drugs, toxins and hyperthermia. *Biochem. Pharmacol.* **40,** 2353–2362.
4. Chu, G. (1994) Cellular responses to cisplatin. The roles of DNA-binding proteins and DNA repair. *J. Biol. Chem.* **269,** 787–790.
5. Henkels, K. M. and Turchi, J. J. (1997) Induction of apoptosis in cisplatin-sensitive and -resistant human ovarian cancer cell lines. *Cancer Res.* **57,** 4488–4492.
6. Fichtinger-Schepman, A. M., van der Veer, J. L., den Hartog, J. H., Lohman, P. H., and Reedijk, J. (1985) Adducts of the antitumor drug *cis*-diamminedichloroplatinum(II) with DNA: formation, identification, and quantitation. *Biochemistry* **24,** 707–713.
7. Comess, K. M. and Lippard, S. J. (1993) Molecular aspects of platinum-DNA interactions, in *Molecular Aspects of Anti-Cancer Drug-DNA Interactions*, vol. 1 (Neidle, S. and Waring, M., eds), Macmillan, London, pp. 134–168.
8. Reedijk, J. (1996) Improved understanding in platinum antitumor chemistry. *Chem. Commun.* 801–806.
9. Lepre, C. A. and Lippard, S. J. (1990) Interaction of platinum antitumor compounds with DNA, in *Nucleic Acids and Molecular Biology*, vol. 4 (Eckstein, F. and Lilley, D. M. J., eds.), Springer-Verlag, Berlin, pp. 9–38.
10. Sip, M. and Leng, M. (1993) DNA, cisplatinum and intercalators: catalytic activity of the DNA double helix, in *Nucleic Acids and Molecular Biology*, vol. 7 (Eckstein, F. and Lilley, D. M. J., eds.), Springer-Verlag, Berlin, pp. 1–15.
11. Frit, P., Calsou, P., Canitrot, Y., Muller, C., and Salles, B. (1996) Damaged-DNA binding proteins and cisplatin resistance. *Anti-Cancer Drugs*, **7,** 101–108.
12. Whitehead, J. P. and Lippard, S. J. (1996) Proteins that bind to and mediate the biological activity of platinum anticancer drug-DNA adducts, in *Metal Ions in Biological Systems* (Sigel, A. and Sigel, H., eds.) Marcel Dekker, New York, pp. 687–720.
13. Stros, M. (1998) DNA bending by the chromosomal protein HMG1 and its high mobility group box domains. Effect of flanking sequences. *J. Biol. Chem.* **273,** 10355–1036.
14. Ohndorf, U. M., Whitehead, J. P., Raju, N. L., and Lippard, S. J. (1997) Binding of tsHMG, a mouse testis-specific HMG-domain protein, to cisplatin-DNA adducts. *Biochemistry* **36,** 14807–14815.
15. Yaneva, J., Leuba, S. H., van Holde, K., and Zlatanova, J. (1997) The major chromatin protein histone H1 binds preferentially to cisplatinum-damaged DNA. *Proc. Natl. Acad. Sci. USA* **94,** 13448–13451.
16. Moggs, J. G., Szymkowski, D. E., Yamada, M., Karran, P., and Wood, R. D. (1997) Differential human nucleotide excision repair of paired and mispaired cisplatin-DNA adducts. *Nucleic Acids Res.* **25,** 480–491.
17. Hoffmann, J. S., Locker, D., Villani, G., and Leng, M. (1997) HMG1 protein inhibits the translesion synthesis of the major DNA cisplatin adduct by cell extracts. *J. Mol. Biol.* **270,** 539–543.
18. Vichi, P., Coin, F., Renaud, J. P., Vermeulen, W., Hoeijmakers, J. H., Moras, D. and Egly, J. M. (1997) Cisplatin- and UV-damaged DNA lure the basal transcription factor TFIID/TBP. *EMBO J.* **16,** 7444–7456.
19. Zhai, X., Beckmann, H., Jantzen, H. M., and Essigmann, J. M. (1998) Cisplatin-DNA

adducts inhibit ribosomal RNA synthesis by hijacking the transcription factor human upstream binding factor. *Biochemistry* **37,** 16307–16315.

20. Farrell, N., ed. (1989) *Transition Metal Complexes as Drugs and Chemotherapeutic Agents*, Kluwer Academic Publishers, Dordrecht.
21. Kelland, L. R., Barnard, C. F., Mellish, K. J., Jones, M., Goddard, P. M., Valenti, M., et al. (1994) A novel transplatinum coordination complex possessing in vitro and in vivo antitumor activity. *Cancer Res.* **54,** 5618–5622.
22. Kelland, L. R., Barnard, C. F., Evans, I. G., Murrer, B. A., Theobald, B. R., Wyer, S. B., et al. (1995) Synthesis and in vitro and in vivo antitumor activity of a series of transplatinum antitumor complexes. *J. Med. Chem.* **38,** 3016–3024.
23. Farrell, N., Kelland, L. R., Roberts, J. D., and Van Beusichem, M. (1992) Activation of the trans geometry in platinum antitumor complexes: a survey of the cytotoxicity of trans complexes containing planar ligands in murine L1210 and human tumor panels and studies on their mechanism of action. *Cancer Res.* **52,** 5065–5072.
24. Zou, Y., Van Houten, B., and Farrell, N. (1993) Ligand effects on platinum binding to DNA. A comparison of DNA binding properties for *cis*- and *trans*-[$PtCl_2$(amine)$_2$] (amine = NH_3, pyridine). *Biochemistry* **32,** 9632–9638.
25. Coluccia, M., Nassi, A., Loseto, F., Boccarelli, A., Mariggio, M. A., Giordano, D., et al. (1993) A transplatinum complex showing higher antitumor activity than the cis congeners. *J. Med. Chem.* **36,** 510–512.
26. Coluccia, M., Boccarelli, A., Mariggio, M. A., Cardellicchio, N., Caputo, P., Intini, F. P., et al. (1995) Platinum(II) complexes containing iminoethers: a transplatinum antitumour agent. *Chem. Biol. Interact.* **98,** 251–266.
27. Farell, N. (1996) DNA binding of dinuclear platinum complexes, in *Advances in DNA Sequence Specific Agents*, vol. 2, JAI, 187–216.
28. Lippert, B. (1996) *Trans*-diammineplatinum(II): what makes it different from *cis*-DDP? Coordination chemistry of a neglected relative of cisplatin and its interaction with nucleic acids, in *Metal Ions in Biological Systems* (Sigel, A. and Sigel, H., eds.) Marcel Dekker, New York, pp. 105–133.
29. Dalbies, R., Payet, D., and Leng, M. (1994) DNA double helix promotes a linkage isomerization reaction in *trans*-diamminedichloroplatinum(II)-modified DNA. *Proc. Natl. Acad. Sci. USA* **91,** 8147–8151.
30. Boudvillain, M., Guerin, M., Dalbies, R., Saison-Behmoaras, T., and Leng, M. (1997) Transplatin-modified oligo(2′-O-methyl ribonucleotide)s: a new tool for selective modulation of gene expression. *Biochemistry* **36,** 2925–2931.
31. Arpalahti, J. (1996) Platinum(II)-nucleobase interactions. A kinetic approach, in *Metal Ions in Biological Systems* (Sigel, A. and Sigel, H., eds.) Marcel Dekker, New York, pp. 379–392.
32. Eastman, A. and Barry, M. A. (1987) Interaction of *trans*-diamminedichloroplatinum(II) with DNA: formation of monofunctional adducts and their reaction with glutathione. *Biochemistry* **26,** 3303–3307.
33. Eastman, A., Jennerwein, M. M., and Nagel, D. L. (1988) Characterization of bifunctional adducts produced in DNA by *trans*-diamminedichloroplatinum(II). *Chem. Biol. Interact.* **67,** 71–80.
34. Bancroft, D. P., Lepre, C. A., and Lippard, S. J. (1990) ^{195}Pt NMR kinetic and mechanistic studies of *cis*- and *trans*-diamminedichloroplatinum(II) binding to DNA. *J. Am. Chem. Soc.* **112,** 6860–6871.
35. Boudvillain, M., Dalbies, R., Aussourd, C., and Leng, M. (1995) Intrastrand crosslinks are not formed in the reaction between transplatin and native DNA: relation with the clinical inefficiency of transplatin. *Nucleic Acids Res.* **23,** 2381–2388.
36. Lemaire, M. A., Schwartz, A., Rahmouni, A. R., and Leng, M. (1991) Interstrand crosslinks are preferentially formed at the d(GC) sites in the reaction between *cis*-diamminedichloroplatinum (II) and DNA. *Proc. Natl. Acad. Sci. USA* **88,** 1982–1985.
37. Brabec, V. and Leng, M. (1993) DNA interstrand crosslinks of *trans*-diamminedichloroplat-

inum(II) are preferentially formed between guanine and complementary cytosine residues. *Proc. Natl. Acad. Sci. USA* **90,** 5345–5349.
38. Brabec, V., Sip, M., and Leng, M. (1993) DNA conformational change produced by the site-specific interstrand crosslink of *trans*-diamminedichloroplatinum(II). *Biochemistry* **32,** 11676–11681.
39. Bernal-Mendez, E., Boudvillain, M., Gonzalez-Vilchez, F., and Leng, M. (1997) Chemical versatility of transplatin monofunctional adducts within multiple site-specifically platinated DNA. *Biochemistry* **36,** 7281–7287.
40. Leng, M. (1990) DNA bending induced by covalently bound drugs. Gel electrophoresis and chemical probe studies. *Biophys. Chem.* **35,** 155–163.
41. Nielsen, P. E. (1990) Chemical and photochemical probing of DNA complexes. *J. Mol. Recognit.* **3,** 1–25.
42. Bellon, S. F. and Lippard, S. J. (1990) Bending studies of DNA site-specifically modified by cisplatin, *trans*-diamminedichloroplatinum(II) and *cis*-$[Pt(NH_3)_2(N_3\text{-cytosine})Cl]^+$. *Biophys. Chem.* **35,** 179–188.
43. Paquet, F., Boudvillain, M., Leng, M., and Lancelot, G., (1999). NMR solution structure of a DNA dodecamer containing a transplatin interstrand GN7/CN3 cross-link. *Nucleic Acids Res.* (in press).
44. Leng, M., unpublished results.
45. Zakovska, A., Novakova, O., Balcarova, Z., Bierbach, U., Farrell, N., and Brabec, V. (1998) DNA interactions of antitumor *trans*-$[PtCl_2(NH_3)(\text{quinoline})]$. *Eur. J. Biochem.* 254, 547–557.
46. Brabec, V., Vrana, O., Novakova, O., Kleinwachter, V., Intini, F. P., Coluccia, M., et al. (1996) DNA adducts of antitumor *trans*-$[PtCl_2$ (E-imino ether$)_2]$. *Nucleic Acids Res.* 24, 336–341.
47. Zaludova, R., Zakovska, A., Kasparkova, J., Balcarova, Z., Vrana, O., Coluccia, M., et al. (1997) DNA modifications by antitumor *trans*-$[PtCl_2(\text{E-iminoether})_2]$. *Mol. Pharmacol.* **52,** 354–361.
48. Boccarelli, A., Coluccia, M., Intini, F. P., Natile, G., Locker, D., and Leng, M. (1998) Cytotoxicity and DNA binding mode of new platinum-iminoether derivatives with different configuration at the iminoether ligands. *Anti-Cancer Drug Des.*, in press.
49. Millard, J. T., Weidner, M. F., Kirchner, J. J., Ribeiro, S., and Hopkins, P. B. (1991) Sequence preferences of DNA interstrand crosslinking agents: quantitation of interstrand crosslink locations in DNA duplex fragments containing multiple crosslinkable sites. *Nucleic Acids Res.* **19,** 1885–1891.
50. Sip, M., Schwartz, A., Vovelle, F., Ptak, M., and Leng, M. (1992) Distortions induced in DNA by cisplatinum interstrand adducts. *Biochemistry* **31,** 2508–2513.
51. Malinge, J. M., Perez, C., and Leng, M. (1994) Base sequence-independent distorsions induced by interstrand cross- links in *cis*-diamminedichloroplatinum(II)-modified DNA. *Nucleic Acids Res.* **22,** 3834–3839.
52. Huang, H., Zhu, L., Reid, B. R., Drobny, G. P., and Hopkins, P. B. (1995) Solution structure of a cisplatin-induced DNA interstrand crosslink. *Science* **270,** 1842–1845.
53. Paquet, F., Perez, C., Leng, M., Lancelot, G., and Malinge, J. M. (1996) NMR solution structure of a DNA decamer containing an interstrand crosslink of the antitumor drug *cis*-diamminedichloroplatinum(II). *J. Biomol. Struct. Dyn.* **14,** 67–77.
54. Coste, F., Malinge, J. M., Serre, L, Sheppard, W., Roth, M., Leng, M., and Zelwer, C., (1999) Crystal structure of a double-stranded DNA containing a cisplatin interstrand cross-link at 1.63 Å resolution: hydration at the platinated site. *Nucleic Acids Res.* **27,** 1837–1846.
55. Perez, C., Leng, M., and Malinge, J. M. (1997) Rearrangement of interstrand crosslinks into intrastrand crosslinks in *cis*-diamminedichloroplatinum(II)-modified DNA. *Nucleic Acids Res.* **25,** 896–903.
56. Mansy, S., Rosenberg, B., and Thomson, A. J. (1978) Binding of *cis*- or *trans*-dichlorodiammineplatinum(II) to nucleosides. 1. Location of binding sites. *J. Am. Chem. Soc.* **95,** 1633–1640.

57. Comess, K. M., Costello, C. E., and Lippard, S. J. (1990) Identification and characterization of a novel linkage isomerization in the reaction of *trans*-diamminedichloroplatinum(II) with 5′-d(TCTACGCGTTCT). *Biochemistry* **29,** 2102–2110.
58. Gehring, K., Leroy, J. L., and Gueron, M. (1993) A tetrameric DNA structure with protonated cytosine.cytosine base pairs. *Nature* **363,** 561–565.
59. Nonin, S., Phan, A. T., and Leroy, J. L. (1997) Solution structure and base pair opening kinetics of the i-motif dimer of d(5mCCTTTACC): a non canonical structure with possible roles in chromosome stability. *Structure* **5,** 1231–1246.
60. Gallego, J., Chou, S. H., and Reid, B. R. (1997) Centromeric pyrimidine strands fold into an intercalated motif by forming a double hairpin with a novel T:G:G:T tetrad: solution structure of the d(TCCCGTTTCCA) dimer. *J. Mol. Biol.* **273,** 840–856.
61. Dalbies, R., Boudvillain, M., and Leng, M. (1995) Linkage isomerization reaction of intrastrand crosslinks in *trans*-diamminedichloroplatinum(II)-modified single-stranded oligonucleotides. *Nucleic Acids Res.* **23,** 949–953.
62. Prevost, C., Boudvillain, M., Beudaert, P., Leng, M., Lavery, R., and Vovelle, F. (1997) Distortions of the DNA double helix induced by 1,3-*trans*-diamminedichloroplatinum(II)-intrastrand crosslink: an internal coordinate molecular modeling study. *J. Biomol. Struct. Dyn.* **14,** 703–714.
63. Anin, M. F. and Leng, M. (1990) Distortions induced in double-stranded oligonucleotides by the binding of *cis*- or *trans*-diamminedichloroplatinum(II) to the d(GTG) sequence. *Nucleic Acids Res.* **18,** 4395–4400.
64. Boudvillain, M., Dalbies, R., and Leng, M. (1996) Evidences for a catalytic activity of the DNA double helix in the reaction between DNA, platinum(II), and intercalators, in *Metal Ions in Biological Systems* (Sigel, A. and Sigel, H., eds.) Marcel Dekker, New York, pp. 87–102.
65. Colombier, C., Boudvillain, M., and Leng, M. (1997) Interstrand crosslinking reaction in transplatin-modified oligo-2′-O-methyl ribonucleotide-RNA hybrids. *Antisense Nucleic Acid Drug. Dev.* **7,** 397–402.
66. Miller, P. S. (1996) Development of antisense and antigene oligonucleotide analogs. *Prog. Nucleic Acid Res. Mol. Biol.* **52,** 261–291.
67. Crooke, S. T. (1996) Progress in antisense therapeutics. *Med. Res. Rev.* **16**, 319–344.
68. Giovannangeli, C. and Hélène, C. (1997) Progress in developments of triplex-based strategies. *Antisense Nucleic Acid Drug. Dev.* **7**,, 413–421.
69. Agrawal, S. (1996) Antisense oligonucleotides: towards clinical trials. *Trends Biotechnol.* **14,** 376–387.
70. Wagner, R. W. and Flanagan, W. M. (1997) Antisense technology and prospects for therapy of viral infections and cancer. *Mol. Med. Today* **3,** 31–38.
71. Chadwick, D. J. and Cardew, G., eds. (1997) *Oligonucleotides as Therapeutic Agents*. Ciba Found. Symp. 209, John Wiley & Sons, Chichester.
72. Colombier, C., Lippert, B., and Leng, M. (1996) Interstrand crosslinking reaction in triplexes containing a monofunctional transplatin-adduct. *Nucleic Acids Res.* **24,** 4519–4524.
73. Bernal-Mendez, E., Sun, J-S., Gonzalez-Vilchez, F., and Leng, M. (1998) Reactivity of transplatin-modified oligonucleotides in triple-helical DNA complexes. *New J. Chem.*, in press.
74. Shirley, L.-M., Auffinger, P., and Westhof, E. (1996) Calculations of nucleic acid conformations. *Curr. Opin. Struct. Biol.* **6,** 289–298.
75. Scherr, M. and Rossi, J. J. (1998) Rapid determination and quantitation of the accessibility to native RNAs by antisense oligodeoxynucleotides in murine cell extracts. *Nucleic Acids Res.* **26,** 5079–5085.
76. Shafer, R. H. (1998) Stability and structure of model DNA triplexes and quadruplexes and their interactions with small ligands. *Prog. Nucleic Acid Res. Mol. Biol.* **59,** 55–94.
77. Zakian, V. A. (1997) Life and cancer without telomerase. *Cell* **91,** 1–3.
78. Crouch, R. J. and J. J. Toulmé, eds. (1998) *Ribonucleases H.*, John Libbey, Paris.

79. Stein, C. A. (1996) Phosphorothioate antisense oligodeoxynucleotides: questions of specificity. *Trends Biotechnol.* **14,** 147–149.
80. Gutierrez, A. J., Matteucci, M. D., Grant, D., Matsumura, S., Wagner, R. W., and Froehler, B. C. (1997) Antisense gene inhibition by C-5-substituted deoxyuridine-containing oligodeoxynucleotides. *Biochemistry* **36,** 743–748.
81. Woolf, T. M. (1995) To cleave or not to cleave: ribozymes and antisense. *Antisense Nucleic Acid Drug Dev.* **5,** 227–232.
82. Pantopoulos, K., Johansson, H. E., and Hentze, M. W. (1994) The role of the 5′ untranslated region of eukaryotic messenger RNAs in translation and its investigation using antisense technologies. *Prog. Nucleic Acid Res. Mol. Biol.* **48,** 181–238.
83. Sierakowska, H., Sambade, M. J., Agrawal, S., and Kole, R. (1996) Repair of thalassemic human beta-globin mRNA in mammalian cells by antisense oligonucleotides. *Proc. Natl. Acad. Sci. USA* **93,** 12840–12844.
84. Nielsen, P. E. (1997) Peptide nucleic acid (PNA) from DNA recognition to antisense and DNA structure. *Biophys. Chem.* **68,** 103–108.
85. Schultz, R. G. and Gryaznov, S. M. (1996) Oligo-2′-fluoro-2′-deoxynucleotide N3′→P5′ phosphoramidates: synthesis and properties. *Nucleic Acids Res.* **24,** 2966–2973.
86. Gryaznov, S. M. and Winter, H. (1998) RNA mimetics: oligoribonucleotide N3′→P5′ phosphoramidates. *Nucleic Acids Res.* **26,** 4160–4167.
87. Gee, J. E., Robbins, I., van der Laan, A. C., van Boom, J. H., Colombier, C., Leng, M., et al. (1998) Assessment of high-affinity hybridization, RNase H cleavage, and covalent linkage in translation arrest by antisense oligonucleotides. *Antisense Nucleic Acid Drug. Dev.* **8,** 103–111.
88. Hélène, C., Giovannangeli, C., Guieysse-Peugeot, A-L., and Praseuth, D. (1997) Sequence-specific control of gene expression by antigene and clamp oligonucleotides, in *Oligonucleotides as Therapeutic Agents* (Chadwick, D. J. and Cardew, G. E., eds.), Ciba Found. Symp. 209, John Wiley & Sons, Chichester.
89. Thuong, N. T. and Hélène, C. (1993) Sequence-specific recognition and modification of double-helical DNA by oligonucleotides. *Angew. Chem. Int. Ed. Engl.* **32,** 666–690.
90. Andrews, P. A., Murphy, M. P., and Howell, S. B. (1985) Differential potentiation of alkylating and platinating agent cytotoxicity in human ovarian carcinoma cells by glutathione depletion. *Cancer Res.* **45,** 6250–6253.
91. Eastman, A. (1987) Glutathione-mediated activation of anticancer platinum(IV) complexes. *Biochem. Pharmacol.* **36,** 4177–4178.
92. Hollis, L.S., Amundsen, A.R., and Stern, E.W. (1989) Chemical and biological properties of a new series of cis-diammineplatinum(II) antitumor agents containing three nitrogen donors: *cis*-$[Pt(NH_3)_2(N\text{-donor})Cl]^+$. *J. Med. Chem.* **32,** 128–136.
93. Lambert, B., Jestin, J. L., Brehin, P., Oleykowski, C., Yeung, A. T., Mailliet, P., et al. (1995) Binding of the *Escherichia coli* UvrAB proteins to the DNA mono- and diadducts of *cis*-[N-2-amino-N-2-methylamino-2,2,1- bicycloheptane]dichloroplatinum(II) and cisplatin. Analysis of the factors controlling recognition and proof of monoadduct-mediated UvrB-DNA crosslinking. *J. Biol. Chem.* **270,** 21251–21257.
94. Manchanda, R., Dunham, S. U., and Lippard, S. J. (1996) Automated solid-phase synthesis of site-specifically platinated oligonucleotides. *J. Am. Chem. Soc.* **118,** 5144–5145.
95. Schiepe, J., Berghoff, U., Lippert, B., and Cech, D. (1996) Automated solid phase synthesis of platinated oligonucleotide phosphonates. *Angew. Chem. Int. Ed. Engl.* **35,** 646–648.
96. Behr, J. P. (1994) Gene transfer with synthetic cationic amphiphiles: prospects for gene therapy. *Bioconjug. Chem.* **5,** 382–389.
97. Zanta, M. A., Boussif, O., Adib, A., and Behr, J. P. (1997) In vitro gene delivery to hepatocytes with galactosylated polyethylenimine. *Bioconjug. Chem.* **8,** 839–844.
98. Zamecnik, P. C. and Stephenson, M. L. (1978) Inhibition of Rous sarcoma virus replication and cell transformation by a specific oligodeoxynucleotide. *Proc. Natl. Acad. Sci. USA* **75,** 280–284.

II PLATINUM BIOCHEMISTRY

4 Cisplatin Accumulation

Paul A. Andrews

CONTENTS

1. INTRODUCTION

Accumulation of a drug is the net effect of drug influx and efflux. Since the first reports of accumulation defects in cells with acquired resistance to cisplatin *(1)*, much effort has been directed toward defining the mechanisms by which cisplatin enters and leaves cells. These mechanisms have been difficult to pinpoint. Several reviews of the literature on cisplatin accumulation have been previously published that document the evidence supporting either passive diffusion or carrier-mediated transport as the dominant mechanism of cisplatin influx *(1–5)*. A definitive case for carrier-mediated transport cannot be made since accumulation is not saturable nor inhibitable with structural analogs *(6–11)*. Likewise, studies demonstrating directly that intact resistant cells have enhanced efflux, presumably via a carrier, are scarce. Conversely, a wide variety of physiologic conditions and pharmacologic treatments modulate cisplatin accumulation, which suggests that a regulatable carrier or channel is an important determinant of cisplatin entry into cells. For example, accumulation is partially Na^+dependent and can be altered by adenosine triphosphate (ATP) depletion, cyclic adenosine monophosphate (cAMP) elevation, protein kinase C agonists, osmotic strength, pH, membrane polarization, calmodulin antagonists,

This article is not an official Food and Drug Administration (FDA) guidance or policy statement. No official support or endorsement by the FDA is intended or should be inferred.

From: *Platinum-Based Drugs in Cancer Therapy*
Edited by: L. R. Kelland and N. Farrell © Humana Press Inc., Totowa, NJ

or *ras* expression *(6,10,12–19)*. The prevalence of defective accumulation phenotypes in cisplatin-resistant cells *(1,2,20–22)* underscores the need to understand more fully how cisplatin enters cells and how such a phenotype is acquired. Such knowledge will potentially allow rational pharmacologic approaches that enhance antitumor efficacy, reverse accumulation-mediated acquired resistance, and reduce toxicity to normal tissues. This chapter will not revisit the many studies on cisplatin accumulation that have been thoroughly reviewed previously, but will focus on the recent literature, which offers new insights into how cisplatin does or does not accumulate in cells, and how certain processes differ in resistant cells.

2. MEMBRANE CARRIERS AND CHANNELS

All known membrane proteins that enable the movement of ions, small solutes, metabolites, or xenobiotics across lipid bilayers do so by forming a passageway through the membrane. Those proteins that form a relatively rigid, water-filled pore are termed channels. Channels can be viewed as sieves that allow movement of substrates based on how well they fit the specificity "rules" for the channel. Channels can be gated, meaning that substrate movement can be controlled by such mechanisms as tethered particles that block a face of the pore or a membrane potential that might cause the channel to twist into a narrower configuration. Carrier proteins also form passageways through membranes, but they differ from channels in that they undergo a conformational change during transport of the substrate(s). The binding site for the substrate in a carrier can be viewed as being alternately exposed to the extracellular and the intracellular sides of the membrane. Carriers can equilibrate the concentration of a substrate between two faces of a membrane (facilitated diffusion) or generate a concentration gradient of the substrate (active transport). Active transport of a substrate requires energy either from direct ATP hydrolysis or by coupling to the concentration gradient of a cotransported substrate, e.g., the sodium gradient generated by the Na^+, K^+-adenosine triphosphatase. Channels can pass 10^6–10^7 molecules per second across the membrane (turnover number), whereas carriers can only move 10^2–10^4 molecules (or atoms) of their substrate per second, presumably due to the temporal limitations imposed by conformational changes.

2.1. Sodium and Potassium Adenosine Triphosphatase

Andrews et al. *(12,16)* first reported changes in Na^+,K^+-ATPase in cisplatin-resistant cells, and this observation has been confirmed in other cell types. Ouabain is a highly specific inhibitor of Na^+,K^+-ATPase. Cisplatin-resistant PC-14 non-small cell lung cancer cells have altered ouabain sensitivity, ouabain binding to whole cells, and ability of ouabain to inhibit cisplatin accumulation *(23)*. The ability of ouabain to inhibit cisplatin accumulation (relative to the parent cell lines) was also diminished in cisplatin-resistant IGROV-1(CDDP) and

41M human ovarian carcinoma cells *(24,25)*. Changes in Na^+,K^+-ATPase are also suspected in mouse lymphoma cells with accumulation defects *(26,27)* and have been found in resistant, accumulation-defective A2780 human ovarian carcinoma cells *(16)*. Bando et al. *(28)* have shown that Na^+,K^+-ATPase activity correlated with cisplatin accumulation in a panel of non-small cell lung carcinoma cell lines, but not in small cell lung carcinoma cell lines. When the Na^+,K^+-ATPase in non-small cell lung carcinoma cell lines was inactivated by incubation with sorbitol, cisplatin accumulation was decreased, and the cells became resistant to cisplatin *(29)*. Cisplatin-resistant, accumulation-defective PC-9 non-small cell lung cancer cells had decreased Na^+,K^+-ATPase activity as measured by $^{86}Rb^+$ influx *(30)*. A thromboxane A_2 receptor antagonist sensitized both the cisplatin-sensitive and -resistant PC-9 cells to cisplatin, increased cisplatin accumulation, and enhanced Na^+,K^+-ATPase activity *(30)*. The mechanistic relationship of the change in Na^+,K^+-ATPase activity to cisplatin accumulation was uncertain *(30)*. The association between Na^+,K^+-ATPase activity and clinical cisplatin resistance has been demonstrated by Tokuchi et al. *(31)*. These investigators showed that $^{201}Tl^+$ retention in patients' small cell lung tumors correlated with response to cisplatin chemotherapy. In a small cell lung cancer cell line, they showed that the Na^+,K^+-ATPase inhibitor ouabain restricted thallium accumulation and decreased cisplatin cytotoxicity. The implication is that $^{201}Tl^+$ accumulation in tumor tissue is a marker for Na^+,K^+-ATPase activity, which modulates cisplatin accumulation and hence sensitivity.

There appears to be a growing, strong association between the Na^+,K^+-ATPase and cisplatin accumulation, but it is unclear how these transport activities are linked. Na^+,K^+- ATPase maintains the sodium gradient across cell membranes, and numerous carriers are coupled to this gradient *(32)*. Cisplatin accumulation is partially Na^+ dependent in 2008 cells, but the altered Na^+,K^+-ATPase in resistant cells did not lead to a change in the Na^+ gradient *(12)*. Cisplatin (up to 4.4 m*M*) cannot inhibit K^+ transport through the Na^+,K^+-ATPase, nor does acute stimulation of Na^+,K^+-ATPase activity with monensin alter cisplatin accumulation, so it is unlikely that cisplatin enters cells directly through Na^+,K^+-ATPase *(16)*. Na^+,K^+-ATPase is known to be affected by both the lipid environment and the underlying cytoskeleton *(33,34)*. It is possible that the changes noted in Na^+,K^+-ATPase in resistant cells are a result of pleiotropic membrane changes that affect the Na^+,K^+-ATPase and cisplatin accumulation independently. Nonetheless, this would not explain why ouabain inhibition of Na^+,K^+-ATPase can decrease cisplatin accumulation in many cell lines.

2.2. Folate Carriers

Cisplatin-resistant cells are often cross-resistant to methotrexate. Bhushan et al. *(35)* reported that cisplatin-resistant L1210 cells with accumulation defects were cross-resistant to methotrexate and had decreased methotrexate transport.

The decreased methotrexate transport was associated with decreased phosphorylation of a 66-kDa membrane protein *(35,36)*. Shen et al. *(37–39)* examined accumulation defects in BEL 7404-CP20 human liver carcinoma cells that had been selected for cisplatin resistance. These cells were selected by chronic exposure to cisplatin, were 34- to 111-fold resistant by growth inhibition assay, and had a 14-fold reduction in cisplatin accumulation *(37,38)*. These investigators also demonstrated that these cells were cross-resistant to methotrexate, had reduced accumulation of [^{3}H]methotrexate, and had dramatically reduced expression of the folate binding protein (FBP), which is a carrier that mediates methotrexate transport. Nonetheless, cisplatin did not compete for methotrexate accumulation in these cells, and BEL 7404 cells with reduced expression of FBP after selection in methotrexate are not cross-resistant to cisplatin *(39)*. Reductions in FBP levels were also noted in cisplatin-resistant IGROV-1 ovarian carcinoma cells with accumulation defects *(40)*. Transfection of SKOV3, CHO, or NIH/3T3 cells with the FBP cDNA did not increase sensitivity to cisplatin *(40)*. These data indicate that FBP does not mediate cisplatin accumulation or resistance. The alterations in methotrexate transport in cisplatin-resistant cells are probably the result of changes in dozens of genes elicited as a general response to this cytotoxin and are not causally responsible for defective cisplatin accumulation *(41–43)*.

2.3. ATP Binding Cassette (ABC) Transporters

2.3.1. MDR-1

Cisplatin has never been shown to be a substrate for the *MDR-1* gene product, the P-glycoprotein. Cells overexpressing the *MDR-1* gene and cross-resistant to a broad range of natural products are not cross-resistant to cisplatin. Cisplatin-resistant cells with accumulation defects do not have increased *MDR-1* expression. P-glycoprotein does not participate in the cellular accumulation of cisplatin and is not responsible for the cisplatin accumulation defect in resistant cells.

2.3.2. MRP-1

Unlike MDR-1, MRP-1 can transport a variety of organic conjugates including glutathione-*S*-conjugates, glucuronides, and sulfated conjugates *(44,45)*. Cells overexpressing MRP-1 following selection with natural product drugs are not cross-resistant to cisplatin *(44)*. Similarly, HeLa cells overexpressing MRP-1 following stable transfection with the *MRP-1* gene do not have a cisplatin-resistant phenotype *(46,47)*. In general, cells with acquired cisplatin resistance in vitro do not overexpress MRP-1 *(48,49)*. MRP-1 expression in unselected cell lines does not correlate with cisplatin sensitivity *(50)*. ATP depletion in sensitive and resistant 2008 human ovarian carcinoma cells expressing MRP-1 led to decreased cisplatin accumulation, the opposite expected if MRP-1 was contributing in any way to net cisplatin accumulation *(6,12,48)*. Bone marrow-derived mast cells from knockout mice missing the *Mrp1* gene were less sensitive to cisplatin, rather than more sensitive, as would be expected if Mrp1 participated in cisplatin efflux *(51)*. These data show quite convincingly that MRP-1 does not confer cisplatin resistance and does not participate in cisplatin accumulation.

2.3.3. cMOAT (MRP-2)

The canalicular multispecific organic anion transporter (cMOAT) is known to export glutathione conjugates from cells and is mainly expressed in the canalicular membrane of hepatocytes *(48,52)*. cMOAT levels have been found to be elevated in a number of cell lines with acquired resistance to cisplatin *(48,52,53)*. Koike et al. *(54)* have shown that downregulation of cMOAT with a phosphorothioate antisense oligonucleotide against cMOAT mRNA reverses the cisplatin-resistant phenotype in HepG2 hepatoma cells. However, ATP depletion in cisplatin-resistant C13* human ovarian carcinoma cells expressing higher levels of cMOAT than sensitive 2008 parent cells led to decreased cisplatin accumulation, the opposite expected if cMOAT was functioning as an efflux pump in the net cisplatin accumulation *(6,12,48)*. If cMOAT exports cisplatin conjugates or mediates cotransport of cisplatin with glutathione, then it is not clear why cisplatin is not excreted in the bile since (1) the hepatocyte canalicular membrane is the primary site of cMOAT expression; (2) the liver has very high levels of glutathione; (3) the liver accumulates high levels of platinum, lagging close behind the kidney *(55,56)*; and (4) a high percentage of the intracellular platinum in rat liver cells is in the form of a glutathione complex within 1 h of drug administration *(57)*. Nonetheless, less than 1% of the administered dose of cisplatin is excreted in the bile of mice, rats, or humans *(58–60)*. The antisense experiment provides strong evidence that cMOAT expression confers cisplatin resistance *(54)*, but the evidence that cMOAT participates in cisplatin accumulation is weak. Perhaps cMOAT confers cisplatin resistance by exporting an organic anion, e.g., a glutathione conjugate such as LTC_4, that mediates a step in the apoptotic cascade *(49,61,62)*. Enhanced efflux of such a hypothetical signaling molecule could blunt apoptosis and decrease the cytotoxicity of cisplatin.

2.3.4. Other ABC Transporters

Whereas MDR-1 and MRP-1 play no role in cisplatin accumulation and the role of cMOAT is uncertain, the possibility exists that other as yet unidentified MRP transporter genes are indeed involved *(63)*. However, Kool et al. *(48,52)* showed no obvious correlation of *MRP-3*, *MRP-4*, or *MRP-5* expression with cisplatin resistance in a panel of cell lines. ATP depletion would be expected to increase cisplatin accumulation if an ATP-dependent efflux pump was a major contributor to the overall accumulation. However, both increases and decreases in accumulation have been reported in various cell types in response to ATP depletion *(6,24,25,64,65)*.

A key assumption in proposing that an MRP-like ABC transporter mediates resistance by exporting cisplatin-glutathione conjugates is that the conjugate is cytotoxic. The cell would appear to gain no survival benefit by exporting noncytotoxic forms of the drug. The cisplatin-glutathione conjugate is generally believed to be a noncytotoxic form of the drug because the nucleophilicity of the glutathione sulfur prevents covalent attachment of the platinum complex to DNA. Ishikawa and Ali-Osman *(66)* have presented data that challenges this belief by showing that the cisplatin-glutathione complex inhibits protein synthesis in a cell-free system. A concentration of 190μ*M* was needed to inhibit synthesis by 50%, however, and this seems too high to be pharmacologically relevant, especially if this complex is efficiently removed from the cytoplasm by an MRP transporter *(66)*.

Another problem in proposing MRP-like transporters as the explanation for defective cisplatin accumulation is that, unless the rate law for cisplatin reactions does not apply within the intracellular milieu, kinetic arguments do not favor the presence of any significant quantities of cisplatin-glutathione conjugates within seconds (or hours) of cisplatin exposure when accumulation defects can already be detected *(7,22,67)*. Ishikawa and Ali-Osman *(66)* reported that up to 60% of the cytoplasmic platinum in L1210 cells was in the form of the cisplatin-glutathione complex. This is much higher than reported by others and it is possible that the extraction method used by these investigators artifactually generated the cisplatin-glutathione complex *(6,68)*. However, it is possible that complexation is not required and that glutathione is cotransported with cisplatin by a putative MRP-related protein that recognizes cisplatin, as has been proposed for drugs that are substrates for MRP-1 *(44)*. Depletion of glutathione levels with buthionine sulfoximine increases the accumulation of drugs that are substrates for MRP-1 *(69,70)*. Nonetheless, glutathione depletion has not been demonstrated to affect cisplatin accumulation, and this hypothesis does not appear to be tenable *(71,72)*. Finally, the accumulation defect in resistant cells can usually be accounted for by reductions in influx *(30,38,73,74)*. Direct measurements of platinum efflux in intact cisplatin-loaded cells have rarely been provided to support claims for increased efflux by specific transporters.

2.4. Arsenical Transporters

Naredi et al. *(74,75)* reported that two pairs of cisplatin-sensitive and -resistant human ovarian carcinoma cell lines and two pairs of human head and neck squamous carcinoma cell lines were cross-resistant to antimony potassium tartrate and sodium arsenite. These cells had reduced accumulation of the cisplatin analog [^{3}H]DEP and of $^{73}AsO_3$, neither of which was due to enhanced efflux. When 2008 cells were selected for resistance to antimony potassium tartrate, the derived subline was cross-resistant to cisplatin and arsenite and had defective accumulation of both [^{3}H]DEP and $^{73}AsO_3$. These data suggest that cisplatin, arsenite, and trivalent antimony share a common influx pathway. Cisplatin-resistant BEL 7404-CP20 human hepatoma and KB-CP20 human cervical carcinoma cells were examined for their arsenical cross-resistance and accumulation *(39)*. The BEL 7404-CP20 cells had much reduced cisplatin accumulation *(38)*. These cisplatin-resistant cells were approx 20-fold cross-resistant to trivalent arsenite and pentavalent arsenate and had reduced accumulation of both ionic forms *(39)*. Data were presented indicating that the phosphate carrier system was probably the transporter that mediated arsenate influx, but that it was not involved in arsenite influx *(39)*. Expression of plasma membrane binding proteins highly specific for arsenite (M_r 48 and 230 kDa) and arsenate (M_r 190 kDa), respectively, were reduced in the resistant cells. An M_r-36-kDa arsenite binding protein was increased in resistant cells. Cisplatin could not compete with the arsenicals for binding to these proteins *(39)*.

Although members of the ABC transporter family are known to mediate the efflux of arsenite and antimonite in bacteria and protozoa, nothing is known about the mechanism of influx of these trivalent metals. MRP-1 overexpression can confer resistance to arsenite and antimonite *(47)*. A single carrier protein may exist for cisplatin, antimonite, and arsenite, which explains the observed accumulation defects and metalloid cross-resistance patterns as reported by Naredi et al. *(74)* and Shen et al. *(39)*. However, a nonspecific regulatory response to selection in these metals that causes a broad downregulation of a variety of membrane transport systems or a change in the passive permeability of the plasma membrane cannot be ruled out as the explanation for these findings.

2.5. Gated Channels

Gately and Howell *(3)* proposed that cisplatin enters cells partly by passive diffusion and partly by a gated channel. It is thus worth considering the dimensions of the channel needed to accommodate cisplatin. A space-filling model of the cisplatin square planar complex indicates that the orthogonal dimensions are approximately 4.0×6.9×6.8 Å (Fig. 1). The smallest opening that could accommodate cisplatin entering edge-on would be a 4.0×6.8 Å rectangular pore, or a circular pore of 8 Å diameter (cross-sectional area of 27–50 $Å^2$). The internal pore dimensions of many channels are known (Table 1). These data show that if cisplatin enters through a gated channel, then the channel must have a pore size larger than many well-described channels known to reside in the plasma membrane.

2.6. Water Channels

The recently discovered aquaporins are a family of highly conserved channels that mediate rapid water transport across plasma membranes *(82–84)*. Aquaporins are homotetramers that form an aggregate in the plasma membrane with four functionally independent pores *(83)*. They are widely distributed

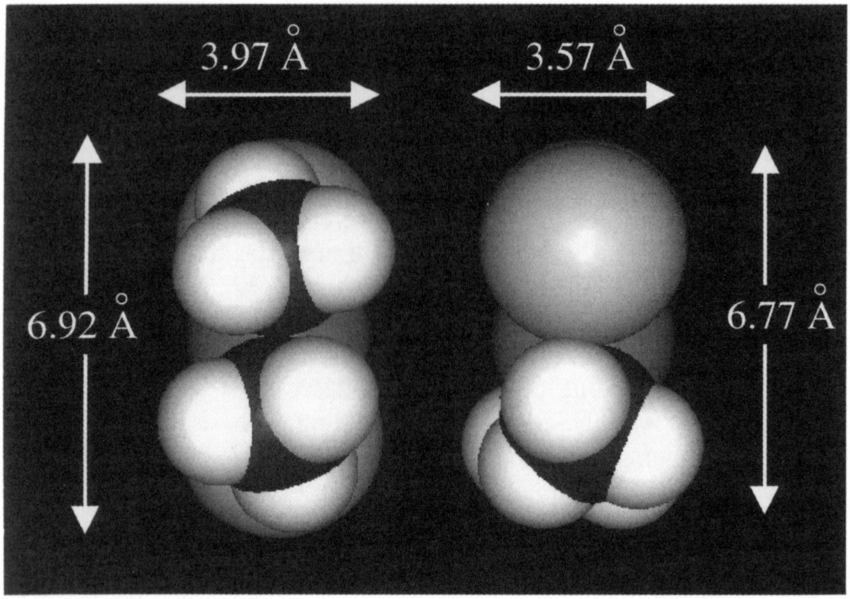

Fig. 1. Space-filling model of cisplatin. The molecule is shown edge-on from either the edge with two ammines (left side) or the edge with an ammine and a chloro ligand (right side). The dimensions were calculated with InsightII version 95.0 (Molecular Simulations, San Diego, CA) and were provided courtesy of Dr. James Weaver (Center for Drug Evaluation and Research, FDA).

throughout mammalian tissues; aquaporin-1 is particularly abundant in the renal proximal tubule *(82–84)*. The kidney accumulates more platinum than any other tissue, and the proximal tubule is the primary site of cisplatin kidney damage *(55,56)*. Aquaporin activity can be modulated by a variety of factors including protein kinase A, which when activated can cause a redistribution of aquaporin from intracellular vesicles to the plasma membrane *(85,86)*. Some of the properties of aquaporins are thus consistent with what is known about cisplatin accumulation (protein kinase A sensitive, nonsaturable, osmotically sensitive). Nonetheless, aquaporin-1 is highly selective for water (it excludes urea and ions), and the internal diameter of the aquaporin-1 pore is estimated to be less than 3 Å. Aquaporin-1 is thus too small to serve as a channel for cisplatin influx (Table 1), but a recent report on the cloning and characterization of a new aquaporin gene product, AQP9, suggests that other members of this family could form a channel large enough to accommodate cisplatin *(87)*. The AQP9 gene product allows the movement of urea, adenine, uracil, glycerol, sorbitol, and mannitol across oocyte membranes, but excludes ions, amino acids, cyclic sugars, and monocarboxylates *(87)*. The molecular radii of some of the compounds that readily permeate AQP9 are greater than that of cisplatin.

Table 1
Inner Diameters of Pores in Various Channels

	Ion diameter[a] *(Å)*	*Inner diameter* *(Å)*	*Cross-sectional area* *(Å²)*	*Ref.*
K^+channel	2.66	3	20	*76*
Na^+channel	1.90	3 × 5	16	*77,* p. 79
Ca^{2+}channel	1.98	6		*77,* p. 359
nAChR[b]	—	6–7	40	*77,* p. 243
Aquaporin-1	—	3		*78, 79*
Amphotericin B	—	4–10		*80, 81*
Gramicidin	—	4	13	*77,* p. 306

[a]Ion diameters are Pauling radii from Hille (ref. 77, p. 276).
[b]Nicotinic acetylcholine receptor.

AQP9 appears to be a promiscuous, neutral solute pore that could also accommodate cisplatin. Exploration of the possible role of aquaporins in cisplatin accumulation need to be undertaken.

2.7. Miscellaneous Effects

Laurencot et al. *(88)* showed that inhibitors of the Na^+/H^+antiporter and HCO_3^-/Cl^- exchanger had no effect on cisplatin accumulation in EMT6 mouse mammary carcinoma cells. Verapamil, which inhibits the calcium channel, does not affect cisplatin accumulation *(89,90)*.

3. MECHANISMS INDEPENDENT OF PROTEINACEOUS CARRIERS AND CHANNEL

3.1. Passive Permeability

3.1.1. Passive Diffusion

Marverti and Andrews *(91)* demonstrated that cisplatin accumulation could be modulated by the isoflavone genistein in 2008 human ovarian carcinoma cells. Changes were also induced in the accumulation of mannitol that exactly mimicked modulations of cisplatin accumulation. Mannitol is not a substrate for any known hexose carrier and is believed to enter cells solely by passive diffusion, perhaps through aqueous pores rather than diffusion through the lipid bilayer *(87,92,93)*. The molecular dimensions of mannitol are 7.4×8.1×11.9 Å *(32)*, which is slightly larger than the dimensions of cisplatin (Fig. 1). Genistein did not modulate the accumulation of cisplatin or mannitol in the resistant C13* subline that has an accumulation defect. These data support the hypothesis that cisplatin enters cells by passive diffusion and that the changes in accumulation mediated by agonists and antagonists of serine/threonine protein kinases and tyrosine kinases do so by modulating the passive permeability properties of the plasma membrane.

Similar to the results with genistein, the polycationic amine spermine increased both cisplatin accumulation and mannitol accumulation *(94)*. Unlike genistein, however, the modulation was similar in both 2008 parent cells and resistant C13* cells. The good correlation of the effects on cisplatin and mannitol accumulation suggests that the spermine effect is due to modulation of the plasma membrane permeability. The effect was specific to spermine; spermidine did not alter cisplatin or mannitol accumulation. Polyamines can bind electrostatically to phospholipids, and it has been speculated that spermine could specifically bridge phospholipid domains with other domains or integral proteins *(94)*. Conceivably this could change the rigidity of the plasma membrane in ways that alter the passive diffusion of cisplatin through the membrane.

In solution, cisplatin exists as an equilibrium of parent drug and various aquated species *(95)*. It has been assumed that the species entering cells is the parent dichloro form. Nonetheless, any of the aquated forms could be the predominant form undergoing influx. Since in the presence of extracellular chloride concentrations these aquated species are present at relatively low levels, the inability to demonstrate saturation of cisplatin accumulation might be explained by the inability ever to raise the concentration of the transported aquated species anywhere close to the K_m for transport. This hypothesis might also explain why carboplatin is accumulated much less effectively than cisplatin despite its higher lipid solubility, i.e., carboplatin aquates much slower than cisplatin and there is much less aquated species present in solution. This might also explain why structural analogs cannot compete for cisplatin accumulation, i.e., an aqua ligand could be critical for recognition by a carrier protein. The role of the form of cisplatin in the accumulation has therefore been investigated. Jennerwein and Andrews *(96)* showed that changing the aquation state in the extracellular medium had no impact on platinum accumulation up to 100 μM cisplatin, but that DNA platination was increased. Zheng et al. *(64)* also demonstrated no affect of aquation state on cisplatin accumulation up to 100 μM; however, they showed that at concentrations above 100 μM, three times more platinum was associated with cells exposed to aquated cisplatin than to cisplatin. The appearance of this differential as the concentration was raised could be the result of membrane damage produced by the more reactive aquated forms. Accumulation at 1 h was not saturable up to 1.6 mM for either native or aquated cisplatin. The energy dependence for accumulation was similar for native and aquated cisplatin. These investigators also showed that the temperature dependence (Q_{10}) for accumulation of aquated cisplatin was different from that of native cisplatin, 2.5 vs 1.6, respectively. However, both Q_{10}s were in a range appropriate for diffusion either through the lipid membrane or through a channel as opposed to a carrier-mediated process. These studies add support to the hypothesis that carrier proteins are not involved in cisplatin accumulation.

3.1.2. Membrane Fluidity

Cisplatin-resistant 2008 cells have the same membrane fluidity as sensitive cells, as measured by fluorescence polarization, despite changes in the cellular phospholipid composition *(97)*. In addition, no changes in membrane fluidity have been detected in these cells using electron paramagnetic resonance and the lipid-soluble spin label probe 5-doxylstearic acid (P.A. Andrews and A. Aszalos, unpublished observations). However, preliminary reports show that several cisplatin-resistant cells with accumulation defects, including the resistant 2008 cells, have increased membrane rigidity compared with the parent cell lines when the cells were analyzed by pressure tuning infrared spectroscopy *(98–100)*. Clearly, more work is needed to investigate whether the passive permeability (as measured by the accumulation of marker molecules) or the fluidity of plasma membranes (as measured by the behavior of interrogating probes) can consistently account for accumulation defects in cisplatin-resistant cells.

3.1.3. Membrane Structure

By studying infrared spectra of dimyristoylphosphatidylserine model membranes as a function of pressure, Taylor et al. *(101)* showed that cisplatin and aquated cisplatin interact with the serine carboxylate head group of this phospholipid. The binding increased the distance between the acyl chains, led to more vibrational motion, and increased the pressure needed to stop these motions. No effect of cisplatin was found on the methylene stretching modes of the acyl chains, implying that cisplatin does not easily diffuse into membranes containing phosphatidylserine *(101)*. Nonetheless, a preliminary report using this infrared method shows that cisplatin does enter the lipid bilayer of cell membranes *(100)*. The reported changes in lipid composition in some cisplatin-resistant cells, including a slight increase in phosphatidylserine, may thus have an important impact on the ability of cisplatin to diffuse through the membrane *(97)*.

The composition of the plasma membrane is known to affect membrane fluidity and permeability *(102)*. Consistent alterations in the composition of the lipid bilayer that might account for an accumulation defect have not been reported in cisplatin-resistant cells. Mann et al. *(97)* found that resistant 2008/DDP cells had increased amounts of phosphatidylcholine and phosphatidylethanolamine. A change in cholesterol content was not observed in these two-fold resistant 2008/DDP cells, but after they were selected for higher levels of resistance Caffrey et al. *(103)* claimed in a preliminary report that the resulting C13* cells had much lower cholesterol content. The differential affect of amphotericin B on cisplatin accumulation in some resistant cells compared with parent cells, as described below in Section 3.2.1, also strongly suggests that these resistant cells have changes in their cholesterol content *(104–106)*.

3.2. Pore Inducers and Detergents

3.2.1. Amphotericin B

Amphotericin B can increase cisplatin accumulation and partially reverse cisplatin resistance. Morikage et al. *(104,107)* reported that amphotericin B selectively reversed the accumulation defect in some resistant non-small cell lung cancer cells, but equally increased cisplatin accumulation in other sensitive and resistant cell pairs. In a panel of 11 lung cancer cell lines, the effect of 10 μg/mL amphotericin B on cisplatin accumulation correlated directly with their intrinsic cisplatin resistance *(104)*. In human larynx carcinoma cells, resistant cells with an accumulation defect were sensitized to cisplatin cytotoxicity by amphotericin B, but the parent HEp2 cells were not affected up to 40 μg/mL amphotericin B *(105)*. The affect on cisplatin accumulation was not determined by these investigators. Amphotericin B has also been shown to increase cisplatin accumulation and cytotoxicity in sensitive and resistant human ovarian carcinoma and malignant mesothelioma cell lines in vitro *(108,109)*. Sharp et al. *(106)* showed that 5–15 μg/mL amphotericin B enhanced cisplatin accumulation and cytotoxicity only in resistant cells (41McisR6, HX62) with accumulation defects. In the parent 41M cells the effect was diminished and in the CH1 pair the effect was absent. Amphotericin B (5 μg/mL) enhanced cisplatin cytotoxicity in six human medullary thyroid carcinoma cell lines *(110)*. Kojima et al. *(111)* demonstrated that amphotericin B and cisplatin were synergistically cytotoxic against human ovarian carcinoma cells in vitro and that amphotericin B increased cisplatin accumulation in these cells. Liang and Bian *(112)* reported that amphotericin B treatment raised cisplatin accumulation and increased Pt-DNA adducts in resistant SKOV3 cells. These studies show that amphotericin B modulates the cellular pharmacology of cisplatin in a variety of cell types. The effect can be substantially greater in some cisplatin-resistant cells compared with the sensitive parent cells.

Investigations exploring the potential of amphotericin B for enhancing cisplatin efficacy in vivo have been reported. Kojima et al. *(111)* showed that simultaneous treatment with ip amphotericin B and cisplatin administered on d 3, 5, 7, and 9 after ip inoculation with HRA human ovarian carcinoma cells significantly prolonged the survival of the athymic mice. Furthermore, they demonstrated that ip amphotericin B at doses ≥1.0 mg/kg increased platinum accumulation in the tumor tissue following a 2-h ip exposure to cisplatin. No changes in hematology or serum chemistry (including blood urea nitrogen and creatinine) were noted in the mice following a cisplatin plus amphotericin B treatment. However, since the 2.0-mg/kg ip cisplatin dose alone was too low to cause any changes in these parameters, it is difficult to conclude that amphotericin B will not enhance cisplatin toxicity in vivo. Sharp et al. *(106)* have commented that amphotericin B enhanced cisplatin-induced nephrotoxicity as detected microscopically. Therefore, instead of using cisplatin, these investigators determined the ability of ip amphotericin B (20 mg/kg) to enhance the antitumor activity of ip carboplatin (80 mg/kg) against HX/62 human ovarian carcinoma cell xenografts when both drugs were administered on an every 7 d×4 schedule. Unfortunately, no significant effect was observed for the combination over carboplatin or amphotericin B alone. Bergström et al. *(113)* treated rats harboring intracerebral glioma implants with ip cisplatin (5 mg/kg) and amphotericin B (5 mg/kg). This treatment caused an increase in Pt-DNA adducts in the kidney but not the tumor, extensive kidney damage, and death within a few days *(113)*. Assem et al. *(81)* reported that, as with other cell lines, amphotericin B increased cisplatin accumulation and cytotoxicity in human HT 29 colon carcinoma cells. However, when HT 29 cells in vitro were exposed to cisplatin added to serum obtained from patients 1 h after an iv infusion of amphotericin B (thus containing 4–7 μg/mL amphotericin B), no enhancement of accumulation was observed. These studies indicate that amphotericin B concentrations high enough to modulate cisplatin accumulation in vitro, approx 15 μg/mL, cannot be achieved using tolerable doses in vivo. Together these reports appear to limit hope for the clinical testing of cisplatin/amphotericin B combinations to intracavitary or regional chemotherapy in which tumors can be exposed to high concentrations of amphotericin B while limiting systemic exposure.

Amphotericin B is a macrolide antifungal that binds to sterols in membranes and forms nonspecific 4–10 Å barrel-shaped pores *(80,81)*. Pore formation leads to dissipation of the K^+ gradient, collapse of the membrane potential, and cell death. Binding affinity of amphotericin B to ergosterol is eightfold higher than to cholesterol *(114)*. Since fungi use ergosterol whereas mammalian cells use cholesterol in their membranes, amphotericin B is thus more cytotoxic to fungi *(80,81,114)*. The mechanism by which amphotericin B enhances cisplatin accumulation is probably the formation of nonspecific pores that accelerate the entry of cisplatin into cells. It can be demonstrated that amphotericin B enhances the accumulation of the passive permeability marker mannitol in a concentration-dependent manner that exactly mimics the effects on cisplatin accumulation in 2008 and C13* human ovarian carcinoma cells (P.A. Andrews, unpublished data). The variability of the effect in different cell lines is probably due to differences in the amphotericin B binding to cholesterol in the plasma membrane, e.g., as a result of differences in cholesterol content. Amphotericin B had a much smaller effect on the accumulation and cytotoxicity of carboplatin, oxaliplatin, and JM216 *(81,104,106,109)*. These platinum agents are all larger than cisplatin and may not be able to enter the pore formed by amphotericin B and cholesterol as readily as cisplatin.

3.2.2. Digitonin

Another compound that permeabilizes membranes in proportion to the cholesterol content is digitonin. Jekunen et al. *(115)* reported that digitonin can increase the accumulation of the cisplatin analog DEP in both cisplatin-sensitive and -resistant 2008 cells. The effect was greater in cisplatin-sensitive cells at 20 μ*M* digitonin, but was equivalent in sensitive and resistant cells at 40 μ*M* digitonin. The increased accumulation led directly to increased DNA platination. To explore the clinical potential of this approach, Lindnér et al. *(116)* coadministered digitonin with carboplatin intraarterially and reported the effect on a syngeneic rat hepatoma inoculated into the central lobe of rat livers. One hour after treatment, digitonin enhanced carboplatin accumulation sixfold into the tumor but had no effect on platinum content in the liver parenchyma. This increased accumulation caused a dramatic affect on tumor size 7 d after a 5-mg/kg dose of carboplatin. No enhancement in carboplatin toxicity was noted. This study demonstrates that modulation of the passive permeability of platinum drugs is a feasible therapeutic approach in vivo.

3.3. Pinocytosis and Endocytosis

Many aspects of cisplatin accumulation are consistent with fluid-phase pinocytosis, e.g., accumulation is energy dependent, temperature dependent, nonsaturable, and modulated by signal transduction pathways *(2,117–120)*. In addition, the accumulation of a compound that enters cells by fluid-phase pinocytosis would not be inhibited by structural analogs. The hypothesis that pinocytosis plays a prominent role in cisplatin accumulation was explored in 2008 human ovarian carcinoma cells using Lucifer yellow as a marker of fluid-phase pinocytosis *(91)*. No difference in Lucifer yellow accumulation was found between 2008 and C13* cells. Although genistein stimulated cisplatin accumulation, it had no effect on pinocytosis in 2008 cells *(91)*. Furthermore, the amount of fluid engulfed as measured by Lucifer yellow could only account for 1–2% of the total platinum accumulated during a cisplatin exposure. Fluid-phase pinocytosis thus appears to play a negligible role in the accumulation of cisplatin.

Similar to pinocytosis, the accumulation of cisplatin exhibits many features consistent with receptor-mediated endocytosis (RME). RME could contribute to cisplatin accumulation as a result of the internalization of medium entrapped during endosome formation. A preliminary report on the importance of RME in mediating cisplatin accumulation in 2008 human ovarian carcinoma cells has appeared *(121)*. RME triggered by low-density lipoprotein (LDL) binding to its receptor(s) was assessed by the accumulation of LDL fluorescently labeled with DiI and was not saturable for up to 6 h in either 2008 or cisplatin-resistant C13* cells. RME of DiI-LDL was over 30% greater in the C13* cells that have a cisplatin accumulation defect. Upregulation of the LDL receptor followed by exposure to 10% fetal bovine serum to stimulate endocytosis did not alter cisplatin accumulation in 2008 cells. These data indicate that RME neither contributes significantly to cisplatin accumulation in 2008 cells nor explains the accumulation defect in C13* cells. Binding of cisplatin to α2-macroglobin (α2M) did not change α2M internalization via RME after binding to the "low-density lipoprotein receptor-related protein" *(122)*. Nonetheless, subsequent rounds of RME were greatly reduced after internalization of the cisplatin-modified α2M. Such an effect does not explain the cisplatin accumulation defect that can be detected 30 s after cisplatin exposure *(7)*.

4. UNCERTAIN MECHANISMS

4.1. Terbium Binding Proteins

Terbium (Tb^{3+}) is a phosphorescent lanthanide metal that behaves very similarly to calcium in biologic systems. Terbium can influence the accumulation of cisplatin in 2008 human ovarian carcinoma cells and MDA-MD-231 human breast carcinoma cells *(89,123)*. Terbium increased cisplatin accumulation in parent, resistant, and revertant cells, but the effect was greater in the resistant and partially revertant cells, which have an accumulation defect *(123)*. The cisplatin accumulation defect was completely reversed at 100 μ*M* terbium in the C13* cells. The number of terbium binding sites was significantly greater on the C13* cells compared with the parent cells. Terbium also increased accumulation in sensitive and resistant MDA-MD-231 human breast cancer cells *(89)*. Unlike 2008 cells, the percent enhancement was similar in the parent and two resistant sublines, but the resistant cells did not have an accumulation defect under the conditions of the experiment. Also in contrast to the 2008 cells, one of the resistant sublines had significantly fewer terbium binding sites while the other subline had the same number as the parent cells. The identity of the terbium binding site that is altered in the resistant cells and that modulates accumulation is not known, nor is the underlying mechanism.

4.2. Cytoskeletal Alterations

Numerous studies have identified changes in cytoskeletal proteins in cisplatin-resistant cells that could possibly be associated with the cisplatin accumulation defects. Resistant 2008 cells express less β-tubulin, have enhanced formation of microtubule bundles, and are hypersensitive to the microtubule stabilizing agent paclitaxel *(124)*. These microtubule changes may contribute to the cisplatin accumulation defect in these cells. In a separate study, these same resistant 2008 cells were found to have five- to sixfold lower levels of cytokeratin-18 protein and mRNA, but no change in cytokeratin-8 expression *(125)*. Transfection of the full-length cytokeratin-18 gene into the resistant C13* cells partially reversed the resistant phenotype in isolated clones. Unfortunately, determinations of cisplatin accumulation were not made in the clones, so an association of cytokeratin expression with accumulation could not be made. Marked reductions of cytokeratin-14 have been found in resistant PC10 human lung squamous-carcinoma cells *(126)*. These cells have a cisplatin accumulation defect relative to the parent PC10 cells *(126)*. It is also known that cisplatin exposure can alter a number of cytoskeletal proteins *(127–130)*. Components of the cytoskeleton can bind to membrane proteins *(131)*. This interaction of the plasma membrane with the cytoskeleton plays a regulatory role in the activity of numerous transporters, e.g., Na^+,K^+-ATPase, Na^+ channels, the Cl^-/HCO_3^- exchanger, and H^+-ATPase *(131)*. In addition to directly modulating membrane transporters, the underlying structure of the cytoskeleton might also affect the rigidity of the membrane as well as the passive permeability of the lipid bilayer to small solutes *(34,132)*. The cytoskeleton can be modified by a variety of signal transduction pathways (e.g., protein kinase C), energy disruptions, osmotic/ionic perturbations, and mechanical disturbances *(131)*. It is therefore possible that the cytoskeleton plays a central role in mediating many of the modulations of cisplatin accumulation observed by these manipulations and that the end result is a nonspecific change in membrane permeability.

5. SUMMARY

Many studies have documented the kinetics of cisplatin influx, efflux, and net accumulation. Many reports have also described the effects of (1) agonists and antagonists of various signaling pathways (protein kinase A, protein kinase C, tyrosine kinases, RAS); (2) ATP depletion; (3) various physiologic manipulations (pH, osmotic strength, ion concentrations); (4) membrane modifications (pore inducers, detergents, lipids); and (5) agonists and antagonists of known carrier-mediated transport systems. From all this work one truth stands out: classic kinetic evidence supporting the hypothesis that cisplatin influx or efflux is carrier mediated has never been found. Such evidence would include saturation, competition from structural analogs, or *trans* stimulation. In the absence of such evidence, one must assume that the best working hypothesis is that cisplatin enters cells by diffusion, either directly through the lipid bilayer, or through water-filled channels, or through both pathways with similar rates. The accumulation of cisplatin is very slow. The accumulation can be estimated to be 10^3–10^4 molecules/s/cell when cells are exposed to 0.1–1.0 m*M* cisplatin. In contrast, the turnover number for many channels is

10^6–10^7 molecules/s/channel. Thus, it appears reasonable to hypothesize that cisplatin enters cells primarily by passive diffusion through the lipoidal regions of the membrane. The variety of pharmacologic and physiologic manipulations that modulate cisplatin accumulation probably either directly or indirectly affect the passive permeability and rigidity of the plasma membrane. Such effects could be transduced through effects of the cytoskeleton, membrane lipids, or integral membrane proteins. More studies testing the correlation of the passive permeability of the plasma membrane with cisplatin accumulation are needed.

The mechanistic basis for defective accumulation in cisplatin-resistant cells has not yet been clearly defined. Most resistant cells have decreased accumulation as a result of decreased influx. Studies demonstrating directly that intact resistant cells have enhanced efflux are scarce. The evidence that some cisplatin-resistant cells have enhanced efflux is based mostly on indirect evidence, e.g., that ATP depletion causes increased accumulation. However, ATP depletion could reasonably be expected to affect a variety of physiologic functions, e.g., the cytoskeleton, which could affect the passive permeability of the plasma membrane. The idea that accumulation defects are due to the enhanced activity of export pumps that remove biotransformation products, such as a cisplatin-glutathione conjugate, is difficult to accept based on chemical kinetic grounds and what is already known about the cellular pharmacology and pharmacokinetic of cisplatin in mammals. Studies examining the membrane composition, membrane fluidity, and permeability to passively diffusing solutes in resistant cells vs sensitive cells are few. The differential effects of amphotericin B on cisplatin accumulation in many resistant cells send a strong signal that these cells have changes in their cholesterol content. Clearly, more work is needed in this area to establish whether changes in membrane structure and permeability can account for cisplatin accumulation defects.

The variety of changes reported in various carriers in the membranes of resistant cells (Na^+,K^+-ATPase, folate binding proteins, arsenical transporters, cMOAT) are most likely the result of a generalized response to cytotoxic damage and are not specifically involved in cisplatin transport (although they could play a functional role in resistance). Whether this pleiotropic affect is due to an alteration in a central signaling pathway *(41–43)* or to changes in multiple regulatory pathways is not known.

ACKNOWLEDGMENTS

I thank Dr. James Weaver from the Center for Drug Evaluation and Research, FDA (Laurel, MD) for providing the space-filling drawing of cisplatin, and Drs. Diana Clark and Hua Zheng from the Center for Drug Evaluation and Research, FDA (Rockville, MD) for providing critical review of this manuscript.

REFERENCES

1. Andrews, P. A. and Howell, S. B. (1990) Cellular pharmacology of cisplatin: perspectives on mechanisms of acquired resistance. *Cancer Cells* **2,** 35–43.
2. Andrews, P. A. (1994) Mechanisms of acquired resistance to cisplatin. *Cancer Treat. Res.* **73,** 217–248.
3. Gately, D. P. and Howell, S. B. (1993) Cellular accumulation of the anticancer agent cisplatin: a review. *Br. J. Cancer* **67,** 1171–1176.
4. Perez, R. P., Hamilton, T. C., and Ozols, R. F. (1990) Resistance to alkylating agents and cisplatin: insights from ovarian carcinoma model systems. *Pharmacol. Ther.* **48,** 19–27.
5. Timmer-Bosscha, H., Mulder, N. H., and de Vries, E. G. E. (1992) Modulation of cis-diamminedichloroplatinum(II) resistance: a review. *Br. J. Cancer* **66**, 227–238.
6. Andrews, P. A., Velury, S., Mann, S. C., and Howell, S. B. (1988) *cis*-Diamminedichloroplatinum(II) accumulation in sensitive and resistant human ovarian carcinoma cells. *Cancer Res.* **48,** 68–73.
7. Mann, S. C., Andrews, P. A., and Howell, S. B. (1990) Short-term *cis*-diamminedichloroplatinum(II) accumulation in sensitive and resistant human ovarian carcinoma cells. *Cancer Chemother. Pharmacol.* **25,** 236–240.
8. Scanlon, K. J., Safirstein, R. L., Thies, H., Gross, R. B., Waxman, S., and Guttenplan, J. B. (1983) Inhibition of amino acid transport by *cis*-diamminedichloroplatinum(II) derivatives in L1210 murine leukemia cells. *Cancer Res.* **43,** 4211–4215.
9. Hromas, R. A., North, J. A., and Burns, C. P. (1987) Decreased cisplatin uptake by resistant L1210 leukemia cells. *Cancer Lett.* **36,** 197–201.
10. Andrews, P. A., Mann, S. C., Velury, S., and Howell, S. B. (1988) Cisplatin uptake mediated cisplatin-resistance in human ovarian carcinoma cells, in *Platinum and Other Metal Coordination Compounds in Cancer Chemotherapy* (Nicolini, M., ed.) Nijhoff, Boston, pp. 248–254.
11. Kelland, L. R., Mistry, P., Abel, G., Loh, S. Y., O'Neill, C. F., Murrer, B. A., and Harrap, K. R. (1992) Mechanism-related circumvention of acquired *cis*-diamminedichloroplatinum(II) resistance using two pairs of human ovarian carcinoma cell lines by ammine/amine platinum(IV) dicarboxylates. *Cancer Res.* **52,** 3857–3864.
12. Andrews, P. A., Mann, S. C., Huynh, H. H., and Albright, K. D. (1991) Role of the Na^+, K^+-adenosine triphosphatase in the accumulation of *cis*-diamminedichloroplatinum(II) in human ovarian carcinoma cells. *Cancer Res.* **51,** 3677–3681.
13. Mann, S. C., Andrews, P. A., and Howell, S. B. (1991) Modulation of *cis*-diamminedichloroplatinum(II) accumulation and sensitivity by forskolin and 3-isobutyl-1-methylxanthine in sensitive and resistant human ovarian carcinoma cells. *Int. J. Cancer* **48,** 866–872.
14. Basu, A., Teicher, B. A., and Lazo, J. S. (1990) Involvement of protein kinase C in phorbol ester-induced sensitization of HeLa cells to *cis*-diamminedichloroplatinum(II). *J. Biol. Chem.* **265,** 8451–8457.
15. Smith, E. and Brock, A. P. (1989) The effect of reduced osmolarity on platinum drug toxicity. *Br. J. Cancer* **59,** 873–875.
16. Andrews, P. A. and Albright, K. D. (1991) Role of membrane ion transport in cisplatin accumulation, in *Platinum and Other Metal Coordination Compounds in Cancer Chemotherapy* (Howell, S. B., ed.) Plenum, New York, pp. 151–159.
17. Kikuchi, Y., Iwano, I., Miyauchi, M., Sasa, H., Nagata, I., and Kuki, E. (1990) Restorative effects of calmodulin antagonists on reduced cisplatin uptake by cisplatin-resistant ovarian cancer cells. *Gynecol. Oncol.* **39,** 199–203.
18. Isonishi, S., Hom, D. K., Thiebaut, F. B., Mann, S. C., Andrews, P. A., Basu, A., et al. (1991) Expression of the c-Ha-*ras* oncogene in mouse NIH 3T3 cells induces resistance to cisplatin. *Cancer Res.* **51,** 5903–5909.

19. Shinohara, N., Ogiso, Y., Arai, T., Takami, S., Nonomura, K., Koyanagi, T., et al. (1994) Differential Na^+, K^+-ATPase activity and cisplatin sensitivity between transformants induced by H-*ras* and those induced by K-*ras*. *Int. J. Cancer* **58,** 672–677.
20. Teicher, B. A., Holden, S. A., Herman, T. S., Sotomayor, E. A., Khandekar, V., Rosbe, K. W., et al. (1991) Characteristics of five human tumor cell lines and sublines resistant to *cis*-diamminedichloroplatinum(II). *Int. J. Cancer* **47**, 252–260.
21. Katabami, M., Fijita, H., Haneda, H., Akita, H., Kuzumaki, N., Miyamoto, H., et al. (1992) Reduced drug accumulation in a newly established human lung squamous-carcinoma cell line resistant to *cis*-diamminedichloroplatinum(II). *Biochem. Pharmacol.* **44,** 394–397.
22. Loh, S. Y., Mistry, P., Kelland, L. R., Abel, G., and Harrap, K. R. (1992) Reduced drug accumulation as a major mechanism of acquired resistance to cisplatin in a human ovarian carcinoma cell line: circumvention studies using novel platinum (II) and (IV) ammine/amine complexes. *Br. J. Cancer* **66,** 1109–1115.
23. Ohmori, T., Morikage, T., Sugimoto, Y., Fujiwara, Y., Kasahara, K., Nishio, K., et al. (1993) The mechanism of the difference in cellular uptake of platinum derivatives in non-small cell lung cancer cell line (PC-14) and its cisplatin-resistant subline (PC-14/CDDP). *Jpn. J. Cancer Res.* **84,** 83–92.
24. Ma, J., Maliepaard, M., Kolker, H. J., Verweij, J., and Schellens, J. H. (1998) Abrogated energy-dependent uptake of cisplatin in a cisplatin-resistant subline of the human ovarian cancer cell line IGROV-1. *Cancer Chemother. Pharmacol.* **41,** 186–192.
25. Sharp, S. Y., Rogers, P. M., and Kelland, L. R. (1995) Transport of cisplatin and bis-acetato-ammine-dichlorocyclohexyl-amine platinum(IV) (JM216) in human ovarian carcinoma cell lines: identifcation of a plasma membrane protein associated with cisplatin resistance. *Clin. Cancer Res.* **1,** 981–989.
26. Kawai, K., Kamatani, N., Georges, E., and Ling, V. (1990) Identification of a membrane glycoprotein overexpressed in murine lymphoma sublines resistant to *cis*-diamminedichloroplatinum(II). *J. Biol. Chem.* **265,** 13137–13142.
27. Kawai, K., Kamatani, N., Kuroshima, S., Nobori, T., Nishioka, K., Kamiya, H., et al. (1987) Cross-resistance to ouabain in a murine leukemia cell variant selected for resistance to *cis*-dichlorodiammineplatinum(II) resistance. *Cancer Lett.* **35,** 147–152.
28. Bando, T., Fujimura, M., Kasahara, K., and Matsuda, T. (1998) Significance of Na_{+},$K_{(+)}$-ATPase on intracellular accumulation of cis-diamminedichloroplatinum(II) in human non-small cell but not in small cell lung cancer cell lines. *Anticancer Res.* **18,** 1085–1089.
29. Bando, T., Fujimura, M., Kasahara, K., Shibata, K., Shirasaki, H., Heki, U., et al. (1997) Exposure to sorbitol induces resistance to cisplatin in human non-small cell lung cancer cell lines. *Anticancer Res.* **17,** 3345–3348.
30. Kasahara, K., Fujimura, M., Bando, T., Shibata, K., Shirasaki, H., and Matsuda, T. (1996) Modulation of sensitivity to *cis*-diamminedichloroplatinum (II) by thromboxane A_2 receptor antagonists in non-small cell lung cancer cell lines. *Br. J. Cancer* **74,** 1553–1558.
31. Tokuchi, Y., Isobe, H., Takekawa, H., Hanada, T., Ishida, T., Ogura, S., et al. (1998) Predicting chemotherapeutic response to small cell lung cancer of platinum compounds by thallium-201 single-photon emission computerized tomography. *Br. J. Cancer* **77,** 1363–1368.
32. Stein, W. D. (1986) *Transport and Diffusion Across Cell Membranes*. Academic, New York.
33. Makarov, V. L. and Kuznetsov, S. R. (1995) Increased Na^+,K^+-pump activity in erythrocytes of rabbits fed cholesterol. *Int. J. Exp. Pathol.* **76,** 93–96.
34. Paller, M. S. (1994) Lateral mobility of Na,K-ATPase and membrane lipids in renal cells. Importance of cytoskeletal integrity. *J. Membr. Biol.* **142,** 127–135.
35. Bhushan, A., Wroblewski, D., Xuan, Y., Tritton, T. R., and Hacker, M. P. (1996) Correlation of altered tyrosine phosphorylation with methotrexate resistance in a cisplatin-resistant subline of L1210 cells. *Biochem. Pharmacol.* **51,** 477–482.

36. Xuan, Y., Hacker, M. P., Tritton, T. R., and Bhushan, A. (1998) Modulation of methotrexate resistance by genistein in murine leukeima L1210 cells. *Oncol. Rep.* **5,** 419–421.
37. Shen, D., Akiyama, S., Schoenlein, P., Pastan, I., and Gottesman, M. M. (1995) Characterisation of high-level cisplatin-resistant cell lines established from a human hepatoma cell line and human KB adenocarcinoma cells: cross-resistance and protein changes. *Br. J. Cancer* **71,** 676–683.
38. Johnson, S. W., Shen, D., Pastan, I., Gottesman, M. M., and Hamilton, T. C. (1996) Cross-resistance, cisplatin accumulation, and platinum-DNA adduct formation and removal in cisplatin-sensitive and -resistant human hepatoma cells. *Exp. Cell Res.* **226,** 133–139.
39. Shen, D., Pastan, I., and Gottesman, M. M. (1998) Cross-resistance to methotrexate and metals in human cisplatin-resistant cell lines results from a pleiotropic defect in accumulation of these compounds associated with reduced plasma membrane binding proteins. *Cancer Res.* **58,** 268–275.
40. Ottone, F., Miotti, S., Bottini, C., Bagnoli, M., Perego, P., Colnaghi, M. I., et al. (1997) Relationship between folate-binding protein expression and cisplatin sensitivity in ovarian carcinoma cell lines. *Br. J. Cancer* **76,** 77–82.
41. Yao, K. S., Godwin, A. K., Johnson, S. W., Ozols, R. F., O'Dwyer, P. J., and Hamilton, T. C. (1995) Evidence for altered regulation of gamma-glutamylcysteine synthetase gene expression among cisplatin-sensitive and cisplatin-resistant human ovarian cancer cell lines. *Cancer Res.* **55,** 4367–4374.
42. Scanlon, K. J., Kashani-Sabet, M., Tone, T., and Funato, T. (1991) Cisplatin resistance in human cancers. *Pharmacol. Ther.* **52,** 385–406.
43. Scanlon, K. J., Jiao, L., Funato, T., Wang, W., Tone, T., Rossi, J. J., et al. (1991) Ribozyme-mediated cleavage of c-fos mRNA reduces gene expression of DNA synthesis enzymes and metallothionein. *Proc. Natl. Acad. Sci. USA* **88,** 10591–10595.
44. Lautier, D., Canitrot, Y., Deeley, R. G., and Cole, S. P. C. (1996) Multidrug resistance mediated by the multidrug resistance protein (MRP) gene. *Biochem. Pharmacol.* **52,** 967–977.
45. Keppler, D., Leier, I., and Jedlitschky, G. (1997) Transport of glutathione conjugates and glucuronides by the multidrug resistance proteins MRP1 and MRP2. *Biol. Chem.* **378,** 787–791.
46. Grant, C. E., Valdimarsson, G., Hipfner, D. R., Almquist, K. C., Cole, S. P. C., and Deeley, R. G. (1994) Overexpression of multidrug resistance-associated protein (MRP) increases resistance to natural product drugs. *Cancer Res.* **54,** 357–361.
47. Cole, S. P. C., Sparks, K. E., Fraser, K., Loe, D. W., Grant, C. E., Wilson, G. M., et al. (1994) Pharmacological characterization of multidrug resistant MRP-transfected human tumor cells. *Cancer Res.* **54,** 5902–5910.
48. Kool, M., de Haas, M., Scheffer, G. L., Scheper, R. J., van Eijk, M. J. T., Julia, A.-M., et al. (1997) Analysis of expression of *cMOAT (MRP2), MRP3, MRP4,* and *MRP5,* homologues of the multidrug resistance-associated protein gene *(MRP1),* in human cancer cell lines. *Cancer Res.* **57,** 3537–3547.
49. Ishikawa, T., Bao, J., Yamane, Y., Akimaru, K., Frindrich, K., Wright, C. D., et al. (1996) Coordinated induction of *MRP/GS-X* pump and gamma-glutamylcysteine synthetase by heavy metals in human leukemia cells. *J. Biol. Chem.* **271,** 14981–14988.
50. Giaccone, G., van Ark Otte, J., Rubio, G. J., Gazdar, A. F., Broxterman, H. J., Dingemans, A. M., et al. (1996) MRP is frequently expressed in human lung-cancer cell lines, in non-small cell lung cancer and in normal lungs. *Int. J. Cancer* **66,** 760–767.
51. Wijnholds, J., Evers, R., van Leusdan, M. R., Mol, C. A. A. M., Zaman, G. J. R., Mayer, U., et al. (1997) Increased sensitivity to anticancer drugs and decreased inflammatory response in mice lacking the multidrug resistance-associated protein. *Nature Med.* **3,** 1275–1279.
52. Borst, P., Kool, M., and Evers, R. (1997) Do cMOAT (MRP2), other MRP homologues, and LRP play a role in MDR? *Cancer Biol.* **8,** 205–213.

53. Taniguchi, K., Wada, M., Kohno, K., Nakamura, T., Kawabe, T., Kawakami, M., et al. (1996) A human canalicular multispecific organic anion transporter (cMOAT) gene is over-expressed in cisplatin-resistant human cancer cell lines with decreased drug accumulation. *Cancer Res.* **56,** 4124–4129.
54. Koike, K., Kawabe, T., Tanaka, T., Toh, S., Uchiumi, T., Wada, M., et al. (1997) A canalicular multispecific organic anion transporter *(cMOAT)* antisense cDNA enhances drug sensitivity in human hepatic cancer cells. *Cancer Res.* **57,** 5475–5479.
55. Litterst, C. L., Gram, T. E., Dedrick, R. L., LeRoy, A. F., and Guarino, A. M. (1976) Distribution and disposition of platinum following intravenous administration of *cis*-diamminedichloroplatinum(II) (NSC 119875) to dogs. *Cancer Res.* **36,** 2340–2344.
56. LeRoy, A. F., Lutz, R. J., Dedrick, R. L., Litterst, C. L., and Gaurino, A. M. (1979) Pharmacokinetic study of *cis*-dichlorodiammineplatinum(II) (DDP) in the beagle dog: thermodynamic and kinetic behavior of DDP in a biologic milieu. *Cancer Treat. Rep.* **63,** 59–71.
57. Mistry, P., Lee, C., and McBrien, D. C. H. (1989) Intracellular metabolites of cisplatin in the rat kidney. *Cancer Chemother. Pharmacol.* **24,** 73–79.
58. Siddik, Z. H., Newell, D. R., Boxall, F. E., and Harrap, K. R. (1987) The comparative pharmacokinetics of carboplatin and cisplatin in mice and rats. *Biochem. Pharmacol.* **36,** 1925–1932.
59. Van der Vijgh, W. J., Verbeek, P. C., Klein, I., and Pindeo, H. M. (1985) Biliary excretion of platinum in rats after administration of cisplatin and aqua 1,1-bis(aminomethyl)-cyclohexane)sulfatoplatinum(II) (spiroplatin, TNO-6). *Cancer Lett.* **28,** 103–109.
60. Shelley, M. D., Fish, R. G., and Adams, M. (1985) Biliary excretion of platinum in a patient treated with cis-dichlorodiammineplatinum(II). *Antimicrob. Agents Chemother.* **27,** 275–276.
61. Akimaru, K., Kuo, M. T., Furuta, K., Suzuki, M., Noyori, R., and Ishikawa, T. (1996) Induction of MRP/GS-X pump and cellular resistance to anticancer prostaglandins. *Cytotechnology* **19,** 221–227.
62. Fujii, R., Mutoh, M., Sumizawa, T., Chen, Z., Yoshimura, A., and Akiyama, S. (1994) Adenosine triphosphate-dependent transport of leukotriene C_4 by membrane vesicles prepared from cisplatin-resistant human epidermoid carcinoma tumor cells. *J. Natl. Cancer Inst.* **86,** 1781–1784.
63. Lee, K., Belinsky, M. G., Bell, D. W., Testa, J. R., and Kruh, G. D. (1998) Isolation of MOAT-B, a widely expressed multidrug resistance-associated protein/canalicular multispecific organic anion transporter-related transporter. *Cancer Res.* **58,** 2141–2147.
64. Zheng, H., Fink, D., and Howell, S. B. (1997) Pharmacological basis for a novel therapeutic strategy based on the use of aquated cisplatin. *Clin. Cancer Res.* **3,** 1157–1165.
65. Fujii, R., Mutoh, M., Niwa, K., Yamada, K., Aikou, T., Nakagawa, M., et al. (1994) Active efflux system for cisplatin in cisplatin-resistant human KB cells. *Jpn. J. Cancer Res.* **85,** 426–433.
66. Ishikawa, T. and Ali-Osman, F. (1993) Glutathione-associated *cis*-diamminedichloroplatinum(II) metabolism and ATP-dependent efflux from leukemia cells. Molecular characterization of glutathione-platinum complex and its biological significance. *J. Biol. Chem.* **268,** 20116–20125.
67. Dedon, P. C. and Borch, R. F. (1987) Characterization of the reactions of platinum antitumor agents with biologic and nonbiologic sulfur-containing nucleophiles. *Biochem. Pharmacol.* **36,** 1955–1964.
68. Mauldin, S. K., Gibbons, G., Wyrick, S. D., and Chaney, S. G. (1988) Intracellular biotransformation of platinum compounds with the 1,2-diaminocyclohexane carrier ligand in the L1210 cell line. *Cancer Res.* **48,** 5136–5144.
69. Versantvoort, C. H. M., Broxterman, H. J., Bagrij, T., Scheper, R. J., and Twentyman, P. R. (1995) Regulation by glutathione of drug transport in multidrug-resistant human lung

tumor cells lines overexpressing multidrug resistance-associated protein. *Br. J. Cancer* **72,** 82–89.

70. Zaman, G. J. R., Lankelma, J., Van Tellingen, O., Beijnen, J., Dekker, H., Paulusma, C., Oude Elferink, R. P. J., Baas, F., and Borst, P. (1995) Role of glutathione in the export of compounds from cells by the multidrug-resistance-associated protein. *Proc. Natl. Acad. Sci. USA* **92,** 7690–7694.
71. Mistry, P., Loh, S. Y., Kelland, L. R., and Harrap, K. R. (1993) Effect of buthionine sulfoximine on PtII and PtIV drug accumulation and the formation of glutathione conjugates in human ovarian-carcinoma cell lines. *Int. J. Cancer* **55,** 848–856.
72. Kurokawa, H., Nishio, K., Ishida, T., Arioka, H., Fukuoka, K., Nomoto, T., et al. (1997) Effect of glutathione depletion on cisplatin resistance in cancer cells transfected with the g-glutamylcysteine synthetase gene. *Jpn. J. Cancer Res.* **88,** 108–110.
73. Jekunen, A. P., Hom, D. K., Alcaraz, J. E., Eastman, A., and Howell, S. B. (1994) Cellular pharmacology of dichloro(ethylenediamine)platinum(II) in cisplatin-sensitive and resistant human ovarian carcinoma cells. *Cancer Res.* **54,** 2680–2687.
74. Naredi, P., Heath, D. D., Enns, R. E., and Howell, S. B. (1995) Cross-resistance between cisplatin, antimony potassium tartrate, and arsenite in human tumor cells. *J. Clin. Invest.* **95,** 1193–1198.
75. Naredi, P., Heath, D. D., Enns, R. E., and Howell, S. B. (1994) Cross-resistance between cisplatin and antimony in a human ovarian carcinoma cell line. *Cancer Res.* **54,** 6464–6468.
76. Doyle, D. A., Cabral, J. M., Pfuetzner, R. A., Kuo, A., Gulbis, J. M., Cohen, S. L., et al. (1998) The structure of the potassium channel: basis of K^+ conduction and selectivity. *Science* **280,** 69–77.
77. Hille, B. (1992) *Ionic Channels of Excitable Membranes*, Sinauer, Sunderland, MA.
78. Heymann, J. B., Agre, P., and Engel, A. (1998) Progress on the structure and function of aquaporin 1. *J. Struct. Biol.* **121,** 191–206.
79. Walz, T., Smith, B. L., Agre, P., and Engel, A. (1994) The three-dimensional structure of human erythrocyte aquaporin CHIP. *EMBO J.* **13,** 2985–2993.
80. Hartsel, S. C., Hatch, C., and Ayenew, W. (1993) How does amphotericin B work?: studies on model membrane systems. *J. Liposome Res.* **3,** 377–408.
81. Assem, M., Bonvalot, S., Beltramo, J. L., Garrido, C., Dimanche-Boitrel, M. T., Genne, P., et al. (1994) Deleterious effect of serum proteins on the amphotericin B-induced potentiation of cisplatin in human colon cancer cells. *Br. J. Cancer* **70,** 631–635.
82. Nielsen, S. and Agre, P. (1995) The aquaporin family of water channels in kidney. *Kidney Int.* **48,** 1957–1068.
83. Verkman, A. S., Shi, L., Frigeri, A., Hasegawa, H., Farinas, J., Mitra, A., et al. (1995) Structure and function of kidney water channels. *Kidney Int.* **48,** 1069–1081.
84. Martin, P. and Schrier, R. W. (1998) Role of aquaporin-2 water channels in urinary concentration and dilution effects. *Kidney Int.* **53(Suppl. 65),** S-57–S-62.
85. Connolly, D. L., Shanahan, C. M., and Weissbeg, P. L. (1998) The aquaporins. A family of water channel proteins. *Int. J. Biochem. Cell Biol.* **30,** 169–172.
86. Valenti, G., Procino, G., Liebenhoff, U., Frigeri, A., Benedetti, P. A., Ahnert-Hilger, G., et al. (1998) A heterotrimeric G protein of the Gi family is required for cAMP-triggered trafficking of aquaporin 2 in kidney epithelial cells. *J. Biol. Chem.* **273,** 22627–22634.
87. Tsukaguchi, H., Shayakul, C., Berger, U. V., Mackenzie, B., Devidas, S., Guggino, W. B., et al. (1998) Molecular characterization of a broad selectivity neutral solute channel. *J. Biol. Chem.* **273,** 24737–24743.
88. Laurencot, C. M., Andrews, P. A., and Kennedy, K. A. (1995) Inhibitors of intracellular pH regulation induce cisplatin resistance in EMT6 mouse mammary tumor cells. *Oncol. Res.* **7,** 363–369.
89. Mack, K. M., Canada, R. G., and Andrews, P. A. (1997) The effects of terbium on the cel-

lular accumulation of cisplatin in MDA-MB-231 human breast tumor cells. *Cancer Chemother. Pharmacol.* 217–222.
90. Hong, W., Saijo, N., Sasaki, Y., Minato, K., Nakano, H., Nakagawa, K., et al. (1988) Establishment and characterization of cisplatin-resistant sublines of human lung cancer cell lines. *Int. J. Cancer* **41,** 462–467.
91. Marverti, G. and Andrews, P. A. (1996) Stimulation of *cis*-diamminedichloroplatinum(II) accumulation by modulation of passive permeability with genistein: an altered response in accumulation-defective resistant cells. *Clin. Cancer Res.* **2,** 991–999.
92. Dawson, D. C. (1977) Na and Cl transport across the isolated turtle colon: parallel pathways for transmural ion movement. *J. Membr. Biol.* **37,** 213–233.
93. Madara, J. L., Barenberg, D., and Carlson, S. (1986) Effects of cytochalasin D on occluding junctions of intestinal absorptive cells: further evidence that the cytoskeleton may influence paracellular permeability and junctional charge selectivity. *J. Cell Biol.* **102,** 2125–2136.
94. Marverti, G., Andrews, P. A., Piccinini, G., Ghiaroni, S., Barbieri, D., and Moruzzi, M. S. (1997) Modulation of *cis*-diamminedichloroplatinum(II) accumulation and cytotoxicity by spermine in sensitive and resistant human ovarian carcinoma cells. *Eur. J. Cancer* **33,** 669–675.
95. Jennerwein, M. and Andrews, P. A. (1995) Effect of intracellular chloride on the cellular pharmacodynamics of *cis*-diamminedichloroplatinum(II). *Drug Metab. Dispos.* **23,** 178–184.
96. Jennerwein, M. and Andrews, P. A. (1994) Drug accumulation and DNA platination in cells exposed to aquated cisplatin species. *Cancer Lett.* **81,** 215–220.
97. Mann, S. C., Andrews, P. A., and Howell, S. B. (1988) Comparison of lipid content, surface membrane fluidity, and temperature dependence of *cis*-diamminedichloroplatinum(II) accumulation in sensitive and resistant human ovarian carcinoma cells. *Anticancer Res.* **8,** 1211–1215.
98. Popovic, P., Wong, P. T. T., Kates, M., Grewall, D., Goel, R., Molep, J. M., et al. (1994) Membrane fluidity and lipids in cisplatin-resistant cells with low cisplatin uptake. *Proc. Am. Assoc. Cancer Res.* **35,** 440
99. Popovic, P., Teicher, B., Wong, P. T. T., Goel, R., and Stewart, D. J. (1993) Pressure tuning infrared spectroscopy of EMT-6 tumor and its cyclophosphamide- and cisplatin-resistant variants. *Proc. Am. Assoc. Cancer Res.* **34,** 405
100. Popovic, P., Wong, P., Goel, R., Evans, W. K., Howell, S. B., and Stewart, D. J. (1993) Pressure-tuning infrared spectra of cisplatin sensitive and resistant human ovarian cancer cells exposed to cisplatin. *Proc. Am. Assoc. Cancer Res.* **34,** 404
101. Taylor, K. D., Goel, R., Shirazi, F. H., Molepo, M., Popovic, P., Stewart, D. J., et al. (1995) Pressure tuning infrared spectroscopic study of cisplatin-induced structural changes in a phosphatidylserine model membrane. *Br. J. Cancer* **72,** 1400–1405.
102. Shinitzky M., ed. (1984) *Physiology of Membrane Fluidity*, CRC, Boca Raton, FL.
103. Caffrey, P. B., Marverti, G., and Andrews, P. A. (1995) Decreased cholesterol content is associated with cisplatin resistant ovarian carcinoma cells. *Proc. Am. Assoc. Cancer Res.* **36,** 401
104. Morikage, T., Ohmori, T., Nishio, K., Fujiwara, Y., Takeda, Y., and Saijo, N. (1993) Modulation of cisplatin sensitivity and accumulation by amphotericin B in cisplatin-resistant human lung cancer cell lines. *Cancer Res.* **53,** 3302–3307.
105. Beketic-Oreskovic, L. and Osmak, M. (1995) Modulation of resistance to cisplatin by amphotericin B and aphidicolin in human larynx carcinoma cells. *Cancer Chemother. Pharmacol.* **35,** 327–333.
106. Sharp, S. Y., Mistry, P., Valenti, M. R., Bryant, A. P., and Kelland, L. R. (1994) Selective potentiation of platinum drug cytotoxicity in cisplatin-sensitive and -resistant human ovarian carcinoma cell lines by amphotericin B. *Cancer Chemother. Pharmacol.* **35,** 137–143.

107. Morikage, T., Bungo, M., Inomata, M., Yoshida, M., Ohmori, T., Fujiwara, Y., et al. N. (1991) Reversal of cisplatin resistance with amphotericin B in a non-small cell lung cancer cell line. *Jpn. J. Cancer Res.* **82,** 747–751.
108. Poulain, L., Sichel, F., Crouet, H., Bureau, F., Gauduchon, P., Gignoux, M., et al. (1997) Potentiation of cisplatin and carboplatin cytotoxicity by amphotericin B in different human ovarian carcinoma and malignant peritoneal mesothelioma cells. *Cancer Chemother. Pharmacol.* **40,** 385–390.
109. Kikkawa, F., Kojima, M., Oguchi, H., Maeda, O., Ishikawa, H., Tamakoshi, K., et al. (1993) Potentiating effect of amphotericin B on five platinum anticancer drugs in human cis-diamminedichloroplatinum (II) sensitive and resistant ovarian carcinoma cells. *Anticancer Res.* **13,** 891–896.
110. Massart, C., Gibassier, J., Le Gall, F., Raoul, M. L., Leclech, G., and Lucas, C. (1996) Modulation of cisplatin cytotoxicity by amphotericin B in six human cell lines of medullary thyroid cancer. *Bull. Cancer* **83,** 619–625.
111. Kojima, M., Kikkawa, F., Oguchi, H., Mizuno, K., Maeda, O., Tamakoshi, K., et al. (1994) Sensitisation of human ovarian carcinoma cells to *cis*-diamminedichloroplatinum (II) by amphotericin B *in vitro* and *in vivo*. *Eur. J. Cancer* **30A,** 773–778.
112. Liang, Z. and Bian, D. (1996) Experimental study on the mechanism of cisplatin resistance and its reversion in human ovarian cancer. *Chin. Med. J.* **109,** 353–355.
113. Bergström, P., Johnsson, A., Cavallin-Stahl, E., Bergenheim, T., and Henriksson, R. (1997) Effects of cisplatin and amphotericin B on DNA adduct formation and toxicity in malignant glioma and normal tissues in rats. *Eur. J. Cancer* **33,** 153–159.
114. Szoka, F. C., Jr. and Tang, M. (1993) Amphotericin B formulated in liposomes and lipid based systems: a review. *J. Liposome Res.* **3,** 363–375.
115. Jekunen, A. P., Shalinsky, D. R., Hom, D. K., Albright, K. D., Heath, D., and Howell, S. B. (1993) Modulation of cisplatin cytotoxicity by permeabilization of the plasma membrane by digitonin *in vitro*. *Biochem. Pharmacol.* **45,** 2079–2085.
116. Lindnér, P. G., Heath, D., Howell, S. B., Naredi, P., and Hafstrom, L. R. (1997) Digitonin enhances the efficacy of carboplatinin liver tumour after intra-arterial administration. *Cancer Chemother. Pharmacol.* **40,** 444–448.
117. Swanson, J. A., Yirinec, B. D., and Silverstein, S. C. (1985) Phorbol esters and horseradish peroxidase stimulate pinocytosis and redirect the flow of pinocytosed fluid in macrophages. *J. Cell Biol.* **100,** 851–859.
118. Besterman, J. M. and Low, R. B. (1983) Endocytosis: a review of mechanisms and plasma membrane dynamics. *Biochem. J.* **210,** 1–13.
119. Bar-Sagi, D. and Feramisco, J. R. (1986) Induction of membrane ruffling and fluid-phase pinocytosis in quiescent fibroblasts by *ras* proteins. *Science* **233,** 1061–1068.
120. Raths, S., Rohrer, J., Crausaz, F., and Riezman, H. (1993) *end3* and *end4*: Two mutants defective in receptor-mediated and fluid-phase endocytosis in *Saccharomyces cerevisiae*. *J. Cell Biol.* **120,** 55–65.
121. Ayesu, K. and Andrews, P. A. (1996) Role of receptor mediated endocytosis in cisplatin accumulation. *Proc. Am. Assoc. Cancer Res.* **37,** 403
122. Howard, G. C., Misra, U. K., DeCamp, D. L., and Pizzo, S. V. (1996) Altered interaction of *cis*-diamminedichloroplatinum(II)-modified (α2M) with the low density lipoprotein recptor-related protein/α2M receptor but not the α2M signaling receptor—evidence for interference with receptor dissociation and recycling. *J. Clin. Invest.* **97,** 1193–1203.
123. Canada, R. G., Andrews, P. A., Mack, K. M., and Haider, A. (1995) The effects of terbium on the accumulation of cisplatin in human ovarian cancer cells. *Biochim. Biophys. Acta* **1267,** 25–30.
124. Christen, R. D., Jekunen, A. P., Jones, J. A., Thiebaut, F., Shalinsky, D. R., and Howell, S. B. (1993) In vitro modulation of cisplatin accumulation in human ovarian carcinoma cells by pharmacologic alteration of microtubules. *J. Clin. Invest.* **92,** 431–440.

125. Parekh, H. K. and Simpkins, H. (1995) The differential expression of cytokeratin 18 in cisplatin-sensitive and -resistant human ovarian adenocarcinoma cells and its association with drug sensitivity. *Cancer Res.* **55,** 5203–5206.
126. Katabami, M., Fujita, H., Honke, K., Makita, A., Akita, H., Miyamoto, H., et al. (1993) Marked reduction of type I keratin (K14) in cisplatin-resistant human lung squamous-carcinoma cell lines. *Biochem. Pharmacol.* **45,** 1703–1710.
127. Köpf-Maier, P. and Mühlhausen, S. K. (1992) Changes in the cytoskeleton pattern of tumor cells by cisplatin *in vitro*. *Chem. Biol. Interact.* **82,** 295–316.
128. Boekelheide, K., Arcila, M. E., and Eveleth, J. (1992) *cis*-Diamminedichloroplatinum (II) (cisplatin) alters microtubule assembly dynamics. *Toxicol. Appl. Pharmacol.* **116,** 146–151.
129. Wedrychowski, A., Schmidt, W. N., Ward, W. S., and Hnilica, L. S. (1986) Cross-linking of cytokeratins to DNA in vivo by chromium salt and *cis*-diamminedichloroplatinum(II). *Biochemistry* **25,** 1–9.
130. Peyrot, V., Briand, C., Crevat, A., Braguer, D., Chauvet-Monges, A. M., and Sari, J. C. (1983) Action of hydrolyzed cisplatin and some analogs on microtubule protein polymerization in vitro. *Cancer Treat. Rep.* **67,** 641–646.
131. Mills, J. W. and Mandel, L. J. (1994) Cytoskeletal regulation of membrane transport events. *FASEB J.* **8,** 1161–1165.
132. Aszalos, A., Yang, G. C., and Gottesman, M. M. (1985) Depolymerization of microtubules increases the motional freedom of molecular probes in cellular plasma membranes. *J. Cell Biol.* **100,** 1357–1362.

5 Cisplatin Resistance in Ovarian Cancer

Mismatch Repair and Engagement of Apoptosis

Robert Brown

CONTENTS

1. INTRODUCTION

Ovarian cancer represents a relatively chemosensitive solid tumor, with responsiveness to a range of agents including platinum compounds *(1)*. However, the overall outcome for patients remains unsatisfactory, with the emergence of drug resistance being a major factor in treatment failure *(2)*. It is generally accepted that DNA is a crucial target for many clinically important anticancer drugs, including cisplatin *(3)*. Inability to couple DNA damage to a signal transduction pathway leading to cell death or biochemical defects in the pathway have been shown to lead to resistance of tumor cell models to many widely used anticancer drugs *(4,5)*. Thus tumors could acquire resistance at clinically achievable drug doses because of either tolerance of DNA damage or failure of tumor cells to transduce the damage signal to an apoptotic response.

Resistance mechanisms operating after induction of DNA damage are not the only mechanisms involved in intrinsic or acquired resistance to cytotoxic

From: *Platinum-Based Drugs in Cancer Therapy*
Edited by: L. R. Kelland and N. Farrell © Humana Press Inc., Totowa, NJ

anticancer drugs. Experimental data show that cells can acquire resistance in vitro by, for example, alterations in drug uptake and metabolism affecting the amount of drug reaching the DNA (for reviews, see refs. *6* and *7*). Nevertheless, what remains unclear is the relative importance of drug delivery vs cellular responses to DNA damage on the clinical response to chemotherapy. A recent clinical trial in advanced ovarian cancer has shown a survival benefit for an increased dose of cisplatin (100 mg/m^2 vs 50 mg/m^2), which, although clearly evident at 2 years, is markedly reduced at longer times *(8)*. One interpretation of this would be that delivering more drug eradicates a higher proportion of tumor cells at the time of initial therapy, but that relapse will occur irrespective of dose, due to drug-resistant cells that survived the initial therapy. Drug resistance that is independent of drug delivery could be due to inability to engage cell death after DNA damage. Indeed, studies using cell lines selected in vitro for resistance to cisplatin show that even under conditions in which equivalent levels of initial DNA damage are induced, i.e., equivalent levels of drug delivery to DNA, the resistant lines fail to undergo apoptosis *(9)*.

2. MISMATCH REPAIR AND DRUG RESISTANCE

Mismatch repair (MMR) plays an important role in maintaining the integrity of the genome and in repairing mispaired bases in DNA *(10)*. In addition, expression of MMR proteins is now associated with sensitivity of mammalian cells to an ever increasing range of DNA-damaging agents *(11)*, and loss of MMR has been correlated with reduced ability of certain tumor cells to undergo drug-induced apoptosis *(9)*. Thus, loss of expression of MMR proteins is correlated with resistance, or tolerance, to methylating agents, 6-thioguanine, cisplatin (and carboplatin), doxorubicin, etoposide, and ionizing radiation *(9,12–15)*. Clearly, many of these agents are clinically important in the treatment of cancer. Inactivation of MMR genes in mice causes cellular resistance to methylating agent and cisplatin *(16,17)*. Restoration of MMR activity by chromosome transfer into MMR-defective human tumors leads to increased sensitivity to a range of drugs *(13)*. These observations argue against resistance being due to increased mutation rates at other drug resistance genes and support a direct involvement of MMR proteins in sensitivity to DNA damage. The absence of MMR in human ovarian tumor models correlates with loss of p53-dependent apoptosis *(9)* and reduced G_2 arrest *(15)* in response to cisplatin, although how MMR-generated signals lead to apoptosis is unclear. In MMR-deficient colon and endometrial tumor models, cisplatin activates JNK (c-Jun NH2-terminal kinase) and the c-Abl nonreceptor tyrosine kinase less efficiently than MMR-proficient cells *(18)*.

The most clearly understood function of MMR is its role in the correction of mismatches occurring during DNA replication or DNA recombination (Fig. 1) *(10)*. Mutations in MMR genes occur in the cancer susceptibility syndrome hereditary nonpolyposis colorectal carcinoma (HNPCC) *(19–21)*, which results

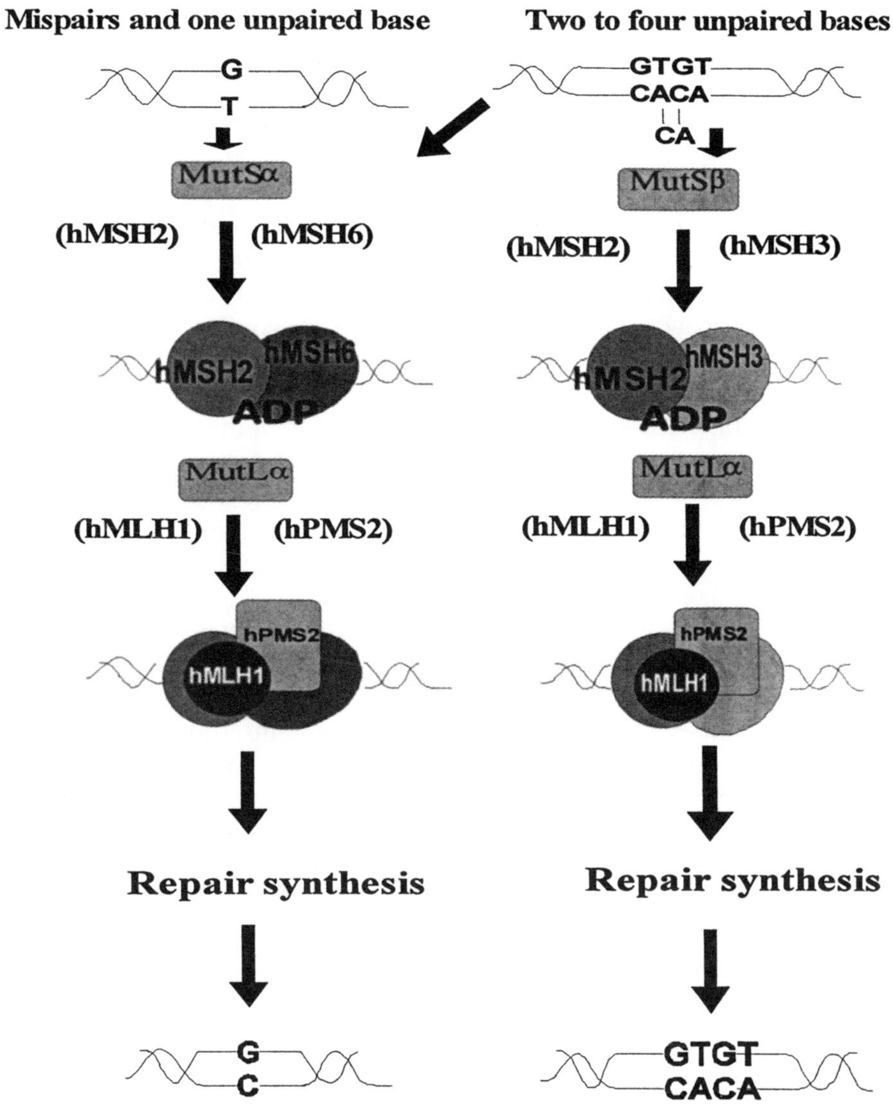

Fig. 1. Model of human mismatch repair. MutSα (a heterodimer of hMSH2 and hMSH6) and MutSβ (a heterodimer of hMSH2 and hMSH3) recognize short insertions of bases, but G/T mismatches appear to be primarily recognized by MutSα. The hMSH2-hMSH6 complex binds mismatched nucleotides in the ADP-bound form and not in the ATP-bound form. ATP hydrolysis has not yet been shown to be necessary for MutSb binding. The hMLH1 protein forms a complex with hPMS2 referred to as MutLα. It has been proposed that the binding of MutS homologs to mismatched DNA allows recruitment of MutLα, which then allows mismatch repair to proceed. Studies so far implicate polδ and possibly polε, as well as PCNA in the repair DNA synthesis step of mismatch repair.

in a predisposition to colorectal carcinoma as well as a number of other tumors, including adenocarcinomas of the endometrium, stomach, and ovary *(22)*. Mutations in the MMR genes *hMLH1*, *hMSH2*, *hPMS2*, and *hPMS1* have all been found to be associated with HNPCC, with the vast majority of mutations being seen in either *hMLH1* or *hMSH2 (23)*. Transgenic mice with genetic inactivation of MMR genes have confirmed the tumor susceptibility associated with defects in *Mlh1*, *Msh2*, and *Pms2 (24)*, although no tumor susceptibility was observed in *Pms1* knockouts *(25)*. One of the striking features of the resulting MMR-defective tumors is their greatly increased rates of mutation at microsatellite sequences, known as microsatellite instability (MIN+) *(26)*. For many tumor types the MIN+ phenotype has also been detected in sporadically occurring disease *(27)*. For example, in ovarian cancer about 15% of sporadic tumors exhibit the MIN+ phenotype. This suggests that these tumors are also MMR-defective; however, mutations of MMR genes have only been observed at low frequency in MIN+ sporadic tumors *(28)*. Recent evidence suggests that methylation of the promoter of MMR genes may play an important role in transcriptional silencing of MMR genes either during acquisition of drug resistance *(29)* or during tumorogenesis *(30)*.

In mammalian cells MMR proteins exist primarily as heterodimeric proteins (Fig. 1). Thus hMSH2 protein associates with hMSH3 and hMSH6. These complexes are referred to as MutSα (hMSH2/hMSH6) and MutSβ (hMSH2/hMSH3). Both complexes recognize short insertions of bases, but G/T mismatches appear to be primarily recognized by MutSα *(31)*. Adenine nucleotide binding and hydrolysis by MutSα have been suggested to act as a molecular switch that determines the timing of downstream MMR events *(32)*. Thus the hMSH2-hMSH6 complex is ON (binds mismatched nucleotides) in the adenosine diphosphate (ADP)-bound form and OFF in the adenosine triphosphate (ATP)-bound form. A central role for the adenine nucleotide binding domain is consistent with the ATP-dependent translocation model of MMR proposed by Modrich and colleagues *(33)*.

The MutL homologs also form heterodimers; thus the hMLH1 protein forms a complex with hPMS2 referred to as MutLα (Fig. 1). Defects in either MutL homolog leads to loss of mismatch correction at or prior to the excision stage of repair *(34)*. It has therefore been proposed that MutS homologs binding to mismatched DNA allows recruitment of MutL homologs, which then allows MMR to proceed. How this occurs is unclear.

3. HOW DOES MMR COUPLE TO APOPTOSIS AND LOSS OF MMR LEAD TO DRUG RESISTANCE?

3.1. Model 1: Futile Repair Cycles

The role of mismatch repair in drug resistance was first identified in the alkylation tolerance phenotype observed in cells selected for resistance to monofunctional alkylating agents such as MNNG and MNU *(35)* (Fig. 2A). The concept of "tolerance" is one in which the damaged base is not removed from the DNA but appears unable to induce cytotoxic effects *(12)*. Agents that methylate DNA, such as MNNG and MNU, are mutagenic and cytotoxic due to the formation of O^6-methylguanine. Under normal circumstances this lesion is directly repaired by the enzyme MGMT. Functional loss of this enzyme, most commonly by epigenetic silencing, results in cellular hypersensitivity to killing and mutagenesis by such agents *(36)*. Resistance (or tolerance) to methylating agents can, however, occur due to inactivation of MMR *(37,38)*. Although the association between defective MMR and tolerance to certain methylating agents is clear, the mechanism underlying this phenomenon remains undefined. It has been proposed that these methylated bases are not a block to replication, but instead the DNA polymerase inserts the best fitting base into the nascent strand opposite the modified guanine. It has been shown that O^6MeG· T introduces the least structural distortion to the DNA *(39)*. In the absence of efficient methyltransferase function, this mismatched O^6MeG· T base pair is recognized by the MMR pathway as abnormal. Repair synthesis, which occurs in the newly synthesized strand opposite O^6MeG, is doomed to failure owing to the inability to find a good complementary match for the methylated base. It is proposed that repeated, futile attempts to repair this mismatch eventually result in cell death, perhaps by the generation of strand breaks *(12)*. Tolerance would therefore arise when the MMR system could no longer initiate these aborted attempts at repair.

3.2. Model 2: MMR-Dependent Replication Stalling

The observation that loss of MMR correlated with acquisition of resistance to cisplatin opened up a much wider examination of the role of MMR in drug resistance beyond monofunctional methylating agents *(9)*. Loss of MMR is now associated with resistance to a diverse range of DNA-damaging agents *(11)*, and hence any model of resistance must take into account this wide variety of types of DNA damage. hMutSα recognizes 1,2-cisplatin crosslinks in a duplex DNA in which the complementary DNA strand contains two C residues opposite a 1,2-diguanyl crosslink *(40)*. However, this is a relatively poor substrate for hMutSα, and a duplex molecule in which the platinated guanine residues are opposite noncomplementary bases is bound with much greater affinity *(41)*. Such structures can arise in the cell if platinum-damaged DNA has undergone replication. Cellular proliferation, and hence presumably DNA replication, is required for induction of apoptosis by cisplatin in sensitive cell types *(42)*. Certain cisplatin-resistant human ovarian cells, which have lost MMR protein expression, appear able to bypass cisplatin DNA intrastrand crosslinks during DNA replication *(43)*. The mechanisms leading to bypass are largely unknown, but if loss of MMR leads to reduced replication stalling and

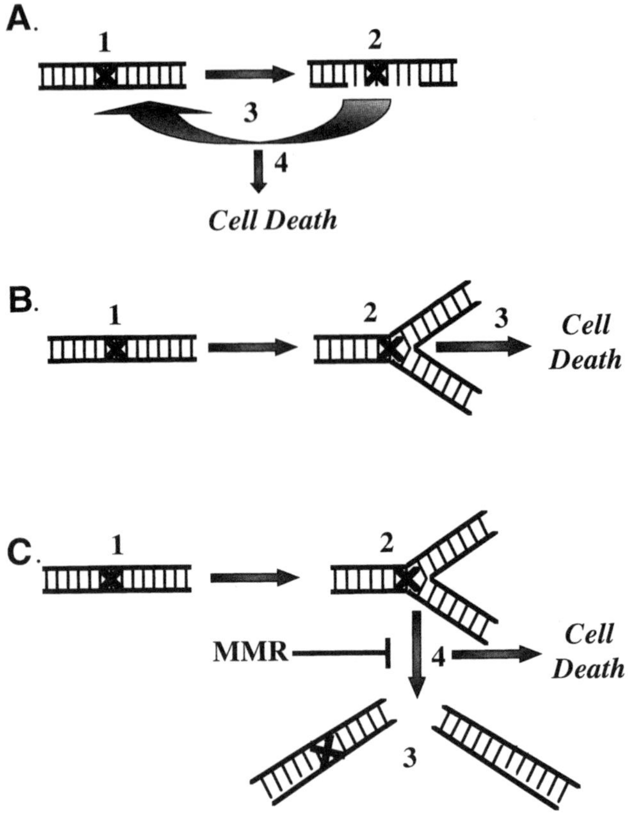

Fig. 2. Models of MMR coupling to cell death. **(A)** Futile repair cycles. 1, In the presence of damage induced in DNA, the DNA polymerase inserts an incorrect base into the nascent strand; 2, this is recognized by the mismatch repair pathway, and repair synthesis occurs in the newly synthesized strand opposite the lesion; 3, MMR, however, does not remove the initial damage, and repeat rounds of MMR cycles ensue; 4, repeated, futile attempts to repair this mismatch result in cell death, perhaps by the generation of strand breaks. **(B)** MMR-dependent replication stalling. 1, Damage induced in DNA is recognized by MMR proteins; 2, this causes stalling of the replication complex; 3, stalled complexes either directly signal cell death, or indirectly signal death by generating DNA strand breaks at the stalled complex. **(C)** Recombination bypass. 1, Damage induced in DNA is recognized by damage recognition proteins; 2, binding of damage recognition proteins induces stalling of the replication complex; 3, the stalled complexes can be bypassed by DNA strand exchange mechanisms, leading to damage tolerance; 4, in the presence of MMR, recombination-dependent bypass is inhibited, inducing cell death.

increased bypass, then this could lead to resistance (Fig. 2B). In general, replicative bypass of 1,2-diguanyl cisplatin adducts has been considered inefficient; however, the replicative polymerases δ and ε are indeed able to bypass these adducts in structures that resemble replication forks, although so far no role for MMR in this process has been demonstrated *(44)*. Thus, one possible mechanism of cisplatin toxicity is that inability to bypass this lesion in MMR-proficient sensitive cells has an intrinsic probability of being lethal or of generating a signal that activates an apoptotic pathway. A direct corollary of this model is that cisplatin resistance may be acquired by reducing the probability of lethal events occurring, or of preapoptotic signals being generated, during replication, allowing replication bypass and cell survival.

3.3. Model 3: Modulation of Recombination Bypass

Recently we have shown that *Saccharomyces cerevisiae* acquire resistance to cisplatin and carboplatin if MMR genes are inactivated *(44a)*. Thus, genetic inactivation of MMR genes *(MLH1, MLH2, MSH2, MSH3, MSH6*, but not *PMS1)* in isogenic strains of *S. cerevisiae* leads to increased resistance to the anticancer drugs cisplatin and/or carboplatin, but has no effect on UV(C) sensitivity. However, inactivation of *MLH1*, *MLH2*, or *MSH2* has no significant effect on drug sensitivities in *rad52* mutant strains. Thus drug resistance mediated by loss of MMR appears to require expression of RAD52, a protein known to be required for recombination *(45)*. As already discussed, bypass of DNA lesions during DNA replication has been suggested as a mechanism for cisplatin-adduct tolerance *(43)*. We propose that loss of MMR proteins can lead to increased *RAD52*-dependent recombinational bypass of adducts (Fig. 2C). The 1,2-intrastrand crosslink induced by cisplatin is poorly repaired, either because it is not recognized by NER *(46)* or because of inhibition of repair, for instance by damage recognition proteins *(47)*. DNA damage persistence or nonrepaired DNA lesions could lead to a cytotoxic signal being generated during DNA replication, perhaps by stalling of the replication complex. Indeed, HMG1 has been shown to bind to cisplatin lesions and has been implicated in replication stalling during in vitro DNA replication *(48)*. RAD52-dependent recombinational bypass during replication would lead to resistance, whereas inhibition of this process by MMR would lead to sensitivity. It is known that MMR proteins can inhibit levels of recombination in yeast and mammalian cells *(49,50)*. Therefore resistance may be acquired by loss of MMR proteins, reducing the probability of lethal signals being generated during replication by allowing increased recombination-dependent bypass and cell survival.

The experimental data discussed earlier and all three of the models discussed above predict that MMR is necessary to engage apoptosis in response to certain types of DNA damage. However, the signal pathways leading from MMR to apoptosis are as yet unclear. In MMR-deficient colon and endometrial tumor models, cisplatin activates JNK and the c-Abl non-receptor tyrosine kinase less efficiently than MMR-proficient cells *(18)*. Furthermore, in tumor cell models selected for cisplatin resistance in vitro, loss of MMR occurs concomitantly with loss of p53 function and ability to undergo p53-dependent apoptosis *(9)*.

However, restoration of MMR activity, while restoring drug sensitivity, does not restore p53 function *(51)*. Loss of MMR correlates with loss of G_2 arrest induced by certain drugs *(52)*, although there is no evidence that the loss of G_2 arrest is functionally linked with the loss of drug-induced apoptosis. Thus loss of MMR in cells affects many signaling pathways, leading to important cellular responses to DNA damage, including apoptosis, although the relative contribution of any given pathway may depend on the cell type being examined.

4. RELEVANCE OF LOSS OF MMR FOR DRUG RESISTANCE OF HUMAN TUMORS

A MIN+ phenotype has been shown to correlate with reduced survival and poor disease prognosis in breast cancer *(53)*. Conversely, MIN+ correlates with good prognosis in colon cancer *(54)*. These differences may reflect the different impact of a mutator phenotype on tumor progression (in the case of colon cancer) vs lack of MMR on drug sensitivity (in the case of breast cancer). MIN+ has been suggested to occur in 15–20% of sporadic ovarian tumors, and two separate studies have raised the possibility that this may have prognostic significance, although possible correlations with response to chemotherapy were not explored *(55,56)*. We observe an increase in ovarian tumors immunologically negative for the hMLH1 subunit of the MMR MutLα heterodimer in samples taken at second-look laparotomy after chemotherapy (36%), compared with untreated tumors (9.5%) *(15)*. Including recent unpublished data from our laboratory, we observe that 5/50 ovarian tumors are negative for hMLH1 before chemotherapy and 6/15 after chemotherapy, which is significantly different ($p < 0.01$ by Fisher's exact test). Together with the data observed in cell line models *(9,14)*, these observations encourage larger studies to be done in ovarian tumors correlating MMR with response to chemotherapy.

It has been shown that tumors release DNA, which can be specifically detected in plasma from patients *(57)*. This provides the possibility of measuring genetic alterations occurring in tumors by taking a simple blood sample from patients. Given that microsatellite instability can be measured by polymerase chain reaction (PCR) using only small amounts of DNA, this opens the exciting possibility of doing large-scale prospective studies using a noninvasive sampling method to correlate MIN status (and indeed other genetic changes) with response to chemotherapy.

5. CIRCUMVENTION OF DRUG RESISTANCE MEDIATED BY LOSS OF MMR

If drug resistance in ovarian tumors is occurring due to mechanisms that occur after induction of DNA damage, then approaches to circumvent resistance that focus on increasing drug delivery and inducing more DNA damage may not be effective. Delivering sufficient damage to induce the appropriate death signals is clearly important. If acquired resistance, however, is due to mechanisms abrogating the death response of the cells to DNA damage, then resistance will not be overcome by strategies that increase intracellular drug accumulation or levels of platinated DNA damage. It can, however, be envisaged that platinum analogs inducing different spectra of DNA damage may be more effective at inducing cell death than cisplatin *(58,59)*. Platinum analogs that induce apoptosis by a mechanism that does not require functional MMR may be more effective in ovarian tumors with defective MMR. The ideal would be to find a drug to which MMR-defective tumors are hypersensitive. So far no such agent has been identified, although it has been suggested that the sensitivity to some drugs is not affected by MMR status *(11)*. For instance, although resistance to cisplatin and carboplatin can be mediated by loss of MMR, the sensitivity of colon tumor cells to the platinum analogs oxaliplatin, tetraplatin, transplatin, JM335, or JM216 appears not to be affected by MMR status *(60)*. This needs to be examined in a wider variety of experimental models.

Drugs that kill tumor cells by mechanisms that are p53 independent may also be effective in subsets of ovarian tumor cells with p53 dysfunction. Indeed, it has been shown that taxoids induce apoptosis independently of p53 *(61)*. Furthermore, ovarian cell lines that lose p53 function induced by gene transfer can acquire resistance to multiple anticancer agents, but retain sensitivity to taxol *(62)*. Such transfectants also retain sensitivity to camptothecin and to clinically usable analogs *(62,63)*. Thus these drugs can use a death-signaling pathway that utilizes neither MMR or p53 and that is separate from cisplatin-induced death pathways. Taxoids and topoisomerase I inhibitors have been reported to be effective in ovarian tumors that recur after cisplatin treatment *(64,65)*.

Genetic therapy approaches may provide a new means of targeting tumors with specific genetic defects. Tumor-specific expression of suicide gene vectors would be one means of killing tumor cells without affecting normal cells *(66)*. For instance, it may be possible to design suicide gene vector systems that utilize defects in MMR to deliver increased levels of a suicide gene to tumor cells. The ability of MMR-defective cells to tolerate damage and allow DNA replication to proceed could be utilized to design vectors containing specific types of damage, such that the suicide gene vector would replicate and express preferentially in MMR-defective cells, but not normal cells. An E1B-attenuated adenovirus that replicates preferentially in tumor cells defective in p53 *(67)* has preferential replication and prevents tumor growth in nude mice of ovarian tumor cells that are cisplatin resistant, have dysfunctional p53, and are defective in MMR *(68)*.

Inhibitors of DNA repair have been widely suggested as possible means of sensitizing resistant tumors *(2,69)*. Effects of such inhibitors on increasing sensitivity of resistant cell line models have been reported; however, it should be noted that such drugs will have pleiotropic effects on the cell, including effects on cell cycle progression and apoptosis. Aphidicolin, an inhibitor of DNA polymerase α, δ, and ε, has been shown to inhibit repair of cisplatin-DNA adducts and to potentate the toxicity of cisplatin in a human ovarian cell line *(70)*. Recently we have been able to show that this sensitization is more marked in ovarian lines that are cisplatin resistant due to loss of MMR *(70a)*.

Reversing the loss of MMR expression in resistant cells should sensitize tumors to anticancer drugs such as cisplatin. We have recently shown that 5-azacytidine treatment of cisplatin-resistant derivatives of ovarian tumor cells resulted in decreased methylation of the *hMLH1* promoter, increased expression of the hMLH1 protein, and a corresponding increase in cisplatin sensitivity *(29)*. Thus tumors that have lost hMLH1 expression due to promoter methylation may be especially sensitive to combined treatment with cisplatin and 5-azacytidine.

6. CONCLUSIONS

In the last few years, there has been an explosion in our understanding of the basic mechanisms of MMR in human cells and an increasing awareness of the possible role of MMR proteins in determining the sensitivity of tumor cells to a wide variety of important chemotherapeutic drugs. The precise mechanisms through which loss of MMR leads to drug resistance remain hypothetical. It is also essential to evaluate properly the relevance of MMR protein expression to clinical drug resistance, both intrinsic and acquired resistance. The MIN status of tumors can be readily assayed using PCR assays and measured not only from tumor biopsies, but also from serum samples from patients *(57)*. Such noninvasive means of monitoring the molecular changes in a tumor provide the exciting possibility of being able to determine the appropriate therapy for a given patient based on molecular genetic determinants of disease progression.

Until recently the main approach to increasing the efficacy of a given drug and to overcoming resistance has been either to synthesize new analogs or to use drugs that modulate the amount of active drug reaching the intracellular target. However, these approaches will not overcome cellular biologic resistance due to post-DNA damage mechanisms. As our understanding of the mechanisms of cell death and cell cycle arrest increases, novel approaches to overcome resistance may become possible. Advances in combinatorial chemistry and molecular approaches may allow the identification of possible resistance modulation molecules. However, it has been argued that one of the reasons for the effectiveness of the clinically useful chemotherapeutic drugs such as cisplatin is that certain tumor types undergo apoptosis readily in response to DNA damage *(71)*. Resistance modulators have to sensitize the tumor cells specifically without affecting normal cells. If resistance is due to inhibition of apoptosis, modulators that increase apoptosis in resistant tumor cells will have the potential to maintain the differential of tumor to normal cell toxicity. This stresses the importance of using appropriate well-defined biologic systems for the identification of a modulator of tumor cell resistance.

ACKNOWLEDGMENTS

I would like to thank all the members, past and present, of the Molecular Mechanisms of Drug Resistance Team in Medical Oncology, Glasgow, and numerous collaborators from other laboratories who have been involved in our work on mismatch repair; Professor S.B. Kaye (Glasgow) for constructive comments on the manuscript; and The Cancer Research Campaign (UK) for funding the majority of our research.

REFERENCES

1. Reed, E., Kohn, E. C., Sarosy, G., Dabholkar, M., Davis, P., Jacob, J., et al. (1995) Paclitaxel, cisplatin, and cyclophosphamide in human ovarian cancer: molecular rationale and early clinical results. *Semin. Oncol.* **22,** 90–96.
2. Johnson, S. W., Ozols, R. F., and Hamilton, T. C. (1993) Mechanisms of drug resistance in ovarian cancer. *Cancer* **71,** 644–649.
3. Epstein, R. J. (1990) Drug-induced DNA damage and tumor chemosensitivity. *J. Clin. Oncol.* **8,** 2062–2084.
4. Bates, S. and Vousden, K. H. (1996) p53 in signalling checkpoint arrest or apoptosis. *Curr. Opin. Gen. Dev.* **6,** 12–19.
5. Oren, M. (1994) Relationship of p53 to the control of apoptotic cell death. *Semin. Cancer Biol.* **5,** 221–227.
6. Andrews, P. A. and Howell, S. B. (1990) Cellular pharmacology of cisplatin: perspectives on mechanisms of acquired resistance. *Cancer Cells* **2,** 35–43.
7. Gately, D. P. and Howell, S. B. (1993) Cellular accumulation of the anticancer agent cisplatin: a review. *Br. J. Cancer* **67,** 1171–1176.
8. Kaye, S. B., Paul, J., Cassidy, J., Lewis, C. R., Duncan, I. D., Gordon, H. K., et al. (1996) Mature results of a randomized trial of two doses of cisplatin for the treatment of ovarian cancer. *J. Clin. Oncol.* **14,** 2113–2119.
9. Anthoney, D. A., McIlwrath, A. J., Gallagher, W. M., Edlin, A. R. M., and Brown, R. (1996) Microsatellite instability, apoptosis and loss of p53 function in drug resistant tumor cells. *Cancer Res.* **56,** 1374–1381.
10. Modrich, P. (1997) Strand-specific mismatch repair in mammalian cells. *J. Biol. Chem.* **272,** 24727–24730.
11. Fink, D., Aebi, S., and Howell, S. B. (1998) The role of DNA mismatch repair in drug resistance. *Clin. Cancer Res.* **4,** 1–6.
12. Karran, P. and Hampson, R. (1996) Genomic instability and tolerance to alkylating agents. *Cancer Surv.* **28,** 69–85.
13. Aebi, S., Fink, D., Gordon, R., Kim, H. K., Zheng, H., Fink, J. L., et al. (1997) Resistance to cytotoxic drugs in DNA mismatch repair-deficient cells. *Clin. Cancer Res.* **3,** 1763–1767.
14. Drummond, J. T., Anthoney, A., Brown, R., and Modrich, P. (1996) Cisplatin and Adriamycin resistance are associated with MutLalpha and mismatch repair deficiency in an ovarian tumor cell line. *J. Biol. Chem.* **271,** 19645–19648.
15. Brown, R., Hirst, G. L., Gallagher, W. M., McIlwrath, A. J., Margison, G. P., van der Zee,

A. G., et al. (1997) hMLH1 expression and cellular responses of ovarian tumor cells to treatment with cytotoxic anticancer agents. *Oncogene* **15,** 45–52.
16. De Wind, N., Dekker, M., Berns, A., Radman, M., and te Riele, H. (1995) Inactivation of the mouse MSH2 gene results in mismatch repair deficiency, methylation tolerance, hyperrecombination and predisposition to cancer. *Cell* **82,** 321–330.
17. Fink, D., Nebel, S., Aebi, S., Nehme, A., and Howell, S. B. (1997) Loss of DNA mismatch repair due to knockout of MSH2 or PMS2 results in resistance to cisplatin and carboplatin. *Int. J. Oncol.* **11,** 539–542.
18. Nehme, A., Baskaran, R., Aebi, S., Fink, D., Nebel, S., Cenni, B., et al. (1997) Differential induction of c-Jun-NH2 terminal kinase and c-abl kinase in DNA mismatch repair proficient and deficient cells exposed to cisplatin. *Cancer Res.* **57,** 3253–3257.
19. Bronner, C. E., Baker, S. M., Morrison, P. T., Warren, G., Smith, L. G., Lescoe, M. K., et al. (1994) Mutation in the DNA mismatch repair gene homolog hMLH1 is associated with hereditary non-polyposis colon cancer. *Nature* **368,** 258–261.
20. Leach, F. S., Nicolaides, N. C., Papadopoulos, N., Liu, B., Jen, J., Parsons, R., et al. (1993) Mutations of a mutS homolog in hereditary nonpolyposis colorectal cancer. *Cell* **75,** 1215–1225.
21. Nicolaides, N. C., Papadopoulos, N., Liu, B., Wei, Y., Carter, K. C., Ruben, S. M., et al. (1994) Mutations of two PMS homologs in hereditary nonpolyposis colon cancer. *Nature* **371,** 75–80.
22. Lynch, H. T. (1993) Genetics, natural history, tumor spectrum and pathology of hereditary nonpolyposis colorectal cancer: an updated review. *Gasteroenterology* **104,** 1535–1549.
23. Liu, B., Parsons, R., Papadopoulos, N., Nicolaides, N. C., Lynch, H. T., Watson, P., et al. (1996) Analysis of the mismatch repair genes in hereditary non-polyposis colorectal cancer patients. *Nature Med.* **2,** 169–174.
24. Reitmair, A. H., Redston, M., Chun, J., Chuang, T. C. Y., Bjerkness, M., Cheng, H., et al. (1996) Spontaneous intestinal carcinomas and skin neoplasms in MSH2-deficient mice. *Cancer Res.* **56,** 3842–3849.
25. Prolla, T. A., Baker, S. M., Harris, A. C., Tsao, J., Yao, X., Bronner, E., et al. (1997) Tumor susceptibility and spontaneous mutation in mice deficient in MLH1, Pms1 and Pms2 DNA mismatch repair. *Nature Genet.* **18,** 276–279.
26. Aaltonen, L. A., Peltomaki, P., Leach, P. S., Sistonen, P., Pylkkanen, L., Maklin, J., et al. (1993) Clues to the pathogenesis of Familial Colorectal Cancer. *Science* **260,** 812–815.
27. Eshleman, J. R. and Markowitz, S. D. (1995) Microsatellite instability in inherited and sporadic neoplasms. *Curr. Opin. Oncol.* **7,** 83–89.
28. Liu, B., Nicolaides, N., Markowitz, S., Wilson, J. K. V., Parsons, R. E., Jen, J., et al. (1995) Mismatch repair defects in sporadic colorectal cancers with microsatellite instability. *Nature Genet.* **9,** 48–54.
29. Strathdee, G., MacKean, M., Illand, M., and Brown, R. (1999) A role for methylation of the *hMLH1* promoter in loss of hMLH1 expression and drug resistance in ovarian cancer. *Oncogene.* **18,** 2335–2341.
30. Kane, M. F., Loda, M., Gaida, G. M., Lipman, J., Mishra, R., Goldman, H., et al. (1997) Methylation of the hMLH1 promoter correlates with lack of expression of hMLH1 in sporadic colon tumors and mismatch repair -defective tumor cell lines. *Cancer Res.* **57,** 808–811.
31. Drummond, J. T., Li, G., Longley, M. J., and Modrich, P. (1995) Isolation of a hMSH2-p160 heterodimer that restores DNA mismatch repair in tumor cells. *Science* **268,** 1909-1912.
32. Gradia, S., Acharya, S., and Fishel, R. (1997) The human mismatch recognition complex hMSH2-hMSH6 functions as a novel molecular switch. *Cell* **91,** 995–1005.
33. Allen, D. J., Makhov, A., Grilley, M., Taylor, J., Thresher, R., Modrich, P., et al. (1997) MutS mediates heteroduplex formation by a translocation mechanism. *EMBO J.* **16,** 4467–4476.
34. Parsons, R., Li, G. M., Longley, M. J., Fang, W. H., Papadopoulos, N., Jen, J., et al. (1993) Hypermutability and mismatch repair deficiency in RER^+ tumor cells. *Cell* **75,** 1227–1236.
35. Branch, P., Aquilina, G., Bignami, M., and Karran, P. (1993) Defective mismatch binding and a mutator phenotype in cells tolerant to DNA damage. *Nature* **362,** 652–654.

36. Hampson, R., Humbert, O., MacPherson, P., Aquilina, G., and Karran, P. (1997) Mismatch repair defects and O-6-methylguanine-DNA methyltransferase expression in acquired resistance to methylating agents in human cells. *J. Biol. Chem.* **272,** 28596–28606.
37. Kat, A., Thilly, W. G., Fang, W., Longley, M. J., Li, G., and Modrich, P. (1993) An alkylating-tolerant, mutator human cell line is deficient in strand-specific mismatch repair. *Proc. Natl. Acad. Sci. USA* **90,** 6424–6428.
38. Koi, M., Umar, A., Chauhan, D. P., Cherian, S. P., Carethers, J. M., Kunkel, T. A., et al. (1994) Human chromosome 3 corrects mismatch repair deficiency and microsatellite instability and reduces N-methyl-N'-nitro-N-nitrosoguanidine tolerance in colon tumor cells with homozygous hMLH1 mutation. *Cancer Res.* **54,** 4308–4312.
39. Wood, R. D. and Shivji, M. K. K. (1997) Which DNA polymerases are used for DNA-repair in eukaryotes? *Carcinogenesis* **18,** 605–610.
40. Duckett, D. R., Drummond, J. T., Murchie, A. I. H., Reardon, J. T., Sancar, A., Lilley, D. M., et al. (1996) Human MutSalpha recognizes damaged DNA base pairs containing O6-methylguanine, O4-methylthymine or the cispaltin-d(GpG) adduct. *Proc. Natl. Acad. Sci. USA* **93,** 6443–6446.
41. Yamada, M., O'Regan, E., Brown, R., and Karran, P. (1997) Selective recognition of a cispaltin-DNA adduct by human mismatch repair proteins. *Nucleic Acids Res.* **25,** 491–495.
42. Evans, D. L., Tilby, M., and Dive, C. (1994) Differential sensitivity to the induction of apoptosis by cisplatin in proliferating and quiescent immature rat thymocytes is independent of the level of drug accumulation and DNA adduct formation. *Cancer Res.* **54,** 1596–1603.
43. Mamenta, E. L., Poma, E. E., Kaufmann, W. K., Delmastro, D. A., Grady, H. L., and Chaney, S. G. (1994) Enhanced replicative bypass of platinum-DNA adducts in cisplatin-resistant human ovarian carcinoma cell lines. *Cancer Res.* **54,** 3500–3505.
44. Hoffmann, J., Pillaire, M., Maga, G., Podust, V., Hubscher, U., and Villani, G. (1995) DNA polymerase b bypasses in vitro a single d(GpG)-cisplatin adduct placed on codon 13 of the HRAS gene. *Proc. Natl. Acad. Sci. USA* **92,** 5356–5360.
44a. Durant, S. T., Morris, M. M., Illand, M., et al. (1999) Dependence on RAD52 and RAD1 for anticancer drug resistance mediated by inactivation of mismatch repair genes. *Current Biology* **9,** 51–54.
45. Petes, T. D., Malone, R. E., and Syminton, L. S. (1991) Recombination in yeast, in *The Molecular and Cellular Biology of the Yeast* Saccharomyces, (Broach, J. R., Pringle, J. R., and Jones, E. W., eds.), Cold Spring Harbor Laboratory Press, Cold Spring Harbor, NY, pp. 407–521.
46. Moggs, J. G., Szymkowski, D. E., Yamada, M., Karran, P., and Wood, R. D. (1997) Differential human nucleotide excision repair of paired and mispaired cisplatin-DNA adducts. *Nucleic Acids Res.* **25,** 480–490.
47. McNulty, M. M. and Lippard, S. J. (1996) The HMG-domain protein Ixr1 blocks excision repair of cisplatin-DNA adducts in yeast. *Mutat. Res.* **362,** 75–86.
48. Hoffmann, J., Locker, D., Villani, G., and Leng, M. (1997) HMG1 protein inhibits the translesion synthesis of the major DNA cisplatin adduct by cell extracts. *J. Mol. Biol.* **270,** 539–543.
49. Alani, E., Reenan, R. A., and Kolodner, R. D. (1994) Interaction between mismatch repair and genetic recombination in Saccharomyces cerevisiae. *Genetics* **137,** 19–39.
50. Ciotta, C., Ceccotti, S., Aquilina, G., Humbert, O., Palombo, F., Jiricny, J., et al. (1998) Increased somatic recombination in methylation tolerant human cells with defective DNA mismatch repair. *J. Mol. Biol.* **276,** 705–719.
51. Brown, R., Ganley, I., Illand, M., and Kim, Y. T. (1998) Preferential replication of an E1B-attenuated adenovirus in drug resistant ovarian tumor lines with defective mismatch repair and loss of p53. *Proc. Am. Assoc. Cancer Res.* **39,** 555 (abstract).
52. Hawn, M. T., Umar, A., Carethers, J. M., Marra, G., Kunkel, T. A., Boland, C. R., et al. (1995) Evidence for a connection between the mismatch repair system and the G2 cell cycle checkpoint. *Cancer Res.* **55,** 3721–3725.
53. Paulson, T. G., Wright, F. A., Parker, B. A., Russack, V., and Wahl, G. M. (1996)

Microsatellite instability correlates with reduced survival and poor disease prognosis in breast cancer. *Cancer Res.* **56,** 4021–4026.

54. Bubb, V. J., Curtis, L. J., Cunningham, C., Dunlop, M. G., Carothers, A. D., Morris, R. G., et al. (1996) Microsatellite instability and the role of hmsh2 in sporadic colorectal-cancer. *Oncogene* **12,** 2641–2649.
55. King, B. L., Carcangiu, M. L., Carter, D., Kiechle, M., Pfisterer, J., Pfleiderer, A., et al. (1995) Microsatellite instability in ovarian neoplasms. *Br. J. Cancer* **72,** 376–382.
56. Fujita, M., Enomoto, T., Yoshino, K., Nomura, T., Buzard, G. S., and Inoue, M. (1995) Microsatellite instability and alterations in the hMSH2 gene in human ovarian cancer. *Int. J. Cancer* **64,** 361–366.
57. Nawroz, H., Koch, W., Anker, P., Stroun, M., and Sidransky, D. (1996) Microsatellite alterations in serum DNA of head and neck cancer patients. *Nature Med.* **2,** 1035–1037.
58. Mellish, K. J., Barnard, C. F. J., Murrer, B. A., and Kelland, L.R. (1995) DNA-binding properties of novel cis and trans platinum-based anticancer agents in 2 human ovarian-carcinoma cell-lines. *Int. J. Cancer* **62,** 717–723.
59. Kelland, L. R., Barnard, C. F. J., Evans, I. G., Murrer, B. A., Theobald, B. R. C., Wyer, S. B., et al. (1995) Synthesis and in-vitro and in-vivo antitumor-activity of a series of trans platinum antitumor complexes. *J. Med. Chem.* **38,** 3016–3024.
60. Vasey, P. A., Jones, N. A., Jenkins, S., Dive, C., and Brown, R. (1996) Cispaltin, camptothecin and taxol sensitivities of cells with p53-associated multidrug resistance. *Mol. Pharmacol.* **50,** 1536–1540.
61. Wahl, A. F., Donaldson, K. L., Fairchild, C., Lee, F. Y. F., Foster, S. A., Demers, G. W., et al. (1996) Loss of normal p53 function confers sensitization to taxol by increasing G2/M arrest and apoptosis. *Nature Med.* **2,** 72–79.
62. Vasey, P. A., Jones, N. A., Jenkins, S., Dive, C., and Brown, R. (1996) Cispaltin, camptothecin and taxol sensitivities of cells with p53-associated multi-agent resistance. *Mol. Pharmacol.* **50,** 1536–1540.
63. McDonald, A. C. and Brown, R. (1998) Topoisomerase-1 inhibitor induced cell cycle changes and cell death may not be related to p53 status. *Br. J. Cancer* **78,** 745–751.
64. McGuire, W. P. (1995) Ovarian cancer, in *Paclitaxel in cancer treatment,* (McGuire, W. P., Rowinsky, E. K., eds.) Marcel Dekker, New York, pp. 201–222.
65. Rowinsky, E., Donehower, R., Rosensheim, N., Walczak, J., and McGuire, W. (1995) A phase II trial of topotecan as salvage therapy in epithelial ovarian cancer. *Proc. Am. Soc. Clin. Oncol.* **36,** 275.
66. Vile, R. G., Sunassee, K., and Diaz, R. M. (1998) Strategies for achieving multiple layers of selectivity in gene therapy. *Mol. Med. Today* **4,** 84–92.
67. Bischoff, J. R., Kirn, D. H., Williams, A., Heise, C., Horn, S., Muna, M., et al. (1996) An adenovirus mutant that replicates selsectively in p53-deficient human tumor cells. *Science* **274,** 373–376.
68. Heise, C., Sampson-Johannes, A., Williams, A., McCormick, F., Von Hoff, D. D., and Kirn, D. H. (1997) Onyx-015, an E1B gene attenuated adenovirus, causes tumor-specific cytolysis and antitumoral efficacy that can be augmented by standard chemotherapeutic agents. *Nature Med.* **3,** 639–645.
69. Burt, R. K., Poirier, M. C., Link, C. J., and Bohr, V. A. (1991) Antineoplastic drug resistance and DNA repair. *Ann. Oncol.* **2,** 325–334.
70. Lai, G. M., Ozols, R. F., Smyth, J. F., Young, R. C., and Hamilton, T. C. (1988) Enhanced DNA repair and resistance to cisplatin in human ovarian cancer. *Biochem. Pharmacol.* **37,** 4597–4600.

70a. Moreland N. J., Illand, M., Kim, Y. T., et al. (1999) Modulation of drug resistance mediated by loss of mismatch repair by the DNA polymerase inhibitor aphidicolin. *Cancer Res.* **59,** 2102–2106.

71. Hickman, J. A. (1992) Apoptosis induced by anticancer agents. *Cancer Metastasis Rev.* **11,** 121–139.

6 DNA Adduct Tolerance and Bypass

Stephen G. Chaney and Alexandra Vaisman

CONTENTS

1. INTRODUCTION

The carrier ligands of platinum anticancer agents appear to play an important role in determining their efficacy against tumors with both intrinsic and acquired resistance to cisplatin. Unfortunately, both cisplatin and carboplatin have *cis*-diammine carrier ligands, and most cisplatin-resistant cell lines and tumors are cross-resistant to carboplatin. Thus, there has been considerable interest in the development of platinum complexes with novel carrier ligands as a means of expanding the range of tumors that will respond to platinum anticancer agents and treating tumors that have acquired resistance to cisplatin as a result of prior chemotherapy. The newer platinum complexes oxaliplatin, JM216, and ZDO473 (ZDO473 has been formerly referred to as JM473 and AMD473) each have different carrier ligands [(*trans*-R,R)1,2-diaminocyclohexane for oxaliplatin, *cis*-ammine, cyclohexylamine for JM216, and *cis*-ammine, 2-methylpyridine for ZDO473] than cisplatin and carboplatin. Each of these platinum complexes appears to offer unique advantages for chemotherapy. For example, oxaliplatin in combination with fluorouracil and folinic acid appears to have efficacy in the treatment of colon cancer, which normally responds poorly to cisplatin- and carboplatin-based chemotherapy *(1–3)*. JM216 is orally active and is effective in cell lines with decreased accumulation of cisplatin, presumably because of its lipophilicity *(4)*. ZDO473 is designed to be unreactive with glutathione and is, therefore, likely to be effective in cell lines with increased glutathione levels *(5)*. However, the driving force for the development of each of these platinum complexes is their potential use in the treat-

From: *Platinum-Based Drugs in Cancer Therapy*
Edited by: L. R. Kelland and N. Farrell © Humana Press Inc., Totowa, NJ

ment of tumors that are resistant to both cisplatin and carboplatin. Unfortunately, although all three platinum complexes offer promise for the treatment of some cisplatin-resistant tumors, other cisplatin-resistant tumors are cross-resistant to one or more of these new drugs. As these and other platinum drugs currently in development enter the clinic, it will become increasingly difficult to predict the optimal platinum-based chemotherapy for each patient. Therefore, the mechanism(s) that determine the carrier ligand specificity of resistance have received a great deal of attention in recent years.

2. CARRIER LIGAND SPECIFICITY OF TUMOR RESPONSE

2.1. Tolerance of Pt-DNA Adducts

Major mechanisms of platinum resistance include decreased accumulation, increased inactivation by glutathione, increased efflux of the platinum drug or the platinum-glutathione complex, increased nucleotide excision repair, and decreased mismatch repair *(6–8)*. Several of these mechanisms are discussed in other chapters of this book. However, a number of laboratories have shown that increased tolerance of Pt-DNA adducts (defined as an increase in the number of adducts required to inhibit cell growth) also plays an important role in resistance *(9–12)*. More importantly, increased tolerance of Pt-DNA adducts appears to play an important role in determining the carrier ligand specificity of resistance.

The carrier ligand specificity of resistance has been most thoroughly investigated with respect to platinum complexes with *cis*-diammine, ethylenediamine (en), and 1,2-diaminocyclohexane (DACH) carrier ligands. For example, the carrier ligand specificity of resistance mechanisms was first studied in mouse L1210 cell lines resistant to either cisplatin and en-Pt complexes (L1210/DDP) or to DACH-Pt complexes (L1210/DACH). These cell lines were characterized by decreased drug accumulation, increased glutathione levels, increased repair, and increased tolerance of Pt-DNA adducts *(13)*. Several laboratories have demonstrated a carrier ligand specificity for platinum drug accumulation in those cell lines *(13–15)*. However, this accounts for only 10% of the carrier ligand specificity of resistance *(13)*. No carrier ligand specificity was observed in those cell lines for inactivation of platinum complexes by glutathione *(13)*, nor was carrier ligand specificity observed for repair of total intrastrand adducts *(13)*, total interstrand crosslinks *(16)* and interstrand crosslinks in the actively transcribed *DHFR* gene *(16)*. However, an increased tolerance of Pt-DNA adducts was observed that was selective for *cis*-diammine-Pt and en-Pt adducts in the L1210/DDP cell line and for DACH-Pt adducts in the L1210/DACH cell line *(13)*. This increased tolerance of Pt-DNA adducts appeared to be the major determinant of the carrier ligand specificity of resistance in those cell lines *(13)*.

Subsequently, similar studies were performed in two pairs of sensitive and cisplatin-resistant human ovarian carcinoma cell lines (2008 and its cisplatin-resistant derivative C13* and A2780 and its cisplatin-resistant derivative A2780/DDP) and one pair of sensitive and cisplatin-resistant human colon carcinoma cell lines (HCT8 and its cisplatin-resistant derivative HCT8/DDP) *(12,17)*. No carrier ligand specificity was observed for decreased accumulation, increased efflux, inactivation by glutathione, and increased repair activity in any of the cisplatin-resistant human carcinoma cell lines *(12,17)*. However, all three cisplatin-resistant cell lines were significantly better able to tolerate *cis*-diammine-Pt adducts than DACH-Pt adducts *(12,17)*. The carrier ligand specificity of resistance mechanisms has been less extensively studied for other platinum complexes such as JM216 and ZDO473. However, in both cases a portion of their efficacy in cisplatin-resistant cell lines appears to be due to their ability to circumvent the increased tolerance of *cis*-diammine-Pt adducts in the cisplatin-resistant cells *(4,5)*.

2.2. Replicative Bypass

The most obvious mechanism for explaining increased tolerance of Pt-DNA adducts is an increase in nucleotide excision repair. However, as described above, nucleotide excision repair does not appear to discriminate between *cis*-diammine-Pt, en-Pt, and DACH-Pt adducts *(12,13,18,19)*. Therefore, one needs to consider other mechanisms that could lead to increased tolerance of unrepaired Pt-DNA adducts. Postreplication repair is an important cellular response that can lead to DNA damage tolerance. It is best defined as replication of damaged DNA without the introduction of potentially lethal secondary lesions (e.g., gaps or discontinuities in the nascent DNA) and/or repair of those secondary lesions following replication *(20–22)*.

The most frequent mechanisms for postreplication repair in mammalian cells appear to be translesion synthesis, gap filling, and template switching during replication (Fig. 1) *(21,22)*. Although recombination plays a major role in postreplication repair in bacteria, its contribution to postreplication repair in mammalian cells appears to be relatively minor *(21)*. Because the mechanisms of postreplication repair are poorly defined in mammalian cells, it may be instructive to consider what is known about postreplication repair in yeast *(20)*, especially since Hartwell et al. *(23)* have recently reported that yeast mutants with defects in postreplication repair display increased sensitivity to cisplatin. In yeast, the RAD6 epistasis group, which is responsible for postreplication repair, can be subdivided into two processes: an error-prone translesion synthesis characterized by *REV1, REV3,* and *REV7* genes and an error-free process that is thought to involve either template switching or gap filling and is characterized by the *RAD5, RAD9,* and *RAD18* genes *(20)*. In yeast the error-prone translesion synthesis appears to make a modest contribution to the tolerance of DNA damage but is responsible for much of the mutagenesis resulting from

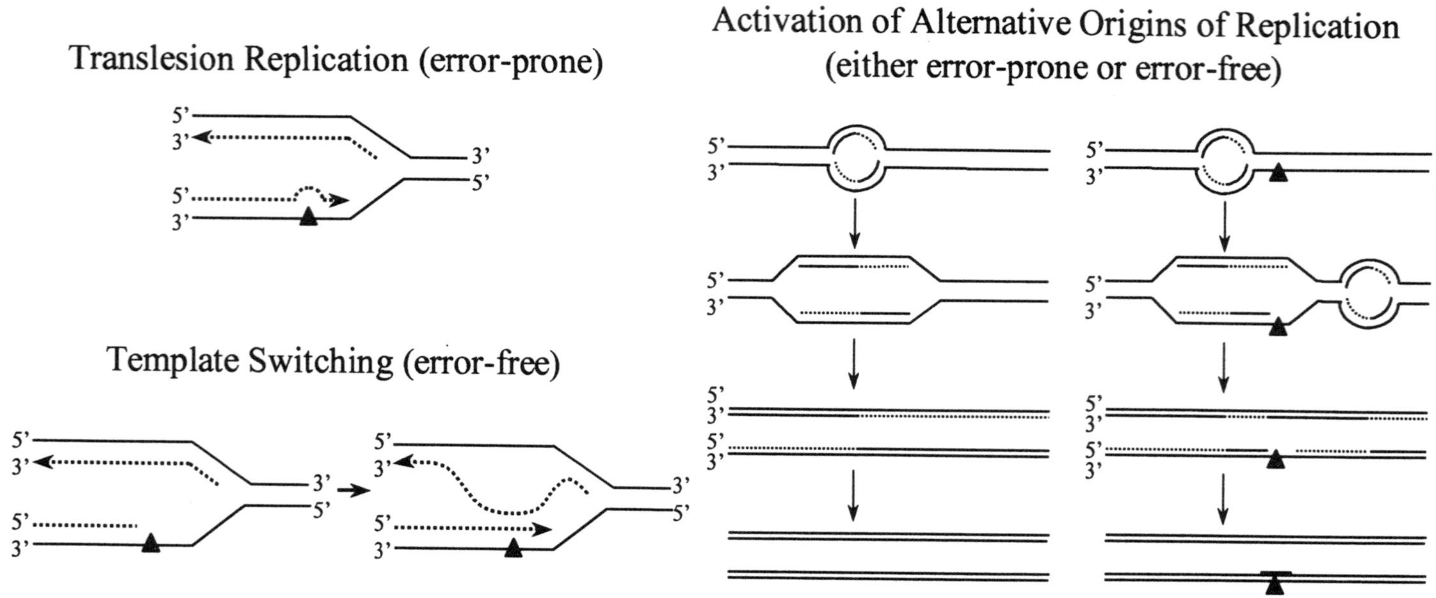

Fig. 1. Proposed mechanisms for replicative bypass (postreplication repair) in mammalian cells. Based on currently available information, The DNA polymerases involved in error-prone translesion synthesis are most likely to be pol β or pol ζ, whereas those involved in strand switching are most likely to be pol δ or pol ε. The other enzymes required for these processes are currently unidentified. The gap filling mechanism could involve either translesion synthesis (which presumably would be error prone) or strand switching (which presumably would be error free).

postreplication repair of DNA containing bulky lesions *(20)*. In contrast, the more complex error-free pathway appears to make a more significant contribution to tolerance of DNA damage and essentially no contribution to mutagenesis *(20)*. The relative contribution of these pathways to DNA damage tolerance in mammalian cells is unknown. Although these postreplication repair pathways have been characterized primarily on the basis of response to ultraviolet (UV) damage, the data of Hartwell et al. *(23)* suggest that they probably apply to platinum anticancer drugs as well.

The term postreplication repair was initially coined to describe the process in bacterial cells in which recombination following replication plays an important role. However, that terminology does not appear to describe the process accurately in mammalian cells. A great deal of what has been called postreplication repair in mammalian cells actually occurs during replication, rather than following it. In addition, this process does not actually remove the primary lesions (e.g., the Pt-DNA adducts) from the DNA, so it is not a repair pathway in the classical sense *(21)*. For that reason the terms "replicative bypass" or "bypass replication" are often used in a broad sense to describe both the error-prone and error-free pathways of postreplication repair in mammalian cells. It is in that sense that we will use the term replicative bypass in this chapter.

As discussed previously, in comparing the carrier ligand specificity of resistance mechanisms, increased tolerance of Pt-DNA adducts was the only resistance mechanism that consistently discriminated between *cis*-diammine-Pt and DACH-Pt adducts *(12,13)*. Because increased replicative bypass (postreplication repair) can lead to tolerance of adducts, the specificity of replicative bypass has been examined in several of the Pt-resistant cell lines described earlier. In the L1210 cell lines, increased replicative bypass of en-Pt adducts was observed in the L1210/DDP cell line, and increased replicative bypass of DACH-Pt adducts was observed in the L1210/DACH cell line *(24)*. In the human ovarian carcinoma cell lines, a 4.5-fold increase in bypass of *cis*-diammine-Pt adducts was observed in the C13* cell line compared with 2008, and a 2.3-fold increase in the A2780/DDP cell line compared with A2780 (Fig. 2) *(17)*. This bypass appeared to be quite specific for *cis*-diammine-Pt DNA adducts. The C13* cell line showed only a 2.1-fold increase in bypass of DACH-Pt adducts and no increase in bypass of UV or BPDE adducts compared with the 2008 line *(17)*. In a subsequent study *(25)*, the A2780/CP, A2780/CP70, and A2780/C30 cell lines have been shown to have a 2–6-fold increase in bypass of *cis*-diammine-Pt adducts compared with A2780, but no increase in bypass of DACH-Pt adducts.

These data suggest that replicative bypass is probably responsible for much of the carrier ligand specificity for tolerance of Pt-DNA adducts that had been observed in earlier studies. Although these studies have been performed in detail only for platinum complexes containing the *cis*-diammine, en, and DACH carrier ligands, it is likely that differences in replicative bypass explain a signifi-

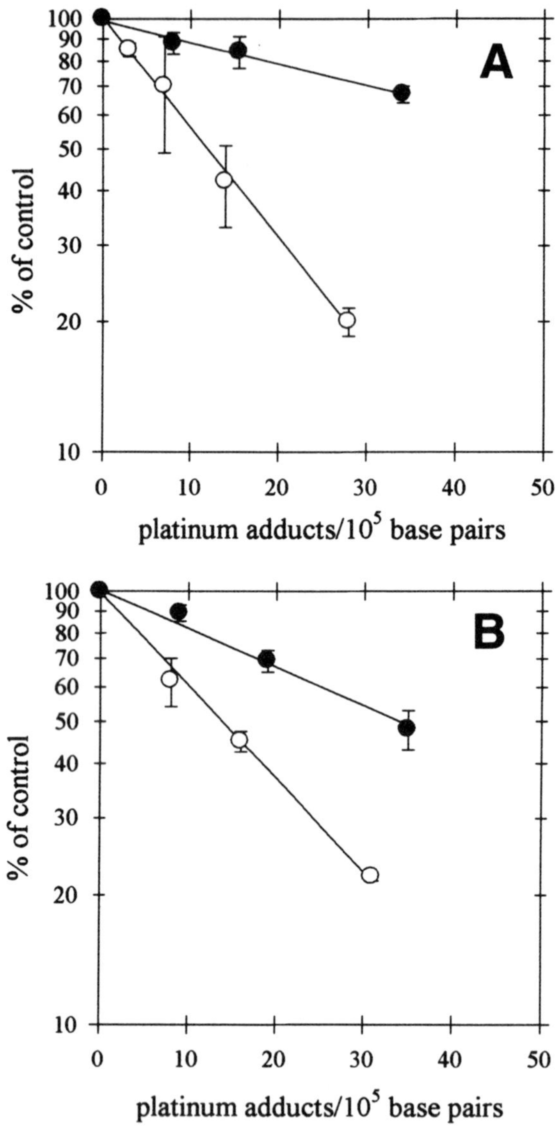

Fig. 2. Inhibition of chain elongation as a function of platinum adducts/10^5 base pairs. Inhibition was determined by sedimentation profiles from steady-state replication assays (*17*), and platinum adducts were determined by atomic absorption. Values are means ± SEM (bars) from at least three different experiments. **(A)** 2008 (○) versus C13* (•). **(B)** A2780 (○) versus A2780/DDP (•). (Reproduced with permission from ref. *17*.)

cant portion of the carrier ligand specificity of resistance for other platinum complexes as well. Thus, it is important to understand the mechanism(s) that impart specificity to the replicative bypass of Pt-DNA adducts. It is obvious that the specificity of replicative bypass could be determined by the DNA polymerases and/or auxiliary enzymes responsible for the bypass of those lesions. However, recent studies have shown that damage recognition proteins that interfere with bypass of Pt-DNA adducts may also play an important role in determining the specificity of replicative bypass. This has been demonstrated most clearly in studies showing that mismatch repair can influence net replicative bypass.

3. SPECIFICITY OF REPLICATIVE BYPASS

3.1. Mismatch Repair

As described in Chapter 8, recent studies have demonstrated that in vitro selection of human ovarian carcinoma cell lines for cisplatin resistance often results in loss of mismatch repair activity *(26,27)*. In addition, mismatch repair defects due to loss of either the hMSH2 or hMSH6 subunits of the hMutSα complex or the hMLH1 or hPMS2 subunits of the hMutL complex have been shown to result in increased cisplatin resistance in cells with no prior history of cisplatin exposure *(28,29)*. Furthermore, the hMutSα complex and the hMSH2 protein by itself bind to *cis*-diammine-Pt adducts on the DNA *(30–33)*. Since the binding to *cis*-diammine-Pt-DNA adducts does not require a sequence mismatch *(31)*, the hMutSα complex can be considered to serve as a damage recognition protein complex as well as a mismatch recognition protein complex.

This effect of mismatch repair activity is quite selective for the carrier ligand of the platinum complex. Whereas mismatch repair activity affects sensitivity to both cisplatin and carboplatin, it does not affect sensitivity to either oxaliplatin or JM216 *(26,34)*. Furthermore, one recent study suggests that mismatch repair proteins do not bind to DACH-Pt adducts *(34)*. The mechanism(s) responsible for the increased resistance to DNA-damaging agents in mismatch repair-defective cells is not known. However, it has been postulated *(35)* that futile cycles of synthesis past the DNA lesion, followed by recognition and removal of the newly synthesized strand by an active mismatch repair system, generate gaps or strand breaks that induce cell death (Fig. 3). According to this "futile cycling" model, cells could acquire resistance to drug killing through loss of mismatch repair activity, thus allowing completion of replication following bypass of the lesion. Thus, if this model were correct, loss of mismatch repair activity should be associated with increased net replicative bypass of Pt-DNA adducts, and the increased replicative bypass should display the same specificity as the mismatch repair system appears to demonstrate for the recognition of Pt-DNA adducts.

A recent study by Vaisman et al. *(25)* has confirmed these predictions of the "futile cycling" model. Three sets of mismatch repair-proficient and -deficient cell lines were evaluated with respect to the specificity of platinum resistance and replicative bypass *(25)*. The human colorectal carcinoma HCT116 cell line

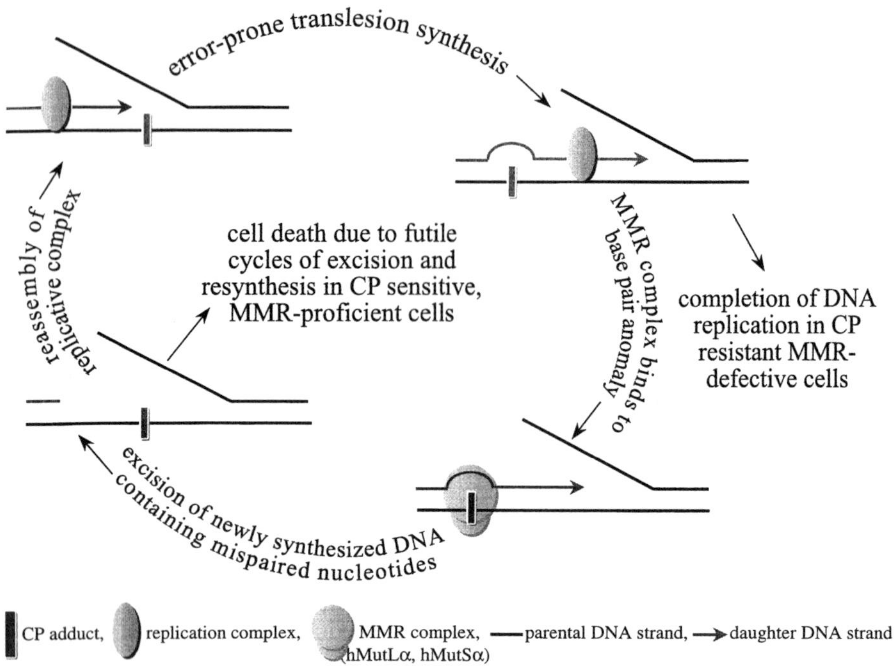

Fig. 3. Futile-cycling model for explaining the contribution of mismatch repair activity to cisplatin cytotoxicity. DNA replication past cisplatin adducts results in imperfect base pairing. This anomaly is recognized by the hMutL/hMutSα mismatch repair complex. This results in removal of the newly synthesized daughter strand while the Pt-DNA adduct in the parental strand remains intact. The continued action of these futile cycles of translesion replication and mismatch repair results in the formation of gaps or strand breaks, which leads to cell death. A defect in mismatch repair would be beneficial to the cell, because these futile cycles would be avoided. (Reproduced with permission from ref. *25*.)

has defective hMLH1 expression. The HCT116 + chr3 cell line contains a transferred chromosome 3, which restores hMLH1 expression *(36)*. The HCT116/MN2 cell line was selected from HCT116 + chr3 for MNNG resistance and has lost expression of hMLH1 from the transferred chromosome 3 *(36)*. The DLD-1 cell line has defective expression of hMSH6, which is restored by the chromosome 2 complement *(37)*. Because the effects of hMutSβ defects on platinum sensitivity had not been previously tested, one cell line with a defect in hMSH3 was also included in the study. The HHUA cell line has defective expression of both hMSH3 and hMSH6. The chromosome 2 complement of HHUA restores expression of hMSH6, and the chromosome 5 complement restores expression of hMSH3 *(38,39)*. The data obtained from these cell lines are summarized in Table 1. Defects in both hMLH1 and hMSH6 resulted in cisplatin resistance and increased net replicative bypass of *cis*-

Table 1
Effect of Mismatch Repair Status on Pt Resistance and Replicative Bypass of Pt-DNA Adducts

Cell line	Mismatch repair status	Fold resistance		Fold increase in replicative bypass	
		CP	OX	CP	OX
HCT116+chr3	WT	1.6	ns	5.5	ns
HCT116	−hMLH1				
HCT116+chr3	WT	1.5	ns	3.4	nd
HCT116/MN2	−hMLH1				
HHUA+chr5	wt/−hMSH6	ns	ns	ns	ns
HHUA	−hMSH3/−hMSH6				
HHUA+chr2	wt/−hMSH3	2.4	ns	2.0	ns
HHUA	−hMSH3/−hMSH6				
DLD-1+chr2	wt	4.8	ns	1.9	nd
DLD-1	−hMSH6				

[a]ns, no significant difference; nd, not done; CP, cisplatin; OX, oxaliplatin.

diammine-Pt adducts, but had no effect on oxaliplatin resistance or bypass of DACH-Pt adducts. In contrast, defects in hMSH3 had no effect on sensitivity to either drug and had no effect on the bypass of either adduct.

These data support the "futile cycling" model for explaining the relationship between mismatch repair activity and sensitivity to cisplatin and suggest that MutSβ may not recognize Pt-DNA adducts with the same affinity as MutSα. These data may also help explain some other recent observations concerning the biologic consequences of mismatch repair defects. For example, Nehme et al. *(40)* have reported that the activation of the JNK and c-abl signal transduction pathways by cisplatin requires an active mismatch repair system. The mechanism of this effect is not presently known. However, according to the futile cycling model, an active mismatch repair system would probably result in the formation of persistent gaps in the DNA during attempts by the cell to replicate past Pt-DNA adducts. Such gaps could serve as a signal for the activation of both the JNK and c-abl signal transduction pathways. In mismatch repair defective cell lines, the increased net replicative bypass of Pt-DNA adducts would result in the formation of fewer gaps to serve as signals for activating these and other damage-inducible pathways.

The data of Vaisman et al. *(25)* clearly demonstrate that mismatch repair imparts specificity to replicative bypass of Pt-DNA adducts. That is, cell lines with defects in the hMutSα or hMutL components of mismatch repair have increased bypass of *cis*-diammine-Pt-DNA adducts, but not of DACH-Pt-DNA adducts. However, some cisplatin-resistant cell lines are not mismatch repair defective. For example, increased replicative bypass that is selective for *cis*-diammine-Pt adducts compared with DACH-Pt adducts has been observed in the C13* human ovarian carcinoma cell line *(17)*, and the C13* line does not appear to be defective in mismatch repair *(26)*. These data suggest that mechanisms other than mismatch repair can also impart specificity to replicative bypass in cisplatin-resistant cell lines. Since mismatch repair defects are only found in 5–15% of most human tumors *(41–43)*, it is essential to understand these other mechanisms as well.

3.2. DNA Polymerases

Because of the complexity of replicative bypass, the polymerases involved in replicative bypass of Pt-DNA adducts in human cells are not known. Nelson et al. *(44)* have recently identified pol ζ, a heterodimer of the REV3 and REV7 gene products, as the polymerase responsible for error-prone translesion synthesis in yeast. Two laboratories *(45,46)* have subsequently identified a REV3 homolog in human cells. The hREV3 mRNA does not appear to be highly expressed in most of the human cancer cell lines examined to date *(46)*, but the relationship between hREV3 mRNA expression and resistance to chemotherapeutic agents has not yet been examined. However, Gibbs et al. *(45)* have shown that expression of hREV3 antisense RNA in human cells increases cytotoxicity and decreases mutagenesis in response to UV irradiation.

Hoffmann et al. *(47)* have also shown that pol β is capable of displacing a stalled pol α or pol δ at the site of a Pt-DNA adduct and performing translesion synthesis in an error-prone manner *(48)*. Thus, pol ζ and pol β must both be considered as candidates for error-prone translesion synthesis past Pt-DNA adducts.

The purified replicative enzymes pol α, pol δ, and pol ε appear to be incapable of replicating past Pt-DNA adducts in vitro *(47,49)*, even in the presence of PCNA *(47)*. However, Torres-Ramos et al. *(50)* have recently used a genetic approach to show that pol δ is likely to be involved in the error-free pathway of replicative bypass in yeast. Finally, Hoffmann et al. *(51)* have recently demonstrated efficient bypass of Pt-DNA adducts in cell extracts using a fork-like template. The enzymes involved in this bypass have not been characterized, but based on sensitivity to *N*-ethylmaleimide and p21, it was suggested that pol δ or pole ε may be involved. The mechanism of this bypass has also not yet been elucidated. However, the inability of purified pol α, pol δ, and pol ε to replicate past Pt-DNA adducts on single-stranded templates in vitro and the evidence that pol δ is involved in the error-free pathway of replicative bypass in yeast and possibly in humans suggest that the DNA polymerases involved in normal DNA replication may utilize a template switching mechanism of replicative bypass.

Since error-prone translesion synthesis may be catalyzed by pol β, we have used the primer extension assay to measure the selectivity of bypass of a single Pt-GG adduct by pol β. At high enzyme concentrations, the DACH-Pt and *cis*-diammine-Pt adducts inhibited translesion synthesis by pol β to the same extent, whereas the ammine, cyclohexylamine-Pt adduct was a much stronger block to chain elongation (Fig. 4). The diethylenetriamine (dien)-Pt monoadduct did not block chain elongation to any significant extent. However, at low enzyme concentrations the order of translesion synthesis was dien-Pt > DACH-Pt > *cis*-diammine-Pt > ammine, cyclohexylamine-Pt (Vaisman et al., *Biochemistry,* in press). Pol ζ showed the same specificity as low concentrations of pol β. Thus, under physiological conditions, pol β and pol ζ appear to discriminate between all four adducts tested.

3.3. Damage Recognition Proteins

The mismatch repair data suggest that the specificity of replicative bypass may also be determined by damage recognition proteins that bind to Pt-DNA adducts and prevent replicative bypass, either by removing the newly synthesized DNA (presumably the mechanism of the mismatch repair complex) or by directly blocking translesion synthesis. As discussed in Chapter 4, a number of cellular proteins have been shown to bind to Pt-DNA adducts with high efficiency compared with undamaged DNA *(52–63).* These proteins have been postulated to increase sensitivity to platinum compounds by blocking nucleotide excision repair of Pt-DNA adducts *(64)* may also sequester those damage recognition proteins that also function as transcription factors and preventing them from binding to their natural promoter sequences *(56,57).* However, Hoffmann et al. *(65)* have also shown that at least one platinum damage recognition protein, HMG1, is capable of blocking replication past Pt-DNA adducts in vitro.

Although HMG1 has been shown to bind to both *cis*-diammine-Pt and DACH-Pt adducts *(66)*, the relative affinity of this protein for *cis*-diammine-Pt, DACH-Pt, and ammine, cyclohexylamine-Pt adducts is not known at present. However, there are theoretical reasons to believe that HMG1 and other HMG-domain damage recognition proteins may bind to at least some these adducts with different affinities. Part of the interaction of HMG-domain proteins with their target DNA involves an insertion of a portion of their *N*-terminal amino acid chain into the minor groove of DNA, which is bent in the direction of the major groove *(67,68).* Both *cis*-diammine-Pt and DACH-Pt adducts appear to bend the DNA in the direction of the major groove *(69).* However, molecular

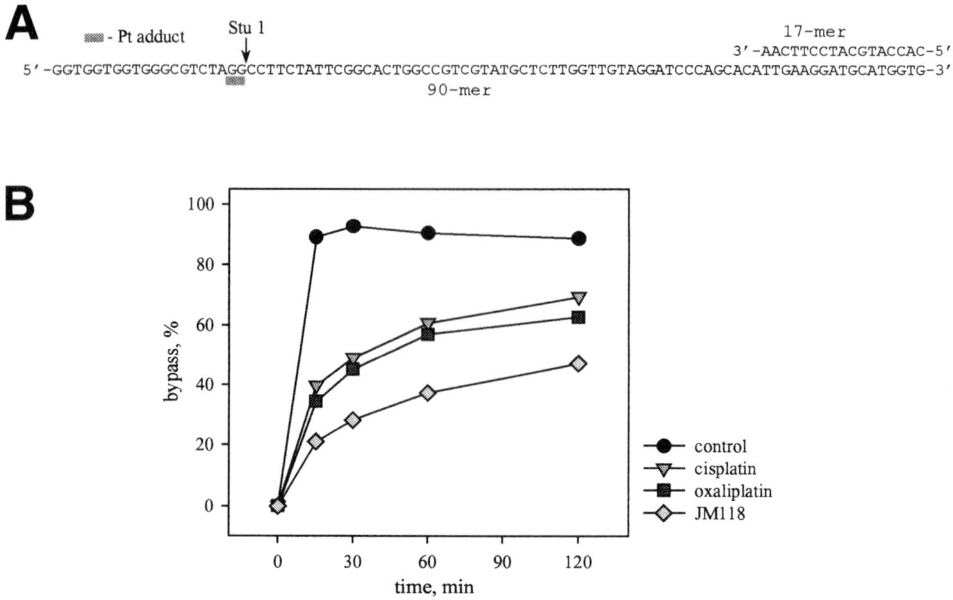

Fig. 4. Replicative bypass of platinum-DNA adducts by high concentrations of pol β. **(A)** The template with a site-specific platinum adduct used in the primer extension assay. **(B)** Quantitative analysis of the time-course experiments for bypass of *cis*-diammine-Pt, DACH-Pt, ammine, cyclohexylamine-Pt, and dien-Pt adducts by pol β. The amount of bypass was calculated as a percentage of total elongated product.

modeling data *(70)* suggest that DACH-Pt adducts alter the conformation of the DNA in such a manner as to create a wider and shallower minor groove than *cis*-diammine-Pt adducts. These data suggest that Pt-DNA adducts with bulky carrier ligands may distort the DNA to a different extent than Pt-DNA adducts with *cis*-diammine carrier ligands and that these differences in distortion could affect the recognition sites for platinum damage recognition proteins such as HMG1.

Vaisman et al. (*Biochemistry,* in press) have evaluated the ability of HMG1 to inhibit replicative bypass of *cis*-diammine-Pt, DACH-Pt, and ammine, cyclohexylamine-Pt adducts by HIV reverse transcriptase. A forked DNA template very similar to one described by Hoffmann et al. *(51)* was used because it contains the Pt-DNA adduct in a double-stranded region of DNA and thus provides a high-affinity binding site for HMG1. HIV reverse transcriptase was used because it efficiently bypasses Pt-DNA adducts on a forked DNA template in vitro (40% bypass of *cis*-diammine-Pt adducts in 2 h at 37° C). In this assay HMG1 was clearly more effective at inhibiting translesion synthesis past *cis*-diammine-Pt adducts than either DACH-Pt adducts or ammine, cyclohexylamine-Pt adducts (Fig. 5). HMG1 did not inhibit replication past dien-Pt

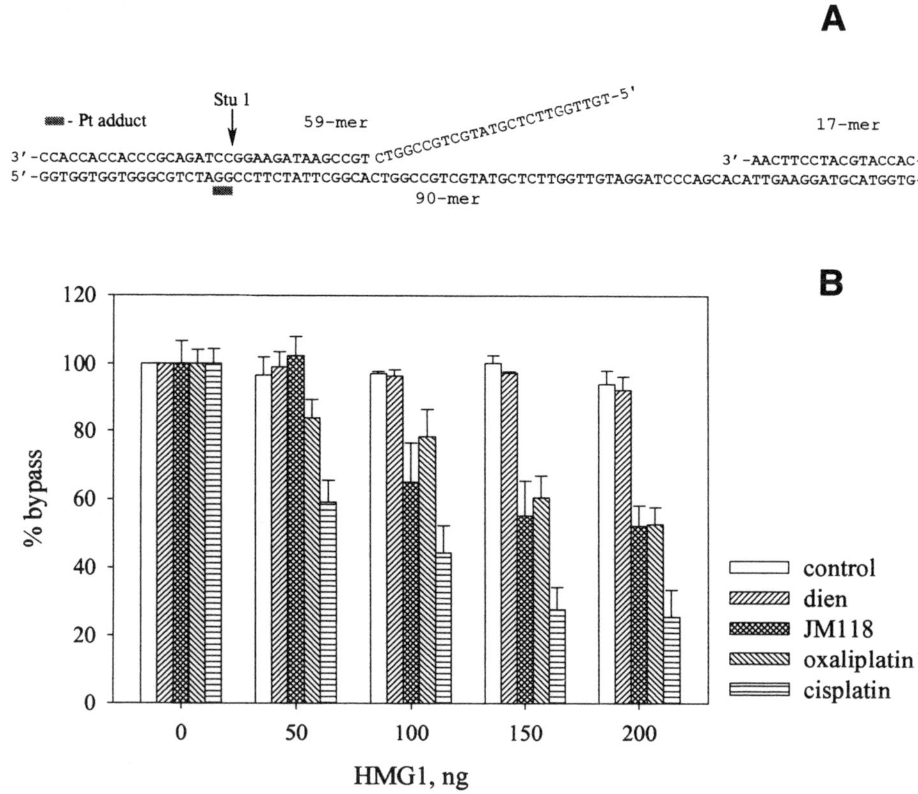

Fig. 5. Effect of HMG1 protein on replicative bypass of platinum-DNA adducts by HIV-1 RT. **(A)** The forked template with a site-specific platinum adduct used in the replication assay. **(B)** Quantitative analysis of the inhibition of the replicative bypass of platinum-DNA adducts by HMG1 protein. In vitro primer extension by HIV-1 RT was performed for 2 h following 40 min of incubation of the template with increasing amounts of HMG1 protein. The frequency of translesion synthesis was calculated as a percent of full-length DNA replicative product on platinated DNA compared with total elongated product. Replication on each template in the absence of HMG1 was assigned to 100%. (Reproduced from Vaisman et al., *Biochemistry*, in press.)

monoadducts to a greater extent than for control (unplatinated) DNA. These data suggest that HMG1 can discriminate between Pt-DNA adducts with different carrier ligands and that this discrimination results in different degrees of inhibition of translesion synthesis past the corresponding Pt-DNA adducts. The mechanism of this effect has not been determined, but it is likely that binding of platinum damage recognition proteins to Pt-DNA adducts on double-stranded DNA acts as a physical barrier to DNA chain elongation. If so, these data suggest a potential mechanism for imparting specificity to both the error-prone translesion synthesis and the error-free strand switching mechanism.

HMG1 itself is a ubiquitous protein and is not likely to be involved in platinum resistance. However, the ability of HMG1 to impart specificity to the replicative bypass of Pt-DNA adducts is unlikely to be unique, since most of the HMG domain proteins appear to interact with Pt-DNA adducts in a similar manner as HMG1. Thus, it is likely that other HMG domain proteins will also prove to be capable of imparting specificity to replicative bypass of Pt-DNA adducts. Furthermore, it is possible that the specificity of other HMG domain proteins for binding to Pt-DNA adducts may be different from that of HMG1. For example, the binding of the HMG domain transcription factors SRY and LEF-1 to their natural promoter sequences has been characterized by nuclear magnetic resonance (NMR) and molecular modeling studies *(67,68)*. In both cases the DNA was bent in the direction of the major groove. However, the width of the minor groove at the site of SRY binding was 9.4 Å, whereas the width of the minor groove at the site of LEF-1 binding was 11 Å. Since the width of the minor groove appears to be different for *cis*-diammine-Pt and DACH-Pt adducts *(70)*, it is possible that these and other HMG domain proteins may differ in their selectivity for Pt-DNA adducts with *cis*-diammine and DACH carrier ligands. Further studies will be needed to determine the ability of the HMG domain proteins and other platinum damage recognition proteins to discriminate between platinum adducts with different carrier ligands and to determine the biologic consequences of the interaction of these proteins with adducts on the DNA. The relationship between platinum damage recognition proteins and the response to platinum-based chemotherapy is discussed in more detail in Chapter 4. However, it should be mentioned that because SRY and some of the other HMG domain proteins display tissue-specific expression, they could be involved in the intrinsic differences in the response of different tumor types to platinum-based chemotherapy.

In addition to the HMG domain proteins, there are a number of other damage recognition proteins that bind with high specificity to Pt-DNA adducts. The conformation of the complex formed by the basal transcription factor TFIID/TBP with its promoter sequence is similar to that of the HMG domain transcription factors *(63)*. However, the TFIID/TBP complex does not appear to discriminate between *cis*-diammine-Pt and DACH-Pt adducts *(71)*. Other platinum damage recognition proteins include RPA *(59,72)*, XPA *(60)*, histone H1 *(61)*, and human KU autoantigen *(62)*. The nature and specificity of their interactions with Pt-DNA adducts are poorly characterized at present. Thus, this appears to be a fertile area for future investigation.

4. CONCLUSIONS

As newer platinum complexes such as oxaliplatin, JM216, and ZDO473 enter the clinic, it will become increasingly important to understand the mechanism(s) that lead to the carrier ligand specificity of tumor response to platinum anticancer agents and to develop assays capable of predicting which of these platinum drugs is most likely to be effective in the treatment of individual patients. Replicative bypass (postreplication repair) appears to be one mechanism of platinum resistance that is strongly dependent on the nature of the carrier ligand. Furthermore, the mechanism(s) that imparts this carrier ligand specificity to replicative bypass are becoming clearer. DNA polymerases such as pol β or pol ζ may be responsible for some of the carrier ligand specificity of error-prone translesion synthesis. In addition, platinum damage recognition proteins such as HMG1 appear to be capable of imparting specificity to both error-prone translesion synthesis and error-free replicative bypass. These mechanisms should apply to both mismatch repair-proficient and -deficient tumors. Finally, the mismatch repair complex appears to represent an unique mechanism. The mismatch repair complex can be thought of as a platinum damage recognition complex, but its interaction with the Pt-DNA adduct probably results in removal of the newly synthesized strand rather than simply forming a physical block to chain elongation. The relative contributions of these three mechanisms to the carrier ligand specificity of replicative bypass in vivo are unknown at present. However, based on current knowledge, it appears likely that the extent and carrier ligand specificity of replicative bypass may be closely associated with some of the other platinum resistance mechanisms (e.g., mismatch repair and platinum damage recognition proteins) discussed elsewhere in this book.

As platinum-based chemotherapy enters its second 25 years and beyond, one important challenge will be to improve further our understanding of the carrier ligand specificity of tumor response and to translate that information effectively into the clinic. Ideally, as our understanding of the mechanisms responsible for the carrier ligand specificity of the response to platinum drugs improves, it should be possible to identify prognostic indicators capable of predicting differential tumor response to cisplatin/carboplatin, oxaliplatin, JM216, ZDO473, and future platinum complexes. Some of the information obtained by these and related studies is already being evaluated clinically. For example, mismatch repair status is currently being evaluated as an independent prognostic indicator for response to platinum-based chemotherapy. The data from our and other laboratories suggest that defects in mismatch repair may predict better response for oxaliplatin and JM216 than for cisplatin and carboplatin. The identification of other markers for predicting the carrier ligand specificity of drug response probably lies further in the future. However, in the near term this remains an exciting and potentially significant area of research.

ACKNOWLEDGMENTS

The authors would like to acknowledge the financial support of Sanofi Pharmaceuticals and the National Institutes of Health (USPHS grant CA34082) for their research. The authors would also like to thank Dr. John Risinger, Dr. J.

Carl Barrett, Dr. Asad Umar, and Dr. Tom Kunkel of the National Institute of Environmental Health Sciences for the mismatch repair defective and chromosome complemented cell lines used in their studies; Dr. Sam Wilson of the National Institute of Environmental Health Sciences for the DNA polymerase β used in their studies; Dr. David Hinkle of the Department of Biology, University of Rochester, and Dr. John Turchi of the Department of Biochemistry and Molecular Biology, Wright State University for the HMG1 used in their studies. Finally, the authors would like to thank Dr. Marila Cordeiro-Stone, Dr. Tom Kunkel, and Dr. William Kaufmann for scholarly discussions and advice.

REFERENCES

1. Gerard, B., Bleiberg, H., Vandaele, D., Gil, T., Hendlisz, A., Dileo, A., et al. (1998) Oxaliplatin combined to 5-fluorouracil and folinic acid—An effective therapy in patients with advanced colorectal cancer. *Anti-Cancer Drugs* **9,** 301–305.
2. Becouarn, Y. and Rougier, P. (1998) Clinical efficacy of oxaliplatin monotherapy—Phase II trials in advanced colorectal cancer. *Semin. Onco.* **25,** 23–31.
3. Bleiberg, H. (1998) Oxaliplatin (l-OHP)—a new reality in colorectal cancer. *Br. J. Cancer* **77,** 1–3.
4. Kelland, L. R., Abel, G., McKeage, M. J., Jones, M., Goddard, P. M., Valenti, M., et al. (1993) Preclinical antitumor evaluation of bis-acetato-ammine-dichloro-cyclohexylamine platinum(IV)—an orally active platinum drug. *Cancer Res.* **53,** 2581–2586.
5. Holford, J., Sharp, S. Y., Murrer, B. A., Abrams, M., and Kelland, L. R. (1998) *In vitro* circumvention of cisplatin resistance by the novel sterically hindered platinum complex AMD473. *Br. J. Cancer* **77,** 366–373.
6. Eastman, A. and Richon, V. M. (1986) Mechanisms of cellular resistance to platinum coordination complexes, in *Biochemical Mechanisms of Platinum Anticancer Drugs* (McBrien, D.C.H. and Slater, T.F., eds.), IRL, Oxford, pp. 91–119.
7. Johnson, S. W., Ozols, R. F., and Hamilton, T. C. (1993) Mechanisms of drug resistance in ovarian cancer. *Cancer* **71**, 644–649.
8. Hill, B. T. (1996) Drug resistance: an overview of the current state of the art. *Int. J. Oncol.* **9,** 197–203.
9. Lanzi, C., Perego, P., Supino, R., Romanelli, S., Pensa, T., Carenini, N., et al. (1998) Decreased drug accumulation and increased tolerance to DNA damage in tumor cells with a low level of cisplatin resistance. *Biochem. Pharmacol.* **55,** 1247–1254.
10. Johnson, S. W., Shen, D. W., Pastan, I., Gottesman, M. M., and Hamilton, T. C. (1996) Cross-resistance, cisplatin accumulation, and platinum-DNA adduct formation and removal in cisplatin-sensitive and—resistant human hepatoma cell lines. *Exp. Cell Res.* **226,** 133–139.
11. Shellard, S. A., Fichtinger-Schepman, A. M.J., Lazo, J. S., and Hill, B. T. (1993) Evidence of differential cisplatin DNA adduct formation, removal and tolerance of DNA damage in three human lung carcinoma cell lines. *Anti-Cancer Drugs* **4,** 491–500.
12. Schmidt, W. and Chaney, S. G. (1993) Role of carrier ligand in platinum resistance of human carcinoma cell lines. *Cancer Res.* **53,** 799–805.
13. Gibbons, G. R., Page, J. D., Mauldin, S. K., Husain, I., and Chaney, S. G. (1990) Role of carrier ligand in platinum resistance in L1210 cells. *Cancer Res.* **50,** 6497–6501.
14. Kraker, A. J. and Moore, C. W. (1988) Accumulation of cis-diamminedichloroplatinum(II) and platinum analogs by platinum-resistant murine leukemia cells in vitro. *Cancer Res.* **48,** 9–13.
15. Richon, V. M., Schulte, N., and Eastman, A. (1987) Multiple mechanisms of resistance to cis-diamminedichloroplatinum(II) in murine leukemia L1210 cells. *Cancer Res.* **47,** 2056–2061.

16. Petersen, L. N., Mamenta, E. L., Stevsner, T., Chaney, S. G., and Bohr, V. A. (1996) Increased gene specific repair of cisplatin induced interstrand crosslinks in cisplatin resistant cell lines, and studies on carrier ligand specificity. *Carcinogenesis* **17,** 2597–2602.
17. Mamenta, E. L., Poma, E. E., Kaufmann, W. K., Delmastro, D. A., Grady, H. L., and Chaney, S. G. (1994) Enhanced replicative bypass of platinum-DNA adducts in cisplatin-resistant human ovarian carcinoma cell lines. *Cancer Res.* **54,** 3500–3505.
18. Jennerwein, M. M., Eastman, A., and Khokhar, A. R. (1991) The role of DNA repair in the resistance of L1210 cells to isomeric 1,2-diaminocyclohexaneplatinum complexes and ultraviolet irradiation. *Mutat. Res.* **254,** 89–96.
19. Page, J. D., Husain, I., Sancar, A., and Chaney, S. G. (1990) Effect of the diaminocyclohexane carrier ligand on platinum adduct formation, repair, and lethality. *Biochemistry* **29,** 1016–1024.
20. Lawrence, C. (1994) The Rad6 DNA repair pathway in *Saccharomyces cerevisiae*—what does it do, and how does it do it. *Bioessays* **16,** 253–258.
21. Naegeli, H. (1994) Roadblocks and detours during DNA replication: mechanisms of mutagenesis in mammalian cells. *Bioessays* **16,** 557–564.
22. Kaufmann, W. K. (1989) Pathways of human cell post-replication repair. *Carcinogenesis* **10,** 1–11.
23. Hartwell, L. H., Szankasi, P., Roberts, C. J., Murray, A. W., and Friend, S. H. (1997) Integrating genetic approaches into the discovery of anticancer drugs. *Science* **278,** 1064–1068.
24. Gibbons, G. R., Kaufmann, W. K., and Chaney, S. G. (1991) Role of DNA replication in carrier-ligand-specific resistance to platinum compounds in L1210 cells. *Carcinogenesis* **12,** 2253–2257.
25. Vaisman, A., Varchenko, M., Umar, A., Kunkel, T. A., Risinger, J. I., Barrett, J. C., et al. (1998) The role of hMLH1, hMSH3, and hMSH6 defects in cisplatin and oxaliplatin resistance: correlation with replicative bypass of platinum-DNA adducts. *Cancer Res.* **58,** *3579–3585.*
26. Aebi, S., Kurdi-Haidar, B., Gordon, R., Cenni, B., Zheng, H., Fink, D., et al. (1996) Loss of DNA mismatch repair in acquired resistance to cisplatin. *Cancer Res.* **56,** 3087–3090.
27. Drummond, J. T., Anthoney, A., Brown, R., and Modrich, P. (1996) Cisplatin and Adriamycin resistance are associated with MutL alpha and mismatch repair deficiency in an ovarian tumor cell line. *J. Biol. Chem.* **271,** 19645–19648.
28. Fink, D., Zheng, H., Nebel, S., Norris, P. S., Aebi, S., Lin, T.-P., et al. (1997) *In vitro* and *in vivo* resistance to cisplatin in cells that have lost DNA mismatch repair. *Cancer Res.* **57,** 1841–1845.
29. Fink, D., Nebel, S., Aebi, S., Nehme, A., and Howell, S. B. (1997) Loss of DNA mismatch repair due to knockout of MSH2 or PMS2 results in resistance to cisplatin and carboplatin. *Int. J. Oncol.* **11,** 539–542.
30. Duckett, D. R., Drummond, J. T., Murchie, A. I.H., Reardon, J. T., Sancar, A., Lilley, D. M., et al. (1996) Human MutS alpha recognizes damaged DNA base pairs containing O- 6-methylguanine, O-4-methylthymine, or the cisplatin-d(GpG) adduct. *Proc. Natl. Acad. Sci. USA* **93,** *6443–6447.*
31. Mu, D., Tursun, M., Duckett, D. R., Drummond, J. T., Modrich, P., and Sancar, A. (1997) Recognition and repair of compound DNA lesions (base damage and mismatch) by human mismatch repair and excision repair systems. *Mol. Cell. Biol.* **17,** 760–769.
32. Yamada, M., Oregan, E., Brown, R., and Karran, P. (1997) Selective recognition of a cisplatin-DNA adduct by human mismatch repair proteins. *Nucleic Acids. Res.* **25,** 491–495.
33. Mello, J. A., Acharya, S., Fishel, R., and Essigmann, J. M. (1996) The mismatch-repair protein hMSH2 binds selectively to DNA adducts of the anticancer drug cisplatin. *Chem. Biol.* **3,** 579–589.
34. Fink, D., Nebel, S., Aebi, S., Zheng, H., Cenni, B., Nehme, A., Christen, R. D., and Howell, S. B. (1996) The role of mismatch repair in platinum drug resistance. *Cancer Res.* **56,** 4881–4886.

35. Goldmacher, V. S., Cuzick, R. A., and Thilly, W. G. (1986) Isolation and partial characterization of human cell mutants differing in sensitivity to killing and mutation by methylnitrosourea and N-methyl-N-nitrosoguanidine. *J. Biol. Chem.* **261,** 12462–12471.
36. Hawn, M. T., Umar, A., Carethers, J. M., Marra, G., Kunkel, T. A., Boland, C. R., and Koi, M. (1995) Evidence for a connection between the mismatch repair system and the G(2) cell cycle checkpoint. *Cancer Res.* **55,** 3721–3725.
37. Umar, A., Koi, M., Risinger, J. I., Glaab, W. E., Tindall, K. R., Kolodner, R. D., et al. (1997) Correction of hypermutability, N-methyl-N'-nitro-N- nitrosoguanidine resistance, and defective DNA mismatch repair by introducing chromosome 2 into human tumor cells with mutations in MSH2 and MSH6. *Cancer Res.* **57,** 3949–3955.
38. Risinger, J. I., Umar, A., Boyd, J., Berchuk, A., Kunkel, T. A., and Barrett, J. C. (1996) Mutation of MSH3 in endometrial cancer and evidence for its functional role in heteroduplex repair. *Nature Genet.* **14,** 102–105.
39. Umar, A., Risinger, J. I., Glaab, W. E., Tindall, K. R., Barrett, J. C., and Kunkel, T. A. (1998) Functional overlap in mismatch repair by human MSH3 and MSH6. *Genetics* **148,** 1637–1646.
40. Nehme, A., Baskaran, R., Aebi, S., Fink, D., Nebel, S., Cenni, B., et al. (1997) Differential induction of c-Jun NH2-terminal kinase and c-Abl kinase in DNA mismatch repair-proficient and deficient cells exposed to cisplatin. *Cancer Res.* **57,** 3253–3257.
41. King, B. L., Carcangiu, M. L., Carter, D., Kiechle, M., Pfisterer, J., and Kacinski, B. M. (1995) Microsatellite instability in ovarian neoplasms. *Br. J. Cancer* **72,** 376–382.
42. Kolodner, R. D. (1995) Mismatch repair: mechanisms and relationship to cancer susceptibility. *Trends Biochem. Sci.* **20,** 397–401.
43. Fujita, M., Enomoto, T., Yoshino, K., Nomura, T., Buzard, G. S., Inoue, M., et al. (1995) Microsatellite instability and alterations in the hMSH2 gene in human ovarian cancer. *Int. J. Cancer* **64,** 361–366.
44. Nelson, J. R., Lawrence, C. W., and Hinkle, D. C. (1996) Thymine-thymine dimer bypass by yeast DNA polymerase zeta. *Science* **272,** 1646–1649.
45. Gibbs, P. E.M., McGregor, W. G., Maher, V. M., Nisson, P., and Lawrence, C. W. (1998) A human homolog of the *Saccharomyces cerevisiae* REV3 gene, which encodes the catalytic subunit of DNA polymerase zeta. *Proc. Natl. Acad. Sci. USA* **95,** 6876–6880.
46. Xiao, W., Lechler, T., Chow, B. L., Fontanie, T., Agustus, M., Carter, K. C., et al. (1998) Identification, chromosomal mapping and tissue-specific expression of hREV3 encoding a putative human DNA polymerase-zeta. *Carcinogenesis* **19,** 945–949.
47. Hoffmann, J.-S., Pillaire, M.-J., Maga, G., Podust, V., Hubscher, U., and Villani, G. (1995) DNA polymerase beta bypasses in vitro a single d(GpG)-cisplatin adduct placed on codon 13 of the HRAS gene. *Proc. Natl. Acad. Sci. USA* **92,** 5356–5360.
48. Hoffmann, J. S., Pillaire, M. J., Garcia-Estefania, D., Lapalu, S., and Villani, G. (1996) *In vitro* bypass replication of the cisplatin-d(GpG) lesion by calf thymus DNA polymerase beta and human immunodeficiency virus type I reverse transcriptase is highly mutagenic. *J. Biol. Chem.* **271,** 15386–15392.
49. Huang, L., Turchi, J. J., Wahl, A. F., and Bambara, R. A. (1993) Effects of the anticancer drug cis-diamminedichloroplatinum(II) on the activities of calf thymus DNA polymerase epsilon. *Biochemistry* **32,** 841–848.
50. Torres-Ramos, C. A., Prakash, S., and Prakash, L. (1997) Requirement of yeast DNA polymerase delta in post-replicational repair of UV-damaged DNA. *J. Biol. Chem.* **272,** 25445–25448.
51. Hoffmann, J. S., Pillaire, M. J., Lesca, C., Burnouf, D., Fuchs, R. P. P., Defais, M., et al. (1996) Fork-like DNA templates support bypass replication of lesions that block DNA synthesis on single-stranded templates. *Proc. Natl. Acad. Sci. USA* **93,** 13766–13769.
52. Hughes, E. N., Engelsberg, B. N., and Billings, P. C. (1992) Purification of nuclear proteins

that bind to cisplatin-damaged DNA—identity with high mobility group protein-1 and protein-2. *J. Biol Chem.* **267,** 13520–13527.

53. Bruhn, S. L., Pil, P. M., Essigmann, J. M., Housman, D. E., and Lippard, S. J. (1992) Isolation and characterization of human cDNA clones encoding a high mobility group box protein that recognizes structural distortions to DNA caused by binding of the anticancer agent cisplatin. *Proc. Natl. Acad. Sci. USA* **89,** 2307–2311.
54. Pil, P. M. and Lippard, S. J. (1992) Specific binding of chromosomal protein HMG1 to DNA damaged by the anticancer drug cisplatin. *Science* **256,** 234–237.
55. Ohndorf, U. M., Whitehead, J. P., Raju, N. L., and Lippard, S. J. (1997) Binding of tsHMG, a mouse testis-specific HMG-domain protein, to cisplatin-DNA adducts. *Biochemistry* **36,** 14807–14815.
56. Treiber, D. K., Zhai, X. Q., Jantzen, H. M., and Essigmann, J. M. (1994) Cisplatin-DNA adducts are molecular decoys for the ribosomal RNA transcription factor hUBF (human upstream binding factor). *Proc. Natl. Acad. Sci. USA* **91,** 5672–5676.
57. Trimmer, E. E., Zamble, D. B., Lippard, S. J., and Essigmann, J. M. (1998) Human testis-determining factor SRY binds to the major DNA adduct of cisplatin and a putative target sequence with comparable affinities. *Biochemistry* **37,** 352–362.
58. Turchi, J. J., Li, M., and Henkels, K. M. (1996) Cisplatin-DNA binding specificity of calf high-mobility group 1 protein. *Biochemistry* **35,** 2992–3000.
59. Clugston, C. K., M. L.ughlin, K., Kenny, M. K., and Brown, R. (1992) Binding of human single-stranded DNA binding protein to DNA damaged by the anticancer drug cis-diamminedichloroplatinum (II). *Cancer Res.* **52,** 6375–6379.
60. Asahina, H., Kuraoka, I., Shirakawa, M., Morita, E. H., Miura, N., Miyamoto, I., et al. (1994) The XPA protein is a zinc metalloprotein with an ability to recognize various kinds of DNA damage. *Mutat. Res. DNA Repair* **315,** 229–237.
61. Yaneva, J., Leuba, S. H., Van Holde, K., and Zlatanova, J. (1997) The major chromatin protein histone H1 binds preferentially to cis-platinum-damaged DNA. *Proc. Natl. Acad. Sci. USA* **94,** 13448–13451.
62. Turchi, J. J. and Henkels, K. (1996) Human Ku autoantigen binds cisplatin-damaged DNA but fails to stimulate human DNA-activated protein kinase. *J. Biol. Chem.* **271,** 13861–13867.
63. Vichi, P., Coin, F., Renaud, J. P., Vermeulen, W., Hoeijmakers, J. H.J., Moras, D., et al (1997) Cisplatin- and UV-damaged DNA lure the basal transcription factor TFIID/TBP. *EMBO J* **16,** 7444–7456.
64. Huang, J. C., Zamble, D. B., Reardon, J. T., Lippard, S. J., and Sancar, A. (1994) HMG-domain proteins specifically inhibit the repair of the major DNA adduct of the anticancer drug cisplatin by human excision nuclease. *Proc. Natl. Acad. Sci. USA* **91,** 10394–10398.
65. Hoffmann, J. S., Locker, D., Viliani, G., and Leng, M.(1997) HMG1 protein inhibits the translesion synthesis of the major DNA cisplatin adduct by cell extracts. *J. Mol. Biol.* **270,** 539–543.
66. Donahue, B. A., Augot, M., Bellon, S. F., Treiber, D. K., Tonry, J. H., Lippard, S. J., et al. (1990) Characterization of a DNA damage-recognition protein from mammalian cells that binds specifically to intrastrand d(GpG) and d(ApG) DNA adducts of the anticancer drug cisplatin. *Biochemistry* **29,** 5872–5880.
67. Love, J. J., Li, X., Case, D. A., Giese, K., Grosschedl, R., and Wright, P. E. (1995) Structural basis for DNA bending by the architectural transcription factor LEF-1. *Nature* **376,** 791–795.
68. Werner, M. H., Huth, J. R., Gronenborn, A. M., and Clore, G. M. (1995) Molecular basis of human 46X,Y sex reversal revealed from the three-dimensional solution structure of the human SRY-DNA complex. *Cell* **81,** 705–714.
69. Takahara, P. M., Frederick, C. A., and Lippard, S. J. (1996) Crystal structure of the anticancer drug cisplatin bound to duplex DNA. *J. Am. Chem. Soc.* **118,** 12309–12321.

70. Scheeff, E. D., and Howell, S. B. (1998) Computer modeling of the primary cisplatin and oxaliplatin DNA adducts and relevance to mismatch repair recognition. *Proc. Am. Assoc. Cancer Res.* **39,** 158.
71. Coin, F., Frit, P., Viollet, B., Salles, B., and Egly, J. M. (1998) TATA binding protein discriminates between different lesions on DNA, resulting in a transcription decrease. *Mol. Cell. Biol.* **18,** 3907–3914.
72. Patrick, S. M. and Turchi, J. J. (1998) Human replication protein A preferentially binds cisplatin-damaged duplex DNA *in vitro*. *Biochemistry* **37,** 8808–8815.

7 How Does Cisplatin Kill Cells?

Daniel Fink and Stephen B. Howell

CONTENTS

1. INTRODUCTION

Cisplatin is widely used as a chemotherapeutic agent. The molecular details of how it causes cells to die are largely unknown, but it is clear that its effectiveness varies quite markedly in different tumor types. Some tumors such as seminoma are highly sensitive, whereas others, such as pancreatic carcinoma, are nearly completely resistant to tolerated doses. A variety of other tumor types, of which ovarian cancer serves as a good example, are typically responsive initially but acquire resistance during the course of therapy. Some insight into the mechanisms by which cisplatin kills cells has been obtained through the identification of factors that control sensitivity to this drug and its close analog carboplatin. Five biochemical alterations have been identified that can cause cisplatin resistance in specific model systems. These include: (1) decreased cellular accumulation of cisplatin; (2) increased levels of glutathione or of glutathione-S-transferase activity; (3) increased levels of intracellular metallothioneins; (4) enhanced DNA repair; and (5) loss of DNA mismatch repair (MMR) activity *(1–5)*. However, it is likely that several of these mechanisms operate together in most resistant cells, and at present the dominant mechanism accounting for either *de novo* or clinically acquired resistance is unknown. It is not even clear that there is a single dominant mechanism even within a single tumor type.

From: *Platinum-Based Drugs in Cancer Therapy*
Edited by: L. R. Kelland and N. Farrell © Humana Press Inc., Totowa, NJ

Novel insights into the mechanisms by which cisplatin kills cells have recently been obtained through advances in the field of cell biology. Elucidation of the steps involved in the apoptotic cell death pathway, and identification of the signal transduction pathways activated during the cellular injury response, have made it possible to sketch a crude diagram of some components of the cellular machinery that must be involved. In addition, the observation that loss of MMR causes cells to become resistant to cisplatin and carboplatin has provided molecular information on at least one pathway involved in the cytotoxic response that will probably prove prototypic of other mechanisms. This chapter will review recent discoveries that have advanced understanding of how cisplatin kills cells, with particular emphasis on the contributions made by studies of the role of MMR in regulating cisplatin sensitivity.

2. CELLULAR PHARMACOLOGY

Cisplatin in its dichloro form is relatively stable and unreactive in high chloride environments such as blood plasma in which the chloride concentration is >100 m*M*. The dichloro form enters cells by mechanisms that probably include both mediated and passive diffusion components *(6)*. In the cytoplasm, the relatively low chloride concentration of approximately 4 m*M* favors displacement of the chlorides by aquation, yielding a highly reactive species whose ionic charge may retard exit from the cell. This reactive electrophile can bind covalently to a variety of thiols and macromolecules. DNA appears to be the most important, although not the exclusive *(7)*, target of cisplatin. For example, the initial studies of Rosenberg et al. *(8,9)* showed that cisplatin induced filamentous growth in *Escherichia coli* while inhibiting cell division, suggesting that cisplatin interferes with DNA replication without affecting normal RNA and protein synthesis. Further evidence for the preeminence of DNA as the most important cellular target for cisplatin comes from the observation that mutations in many of the genes whose products participate in the nucleotide excision repair mechanism cause dramatic degrees of hypersensitivity *(10)*. Pharmacologic inhibition of nucleotide excision repair with fludarabine also increases sensitivity to cisplatin *(11)*.

Cisplatin can form adducts with all DNA bases, but in intact DNA there is preferential binding to the N^7 positions of guanine and adenine *(12)*. This may be due to the high nucleophilicity of the imidazole ring, particularly at the N^7 position *(13)*. The predominant lesions produced by cisplatin and carboplatin DNA are the G-G, A-G, and G-X-G intrastrand crosslinks, and these account for approximately 60, 15, and 20% of the total platinum-DNA adducts, respectively *(14)*. These 1,2-intrastrand adducts produce a local kinking and unwinding of duplex DNA, and this is thought to contribute importantly to the cytotoxic effect of cisplatin based on the observation that the *trans* isomer *trans*-diamminedichloroplatinum(II), which cannot form 1,2-intrastrand adducts, exhibits little antitumor activity. The other, less frequently observed platinum-DNA adducts include monoadducts and G-G interstrand crosslinks. The interstrand crosslink, which constitutes less than 5% of the total platinum-DNA adducts, has also been implicated in cisplatin cytotoxicity as a result of the obvious impedance it presents to DNA replication and transcription processes. Carboplatin contains a 1,1-cyclobutanedicarboxylato-leaving group and undergoes aquation more slowly, but the structures of the aquated forms of cisplatin and carboplatin are the same, as are the types of adducts produced in DNA. The relative frequencies of the individual lesions observed in carboplatin-treated cells are somewhat different from those of cisplatin. The G-X-G intrastrand adduct is the most prevalent (40%), followed by the G-G (30%) and A-G (15%) intrastrand adducts, respectively *(15)*.

3. SIGNAL TRANSDUCTION PATHWAYS INVOLVED IN THE CISPLATIN-INDUCED CELLULAR INJURY RESPONSE

The available evidence is consistent with the hypothesis that, over the clinically relevant concentration range, cisplatin kills most types of cells by activating apoptosis. In many cell types, exposure to cytotoxic concentrations of cisplatin produce fragmentation of DNA into multimers of 180 base pairs, consistent with internucleosomal cleavage of chromatin by an endonuclease, followed by loss of membrane integrity and cell shrinkage *(16,17)*. This process is inhibited by cycloheximide, suggesting that cell death requires new protein synthesis, which is also characteristic of apoptosis. In both sensitive and resistant cells, cisplatin treatment results in the cleavage of proteins known to be substrates for the caspases *(18)*. Further evidence that cisplatin kills via apoptosis has emerged from studies of bcl-2 and bcl-x_L, proteins whose expression antagonizes this pathway. The overexpression of the bcl-2 and bcl-x_L proteins prevents apoptosis in cells treated with cisplatin *(19,20)*.

The fact that cisplatin kills via apoptosis implies the existence of specific mechanisms for detecting the injury and for signaling the presence of injury to the apoptotic machinery of the cell. Little is known of the details of any of the signal transduction pathways activated by cisplatin, but it is possible to identify the general nature of some components that must be present. The detector must be able to generate a signal, and there must be a mechanism that integrates this signal with those coming from a variety of cell surface and intracellular receptors. For example, the cytotoxicity of cisplatin is modulated in many types of cells by activation of the epidermal growth factor (EGF) receptor at the cell surface *(21)* or activation of the protein kinase C (PKC) receptor intracellularly *(22)*. The facility with which cisplatin activates the apoptotic cascade also depends on the proliferative status of the cells at the time of drug exposure *(23)*. In some types of cells, p53 appears to play a central role in cisplatin-induced apoptosis *(24)*, but in others the level of expression of wild-type p53 has little effect on sensitivity *(25)*. Increased levels of p53 have been demonstrated in several cisplatin-resistant human ovarian cancer cell lines *(26,27)*.

In addition to the activation of apoptosis, the cisplatin injury response is accompanied by changes in a large number of other cellular parameters. Each perturbation develops with a specific time-course and returns to baseline as the cell population recovers exponential growth. For example, cisplatin injury activates cell cycle control checkpoints. At clinically relevant concentrations this is largely a G_2 arrest, although variable degrees of S phase and G_1 arrest occur at higher concentrations. The cytotoxicity of cisplatin correlates more closely with the arrest of cells in G_2 than with the degree of inhibition of DNA synthesis *(28)*. The G_2 arrest is accompanied by the accumulation of inactive, phosphorylated $p34^{cdc2}$ protein. A number of agents that abrogate the G_2 checkpoint and induce premature mitosis have been shown to enhance the cytotoxicity of cisplatin *(29)*. Cisplatin treatment also increases or decreases the level of a large number of mRNAs, some of which correspond to known early response genes but most of which are not yet identified. Whether such changes are required for the activation of apoptosis or simply occur in parallel is unknown.

4. GENOMIC INSTABILITY AND DNA MISMATCH REPAIR

Among the types of genetic defects that can cause genomic instability, the loss of MMR is of particular interest both because it occurs commonly in several types of sporadic cancers as well as hereditary nonpolyposis colon cancer syndrome (reviewed in ref. 30), and because it has the potential to predispose markedly to the development of drug-resistant variants in the tumor cell population *(31)*. A cell normally makes a number of mistakes during the replication of DNA that create mismatched bases. Misincorporation of a base or "slippage" of DNA polymerase on the template can create a short segment of mismatch. These types of errors are repaired by the MMR system, which is homologous to the mutHLS system in bacteria *(32–34)*. In bacteria and yeast, a minimum of 10 proteins participate in the mutHLS-related complex that repairs single bases and small loops *(35)*. Of these proteins, three are involved in the initiation of excision *(36)*. Thus far, the products of at least five human genes have been shown to play a role in MMR including hMSH2, hMSH3, hMSH6, hMLH1, and hPMS2. A sixth human gene, hPMS1, is also believed, on the basis of genetic evidence, to be important for MMR, although biochemical studies supporting its involvement in MMR are not yet available *(37)*. The first step involves the binding of a hMSH2-hMSH6 or a hMSH2-hMSH3 heteroduplex *(38,39)* to the segment of DNA containing the mismatched base. This is followed by binding of the hMLH1-hPMS2 heteroduplex *(40)*, cutting of the strand containing the mismatch, exonuclease-mediated removal of the segment between the nick and the mismatch, filling in the gap by DNA polymerase δ, and ligation that renders the strand whole again. Analysis of the mismatched nucleotide-binding specificity of the hMSH2-hMSH3 and hMSH2-hMSH6 protein complexes showed that they have overlapping but not identical binding specificity *(39)*.

Loss of MMR results in the appearance of nucleotide additions or deletions, as well as transitions and transversions in both repetitive and nonrepetitive sequences scattered throughout the genome *(31,41)*. One consequence of the loss of MMR shows up in DNA sequences called microsatellites *(42–44)*. Microsatellites are stretches of DNA in which the same sequence of two, three, or four bases is repeated many times. Microsatellites and stretches of DNA in which a single nucleotide is repeated many times appear to cause DNA polymerase to "slip" during replication, creating a mismatched base or short loop that is normally recognized and repaired by the MMR system *(45)*. If the MMR system is defective, then the mismatched bases persist, and during the next round of DNA replication generate two daughter chromosomes with different numbers of mono-, di-, tri-, or tetranucleotide repeats in allelic sequences, a phenomenon known as microsatellite instability.

There is now good evidence to show that loss of MMR increases the rate of mutation in many genes *(31,41)*. The genes at greatest risk appear to be those rich in reiterated short mononucleotide sequences, such as the *HPRT* and *p53* genes, or microsatellite sequences within or near coding regions such as the *BRCA1* and *c-myc* genes *(46)*. In fact, MMR-deficient cells have high mutation rates both in noncoding microsatellite sequences and in the coding sequences of a number of genes including *HPRT (31)*, *APRT (47)*, *APC (48)*, type II *TGF-β (49)*, and *BAX (50)*. Loss of MMR due to mutation of hMSH2, hMLH1, and hPMS2 is known to underlie most cases of hereditary nonpolyposis colon cancer *(51–54)*. Whereas the MMR system appears to be normal in the heterozygote cells containing a single functional gene copy, during carcinogenesis the remaining wild-type allele is somatically mutated, resulting in the complete loss of MMR function in the tumor *(53)*. The resulting genomic instability probably plays a role in causing the series of genetic changes involving inactivation of the *p53* gene and other genetic changes that are required to create a fully malignant colon cancer *(55)*. The mutation rate at microsatellite sequences can be extremely high *(31)*, and it is increased 100- to 1000-fold at selectable markers such as the *HPRT* and ouabain resistance loci *(31,56)*.

In addition to hereditary nonpolyposis colon cancer, loss of MMR occurs frequently in many types of sporadic cancers, including endometrial, small and non-small cell lung, pancreatic, gastric, ovarian, cervix, and breast cancer *(56–61)*. Mice that are deficient in either MLH1, MSH2, MSH6, or PMS2 have microsatellite instability in many tissues and a predisposition to form tumors, especially lymphomas *(62–65)*. This suggests that loss of MMR is an important component of the transformation or progression process in many kinds of cancer.

5. DRUG RESISTANCE DUE TO LOSS OF DNA MISMATCH REPAIR

5.1. Resistance to 6-Thioguanine

In addition to being involved in tumorigenesis, loss of MMR activity is of concern with respect to the use of chemotherapeutic agents to treat established tumors. In one example of this, loss of MMR may result in drug resistance directly by knocking out the ability of the cell to detect adducts in its DNA that mimic base mismatches. Loss of MMR has been reported to cause resistance to a variety of drugs that cause lesions in DNA. It causes high-level resistance to the antimetabolite 6-thioguanine *(66)* and moderate levels of resistance to the methylating agents *N*-methyl-*N′*-nitro-*N*-nitrosoguanidine (MNNG; see ref. *67*). After incorporation into DNA, 6-thioguanine can be chemically methylated by *S*-adenosylmethionine to form S^6-methylthioguanine. This adduct is not a good substrate for alkylmethyltransferase and therefore would be expected to persist in the DNA *(68)*. Particularly when preceded by a 5′cytosine, S^6-methylthioguanine paired with cytosine is recognized by hMutSα *(66,69)*. During DNA replication, S^6-methylthioguanine can pair with thymine as well as its normal partner cytosine, and the resultant S^6-methylthioguanine-thymine pairs are also identified by the MMR system as replication errors *(68)*. The currently available data support the argument that it is the ability of the MMR system to recognize the abnormalities in the DNA produced by the incorporation of 6-thioguanine and attempt repair that triggers cytotoxicity.

5.2. DNA Mismatch Repair-Deficient Cell Lines Are Resistant to Cisplatin and Carboplatin

The first indication that MMR might be a determinant of sensitivity to cisplatin was the observation that introduction of *mutS* or *mutL* mutations into *E. coli* already hypersensitive to cisplatin due to the presence of a *dam* mutation caused them to become resistant *(70)*. We examined the effect of loss of MMR on sensitivity to cisplatin and carboplatin using pairs of cell lines that were MMR proficient and deficient due to lesions in both alleles of either the *hMSH2*, *hMLH1*, or *PMS2* genes. The human colorectal adenocarcinoma cell line HCT116, which is hMLH1 deficient due to a hemizygous mutation in *hMLH1*, resulting in a truncated and nonfunctional protein, exhibits microsatellite instability and does not correct mismatches in cell-free extracts *(71)*. In the HCT116+ch3 subline, the hMLH1 deficiency was complemented by transfer of chromosome 3 containing a wild-type copy of *MLH1* into the cell; the HCT116+ch2 subline into which chromosome 2 had been transferred served as a control *(72)*. The human endometrial adenocarcinoma cell line HEC59 is hMSH2 deficient due to different mutations in each of the two *MSH2* alleles. Similarly, in the HEC59+ch2 subline, the hMSH2 deficiency was complemented by transfer of a full-length chromosome 2 containing a wild-type copy of *MSH2 (73)*. Since neither of these two pairs of cell lines was truly isogenic, additional studies were carried out in cells in which *MSH2* and *PMS2* had been molecularly "knocked out," including the isogenic wt-2 ($MSH2^{+/+}$) and the double knockout dMsh2–9 ($MSH2^{-/-}$) embryonic stem cell lines *(62)*, and the $PMS2^{+/+}$ and $PMS2^{-/-}$ mouse embryo fibroblast lines *(64)*. In all four cell systems the MMR-deficient cells were approximately twofold more resistant to cisplatin than the MMR-proficient cells. Likewise, low-level resistance to cisplatin and carboplatin was found for all MMR-deficient cell lines tested *(74–76)*. The fact that loss of MMR results in resistance to both cisplatin and carboplatin was not unexpected, since, although carboplatin contains a 1,1-cyclobutanedicarboxylato-leaving group and undergoes aquation more slowly, the structures of the aquated forms of cisplatin and carboplatin are the same as are the types of adducts. In contrast, no difference was observed in either the HCT116 or HEC59 systems between MMR-deficient and -proficient cells with respect to sensitivity to oxaliplatin *(74)*, a platinum compound that forms structurally different types of adducts in DNA. The similarity in the degree of resistance between four such disparate types of cells suggests a lack of cell line-specific factors that can modulate the impact of loss of MMR.

The difference in the sensitivity of the MMR-deficient HCT116 and HEC59 cells was not due to a decrease in the uptake of cisplatin or the extent of DNA platination. Likewise, MMR deficiency due to loss of hMLH1 function did not change the kinetics of platinum removal from total cellular DNA *(77)*. Since lesions that alter nucleotide excision repair activity produce large changes in the kinetics of platinum removal *(78)*, this result suggests that loss of MMR does not increase the ability of the nucleotide excision repair system to remove adducts, and that the observed resistance to cisplatin is not due to enhanced nucleotide excision repair activity.

A separate observation of importance is that the in vitro selection of cells for resistance to cisplatin yields clones and populations that have lost MMR. The human ovarian cell line 2008/A *(79)*, selected from the parental 2008 cells for resistance to cisplatin, had completely lost expression of hMLH1 in immunoblots, and exhibited the phenotype typical of MMR deficiency including microsatellite instability *(80)*. Likewise, acquisition of a replication error phenotype as well as defects in strand-specific MMR has been reported in other cell lines selected for resistance to cisplatin *(81,82)*. Although this could have resulted from either cisplatin selection of preexisting MMR-deficient cells in the population or *de novo* cisplatin mutagenesis of the *hMLH1* gene followed by enrichment, it provides further evidence that loss of MMR results in resistance to cisplatin.

Although one might have expected that loss of MMR would cause the cells to be more sensitive to cisplatin due to the persistence of DNA damage, loss of this repair function paradoxically causes the cell to become more resistant. The best explanation for the resistance to cisplatin relates to the fact that this agent, as well as most other anticancer drugs, causes cell death by apoptosis. Triggering apoptosis requires the cell to be able to recognize the presence of the damage in DNA, and it may be lack of detection or lack of attempted repair that causes failure to generate an apoptotic signal in MMR-deficient cells.

5.3. DNA Mismatch Repair Proteins Bind to Cisplatin-DNA Adducts

The ability of MMR proteins to recognize different types of platinum adducts was examined with mobility shift assays using nuclear extracts from the human ovarian cell line 2008. The formation of protein complexes on platinated DNA was demonstrated by gel mobility shift assay using a 123-bp double-stranded oligonucleotide platinated with either cisplatin or oxaliplatin, and the presence of hMSH2 and hMLH1 proteins in the complexes was documented by supershift using antibodies directed against hMSH2 or hMLH1. When an oxaliplatinated probe was used, different complexes were formed, and no supershift was produced by anti-hMSH2 or anti-hMLH1 antibody, indicating that the MMR complex that forms on cisplatin adducts does not form on oxaliplatin adducts *(74)*. This specificity parallels the fact that loss of MMR resulted in resistance to cisplatin but not oxaliplatin *(74)*, suggesting that the components of the MMR system responsible for the difference in sensitivity are quite specific in their ability to discriminate between different types of closely related DNA adducts. Likewise, pure hMSH2 has been reported to bind to platinated DNA in mobility shift assays *(83)*. The human MSH2-MSH6 heterodimer also binds to cisplatin intrastrand adducts *(84)* and has the greatest affinity for lesions in which a thymine has been misincorporated opposite a *3′* guanine *(85)*. Both the GG adduct itself (simple adduct), and the lesion consisting of an adduct and a misincorporated base on the opposite strand (compound adduct), are recognized and possibly processed by the MMR system *(86)*. It is not yet clear how the platinum adducts are recognized by the MMR proteins. It has been demonstrated biochemically that hMSH2 can bind to a 1,2 d(GpG) adduct, but it is also possible that the MMR system recognizes monoadducts, monoadducts modified by reaction with glutathione, or interstrand adducts as well. It is possible that cisplatin adducts distort the DNA in a manner that mimics the presence of either a single-base mismatch or an insertion/deletion mispair.

The current paradigm is that the MMR system serves as a detector for cisplatin-damaged DNA; resistance is thought to result from failure of the cell to recognize the adducts and to activate signaling pathways that trigger apoptosis. If this paradigm is correct, then the detector must be able to initiate activation of signaling pathways. Indeed, recently it has been reported that cisplatin activates c-jun NH_2-terminal kinase1 (JNK1) by a p21-activated kinase protein 65 and mitogen-activated protein kinase kinase 4-independent mechanism more efficiently in MMR-proficient than -deficient cells, and that cisplatin activates c-Abl kinase in the MMR-proficient cells, whereas this response is completely absent in MMR-deficient cells *(87)*. This reveals that activation of JNK1 and c-Abl by cisplatin is in part dependent on the integrity of the MMR function, suggesting that these kinases are part of the signal transduction pathway activated when MMR proteins recognize cisplatin adducts in DNA. Furthermore, it has been suggested that the MMR system is involved in promoting G_2 cell cycle arrest and cell death after treatment with MNNG or 6-thioguanine in cells that are MMR proficient *(88,89)*. Recently it has been reported that MLH1-deficient human tumor cell lines fail to engage G_2 cell cycle arrest after cisplatin damage *(90)*. The link between the MMR system and G_2 arrest suggests that the MMR system is involved not only in the repair of true mismatches, but also in processes that limit the replication of cells when DNA damage is detected. The arrest at the G_2 cell cycle checkpoint may permit the cell to attempt repair of DNA mismatches and prevent the replication of mutated DNA, similar to the arrest at the G_1/S checkpoint mediated by p53 and p21 in response to DNA damage.

The studies reviewed above support the conclusion that the binding of MLH1-PMS2, MSH2-MSH6, or MSH2-MSH3 heterodimers alone is not sufficient for full detector function since cells containing normal amounts of MLH1 and MSH2 but lacking PMS2, and cells containing normal amounts of MLH1 and PMS2 but lacking MSH2 were still resistant to cisplatin. This is consistent with the hypothesis that the assembly on the damaged DNA of at least either the MSH2-MSH6 *(38,39)* or MSH2-MSH3 *(39,91)* heterodimers together with the MLH1-PMS2 heterodimer *(40)* is required before a damage signal can be generated.

5.4. Treatment with Cisplatin Enriches for DNA Mismatch Repair-Deficient Cells In Vitro and In Vivo

Human cells expressing green fluorescent protein, the product of the *GFP* gene, can be readily identified by their high level of fluorescence. Parental MMR-deficient HCT116 cells were infected with a retrovirus containing the *GFP* gene driven by a cytomegalovirus (CMV) promoter. Infected cells were selected with geneticin, and the resulting cell population was identified as HCT116-GFP. GFP was expressed in high levels in 90–95% of these cells. The HCT116 and HCT116-GFP cells were tested by clonogenic assay, and no difference in sensitivity to cisplatin was found. A population containing 5% MMR-deficient GFP-expressing cells and 95% MMR-proficient HCT116+ch3 cells was prepared by mixing and subjected to four cycles of a 1-h exposure to cisplatin or oxaliplatin followed by a 5-d recovery period. Five days after a single 1-h exposure to an inhibitory concentration of 50% (IC_{50}) concentration of cisplatin, the treated population contained 53% more MMR-deficient GFP-expressing cells than the untreated population; after the second, third, and fourth cycles there were 68, 72, and 77% more GFP-expressing cells in the treated population, respectively. Enrichment was more dramatic when the cells were exposed to an IC_{90} concentration of cisplatin. After the fourth cycle of exposure, there were 163% more GFP-expressing cells in the treated than in the untreated control population ($p < 0.0001$, ANOVA). In contrast, when the cells were treated with either an IC_{50} or IC_{90} concentration of oxaliplatin, there was no progressive enrichment for the MMR-deficient GFP-expressing cells. Thus, treatment with cisplatin, to which the MMR-deficient cells were 2.1-fold resistant, resulted in rapid enrichment for the resistant cells in the population, whereas treatment with oxaliplatin, to which the MMR-deficient cells were not resistant, produced no enrichment *(92)*.

Since the behavior of tumor cell populations growing under different conditions of density can be markedly different *(93)*, these studies were extended to a Chinese hamster ovary model that permits in vitro and in vivo experiments with the same cells *(94)*. The degree of enrichment in vitro was dependent on the cisplatin concentration but not on the fraction of mismatch repair-deficient cells preexisting in the tumor cell population *(95,96)*. When grown as a xenograft in vivo, a single lethal dose for 10% of subjects (LD_{10}) of cisplatin enriched the tumors by 48% from 4.6 to 6.8% repair-deficient cells ($p = 0.04$).

These results provide further support for the hypothesis that the presence of even small numbers of DNA mismatch repair-deficient cells in a tumor may adversely affect therapeutic outcome. Not only are such cells intrinsically resistant to cisplatin and 6-thioguanine, and enriched for by treatment with these agents, but they also have an increased rate of spontaneous mutation to resistance to other chemotherapeutic agents including etoposide *(31,97)*. Also, to the extent that treatment enriches for these cells, one would expect an increase in the number of cells developing mutations in other genes that cause tumor progression *(98)*. What fraction of tumor cells must have lost mismatch repair before a therapeutically adverse outcome can be detected is unknown. However, in experiments that involved mixtures of cells that differed only in their drug sensitivity, and not also in their genomic stability, Skipper et al. *(99)* found that the presence of only 1% resistant cells was sufficient to cause clinical failure of treatment. These results demonstrate that, even though loss of mismatch repair yields only modest levels of cisplatin resistance, even a single exposure to cisplatin produces quite a marked enrichment for repair-deficient cells in vitro and in vivo.

5.5. Effect of Loss of DNA Mismatch Repair on Sensitivity In Vivo

Nude mice were inoculated sc with either the MMR-proficient wt-2 ($MSH2^{+/+}$) or the MMR-deficient dMsh2–9 ($MSH2^{-/-}$) embryonic stem cells *(62)* and treated 48 h after implantation with either isotonic saline or an LD_{10} dose of cisplatin or oxaliplatin. In the control animals the doubling time was similar for the $MSH2^{+/+}$ and $MSH2^{-/-}$ tumors. The LD_{10} dose of cisplatin produced a greater response in the $MSH2^{+/+}$ than in the $MSH2^{-/-}$ tumors; the MMR-proficient tumors shrank in size over the first 10 days after treatment, reaching a nadir volume that averaged only 13% of their starting volume before growth resumed. In contrast, the MMR-deficient tumors suffered a growth delay of only 4 d before resuming growth. The mean tumor volumes on d 18 after tumor implantation for the $MSH2^{-/-}$ tumors treated with cisplatin were statistically significantly greater than those of the $MSH2^{+/+}$ tumors ($p = 0.0001$). There was no difference in either the control ($p = 0.86$) or the oxaliplatin-treated group ($p = 0.87$). Thus, the 2.1-fold difference in cisplatin sensitivity between the $MSH2^{+/+}$ and $MSH2^{-/-}$ cells measured in vitro translated into a marked difference in tumor responsiveness in vivo *(92)*, arguing that this degree of resistance is likely to have clinical significance.

The issue of when loss of MMR occurs during oncogenesis remains controversial, even for hereditary nonpolyposis colon cancer, which represents the best defined clinical situation *(100)*. However, once such cells are present in the tumor, their genomic instability may result in the accumulation of additional mutations that contribute to the phenomenon of tumor progression. Enrichment of these cells as a result of chemotherapy would be expected to accelerate this process. Indeed, microsatellite instability, a hallmark of the genomic instability due to the loss of MMR *(101)*, has been reported to be present in up to 94% of the patients with therapy-related leukemia or myelodysplastic syndromes, consistent with drug-induced enrichment for genetically unstable cells *(102)*.

5.6. Loss of hMLH1 Expression in Human Ovarian Cancers Treated with Cisplatin or Carboplatin

The observation that loss of MMR results in resistance to cisplatin, and that cisplatin enriches for MMR-deficient cells, has raised the question of whether enrichment for MMR-deficient cells occurs during the course of treatment of ovarian cancers with standard cisplatin- or carboplatin-containing chemotherapy regimens. Microsatellite instability has been reported in 15–20% of sporadic ovarian cancers at the time of diagnosis *(61,103)*, and because of limited assay sensitivity it is possible that a larger fraction contains at least some MMR-deficient cells. The tools with which to assess this in tumor samples from patients are limited to immunohistochemical staining for the expression of the MMR-related proteins and microsatellite analysis. We *(104)* and others

(105,106) have suggested that immunohistochemistry could be used to detect major defects rapidly in the expression of MMR genes.

To determine whether enrichment for MMR-deficient cells occurs during the treatment of human ovarian cancer patients, paired tumor samples were obtained from 38 patients before and after treatment with a minimum of three cycles of platinum drug-based primary chemotherapy and analyzed immunohistochemically for changes in the fraction of tumor cells expressing hMHL1 *(94)*. Following treatment there was a reduction in hMLH1 staining in 66% of the cases ($p = 0.0005$). This result is consistent with the concept that treatment with cisplatin or carboplatin selects for preexisting MMR-deficient cells, and that this contributes to the frequent development of clinical resistance.

6. OVERVIEW

Loss of MMR results in cisplatin resistance directly by impairing the ability of the cell to detect DNA damage and activate apoptosis, and indirectly by increasing the mutation rate throughout the genome *(107)*. The MMR system recognizes the damaged bases or the mismatch that results from attempted replication across the damaged base. Recognition is followed by events, not yet well defined, that generate a signal capable of activating apoptosis (Fig. 1). Operationally, the MMR system is thus functioning as a detector. The paradigm is that when this detector is disabled the cell cannot sense the damage present in its DNA, the apoptotic cascade is not activated as proficiently, and the cell is phenotypically drug resistant. The fact that higher concentrations of cisplatin can still trigger apoptosis in MMR-deficient cells suggests the existence of either additional types of DNA adduct detectors, or an effect of cisplatin on other non-DNA targets that are also capable of engaging the apoptotic mechanism.

Although by the direct route, loss of MMR results only in relatively small degrees of resistance to cisplatin and carboplatin, several lines of evidence suggest that this resistance is nevertheless of substantial biologic and clinical significance: (1) this low-level resistance to cisplatin is sufficient to produce enrichment for MMR-deficient tumor cells during treatment in vitro and in xenografts in vivo *(92,95,96)*; (2) $MSH2^{+/+}$ embryonic stem cells grown as xenografts are responsive to treatment with a single LD_{10} dose of cisplatin, whereas isogenic $MSH2^{-/-}$ tumors are not, suggesting that the degree of cisplatin resistance conferred by loss of MMR is sufficient to produce a large difference in biological responsiveness in vivo *(92)*; (3) loss of MMR has been reported in tumor cell lines selected for resistance to cisplatin *(80,90)*; and (4) following treatment there was a reduction in immunohistochemical staining of hMLH1 in 66% of the cases of ovarian cancer examined *(95)*. Likewise, the frequency of positive immunoblot analysis for hMLH1 protein in ovarian carcinomas obtained following chemotherapy with a cisplatin- or carboplatin-containing regimen was shown to be substantially lower than the frequency

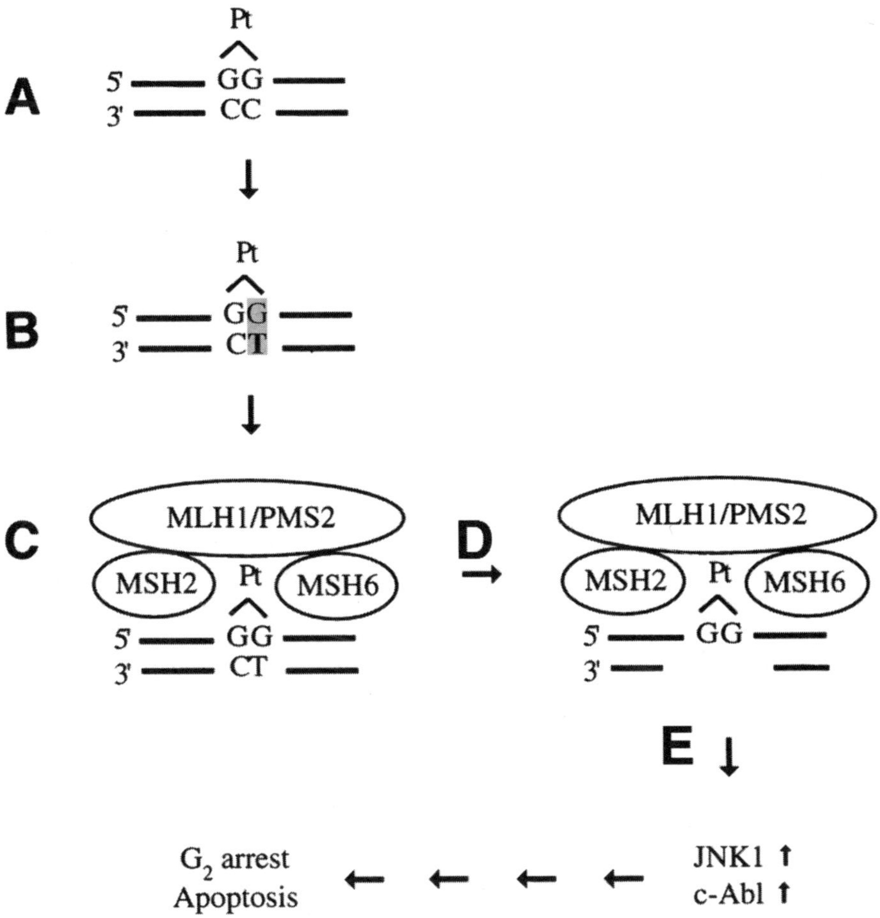

Fig. 1. Proposed sequence of events mediating the cytotoxicity of carboplatin and cisplatin via MMR. **(A)** Formation of the adduct. **(B)** Misincorporation of a base opposite the adduct at the next round of replication. **(C)** Recognition of the adduct/mispair by the MMR system. **(D)** Attempted futile repair. **(E)** Generation of a signal that triggers apoptosis. An intrastrand 1,2d(GpG) adduct is depicted by "Pt." (Reproduced with permission from ref. *107*.)

among tumors sampled prior to treatment *(90)*. Therefore, clinical studies of the significance of MMR-deficient cells in tumors with respect to the rate of development of platinum drug resistance are now urgently needed.

ACKNOWLEDGMENTS

Research funding was provided in part by the Swiss National Science Foundation (NF 31-52531-97). The research work referred to in this review was conducted in part by the Clayton Foundation for Research-California Division. Dr. Howell is a Clayton Foundation Investigator.

REFERENCES

1. Andrews, P. A. and Howell, S. B. (1990) Cellular pharmacology of cisplatin: perspectives on mechanisms of acquired resistance. *Cancer Cells* **2,** 35–43.
2. Perez, R. P., Hamilton, T. C., and Ozols, R. F. (1990) Resistance to alkylating agents and cisplatin: insights from ovarian carcinoma model systems. *Pharmacol. Ther.* **48,** 19–27.
3. Timmer-Bosscha, H., Mulder, N. H., and de Vries, E. G. E. (1992) Modulation of *cis*-diamminedichloroplatinum(II) resistance: a review. *Br. J. Cancer* **66,** 227–238.
4. Anthoney, D. A., McIlwrath, A. J., Gallagher, W. M., Edlin, A. R. M., and Brown, R. (1996) Microsatellite instability, apoptosis, and loss of p53 function in drug-resistant tumor cells. *Cancer Res.* **56,** 1374–1381.
5. Aebi, S., Kurdi-Haidar, B., Gordon, R., Cenni, B., Zheng, H., Fink, D., et al. (1996) Loss of DNA mismatch repair in acquired resistance to cisplatin. *Cancer Res.* **56,** 3087–3090.
6. Gately, D. P., and Howell, S. B. (1993) Cellular accumulation of the anticancer agent cisplatin: a review. *Br. J. Cancer* **67,** 1171–1176.
7. Heminger, K. A., Hartson, S. D., Rogers, J., and Matts, R. L. (1997) Cisplatin inhibits protein synthesis in rabbit reticulocyte lysate by causing an arrest in elongation. *Arch. Biochem. Biophys.* **344,** 200–207.
8. Rosenberg, B., Renshaw, E., Van Camp, L, Hartwick, J., and Drobnik, J. (1967) Platinum-induced filamentous growth in *Escherichia coli. J. Bacteriol.* **93,** 716–721.
9. Rosenberg, B., Van Camp, L, Grimley, E. B., and Thompson, A. J. (1967) The inhibition of growth or cell division in *Escherichia coli* by different ionic species of platinum(IV) complexes. *J. Biol. Chem.* **242,** 1347–1352.
10. Damia, G., Imperatori, L., Stefanini, M., and D'Incalci, M. (1996) Sensitivity of CHO mutant cell lines with specific defects in nucleotide excision repair to different anti-cancer agents. *Int. J. Cancer* **66,** 779–783.
11. Li, L., Keating, M. J., Plunkett, W., and Yang, L. Y. (1997) Fludarabine-mediated repair inhibition of cisplatin-induced DNA lesions in chronic myelogenous leukemia-blast crisis K562 cells: induction of synergistic cytotoxicity independent of reversal of apoptosis resistance. *Mol. Pharmacol.* **52,** 798–806.
12. Pinto, A. L. and Lippard, S. J. (1985) Binding of the antitumor drug *cis*-diamminedichloroplatinum(II) (cisplatin) to DNA. *Biochim. Biophys. Acta* **780,** 167–180.
13. Johnson, N. P., Hoeschele, J. D., and Rahn R. O. (1980) Kinetic analysis of the *in vitro* binding of radioactive *cis*- and *trans*-dichlorodiammineplatinum(II) to DNA. *Chem. Biol. Interact.* **30,** 151–169.
14. Fichtinger-Schepman, A. M., van der Veer, J. L., den Hartog, J. H., Lohman, P. H., and Reedijk, J. (1985) Adducts of the antitumor drug *cis*-dichlorodiammineplatinum(II) with DNA: formation, identification, and quantitation. *Biochemistry* **24,** 707–713.
15. Blommaert, F. A., van Dijk-Knijnenburg, H. C., Dijt, F. J., den Engelse, L., Baan, R. A., Berends, F., et al. (1995) Formation of DNA adducts of the antitumor drug carboplatin: different nucleotide sequence preferences *in vitro* and in cells. *Biochemistry* **34,** 8474–8480.
16. Sorenson, C. M., Barry, M. A., and Eastman, A. (1990) Analysis of events associated with cell cycle arrest at G_2 phase and cell death induced by cisplatin. *J. Natl. Cancer Inst.* **83,** 749–755.
17. Barry, M. A., Behnke, C. A., and Eastman, A. (1990) Activation of programmed cell death (apoptosis) by cisplatin, other anticancer drugs, toxins and hyperthermia. *Biochem. Pharmacol.* **40,** 2353–2362.
18. Henkels, K. M. and Turchi, J. J. (1997) Induction of apoptosis in cisplatin-sensitive and -resistant human ovarian cancer cell lines. *Cancer Res.* **57,** 4488–4492.
19. Miyashita, T. and Reed, J. C. (1993) Bcl-2 oncoprotein blocks chemotherapy-induced apoptosis in a human leukemia cell line. *Blood* **81,** 151–157.

20. Minn, A. J., Rudin, C. M., Boise, L. H., and Thompson, C. B. (1995) Expression of bcl-x_L can confer a multidrug resistance phenotype. *Blood* **86,** 1903–1910.
21. Christen, R. D., Hom, D. K., Porter, D. C., Andrews, P. A., MacLeod, C. L., Hafstrom, L., et al. (1990) Epidermal growth factor regulates the *in vitro* sensitivity of human ovarian carcinoma cells to cisplatin. *J. Clin. Invest.* **86,** 1632–1640.
22. Isonishi, S., Andrews, P. A., and Howell, S. B. (1990) Increased sensitivity to *cis*-diamminedichloroplatinum(II) in human ovarian carcinoma cells in response to treatment with 12-O-tetradecanoylphorbol-13-acetate. *J. Biol. Chem.* **265,** 3623–3627.
23. Evans, D. L., Tilby, M., and Dive, C. (1994) Differential sensitivity to the induction of apoptosis by cisplatin in proliferating and quiescent immature rat thymocytes is independent of the levels of drug accumulation and DNA adduct formation. *Cancer Res.* **54,** 1596–1603.
24. Lowe, S. W., Bodis, S., McClatchey, A., Remington, L., Ruley, H. E., Fisher, D. E., et al. (1994) p53 status and the efficacy of cancer therapy *in vivo*. *Science* **266,** 807–810.
25. Gibson, A. A., Harwood, F. G., Tillman, D. M., and Houghton, J. A. (1998) Selective sensitization to DNA-damaging agents in a human rhabdomyosarcoma cell line with inducible wild-type p53 overexpression. *Clin. Cancer Res.* **4,** 145–152.
26. Brown, R., Clugston, C., Burns, P., Edlin, A., Vasey, P., Vojtesek, B., et al. (1993) Increased accumulation of p53 protein in cisplatin-resistant ovarian cell lines. *Int. J. Cancer* **55,** 678–684.
27. Fajac, A., Da Silva, J., Ahomadegbe, J. C., Rateau, J. G., Bernaudin, J. F., Riou, G., et al. (1996) Cisplatin-induced apoptosis and *p53* gene status in a cisplatin-resistant human ovarian carcinoma cell line. *Int. J. Cancer* **68,** 67–74.
28. Sorenson, C. M. and Eastman, A. (1988) Influence of *cis*-diamminedichloroplatinum(II) on DNA synthesis and cell cycle progression in excision repair proficient and deficient Chinese hamster ovary cells. *Cancer Res.* **48,** 6703–6707.
29. Shi, Y., Frankel, A., Radvanyi, L. G., Penn, L. Z., Miller, R. G., and Mills, G. B. (1995) Rapamycin enhances apoptosis and increases sensitivity to cisplatin *in vitro*. *Cancer Res.* **55,** 1982–1988.
30. Fishel, R. and Kolodner, R. D. (1995) Identification of mismatch repair genes and their role in the development of cancer. *Curr. Opin. Genet. Dev.* **5,** 382–395.
31. Bhattacharyya, N. P., Skandalis, A., Ganesh, A., Groden, J., and Meuth, M. (1994) Mutator phenotypes in human colorectal carcinoma cell lines. *Proc. Natl. Acad. Sci. USA* **91,** 6319–6323.
32. da Costa, L., Liu, B., El-Deiry, W. S., Hamilton, S. R., Kinzler, K. W., Vogelstein, B., et al. (1995) Polymerase δ variants in RER colorectal tumours. *Nature Genet.* **9,** 10–11.
33. Modrich, P. (1994) Mismatch repair, genetic stability, and cancer. *Science* **266,** 1959–1960.
34. Johnson, R. E., Kovvali, G. K., Prakash, L., and Prakash S. (1994) Requirement of the yeast *RTH1* 5′ to 3′ exonuclease for the stability of simple repetitive DNA. *Science* **269,** 238–240.
35. Parsons, R., Li, G-M., Longley, M. J., Fang, W-H., Papadopoulos, N., Jen, J., et al. (1993) Hypermutability and mismatch repair deficiency in RER^+ tumor cells. *Cell* **75,** 1227–1236.
36. Grilley, M., Griffith, J., and Modrich, P. (1993) Bidirectional excision in methyl-directed mismatch repair. *J. Biol. Chem.* **268,** 11830–11837.
37. Kolodner, R. (1996) Biochemistry and genetics of eukaryotic mismatch repair. *Genes Dev.* **10,** 1433–1442.
38. Palombo, F., Gallinari, P., Iaccarino, I., Lettieri, T., Hughes, M., D'Arrigo, A., et al. (1995) GTBP, a 160-kilodalton protein essential for mismatch-binding activity in human cells. *Science* **268,** 1912–1914.
39. Acharya, S., Wilson, T., Gradia, S., Kane, M. F., Guerrette, S., Marsischky, G. T., et al. (1996) hMSH2 forms specific mispair-binding complexes with hMSH3 and hMSH6. *Proc. Natl. Acad. Sci. USA* **93,** 13629–13634.

40. Li, G-M. and Modrich, P. (1995) Restoration of mismatch repair to nuclear extracts of H6 colorectal tumor cells by a heterodimer of human MutL homologs. *Proc. Natl. Acad. Sci. USA* **92,** 1950–1954.
41. Modrich, P. (1991) Mechanisms and biological effects of mismatch repair. *Annu. Rev. Genet.* **25,** 229–253.
42. Ionov, Y., Peinado, M. A., Malkhosyan, S., Shibata, D., and Perucho, M. (1993) Ubiquitous somatic mutations in simple repeated sequences reveal a new mechanism for colonic carcinogenesis. *Nature* **363,** 558–561.
43. Thibodeau, S. N., Bren, G., and Schaid, D. (1993) Microsatellite instability in cancer of the proximal colon. *Science* **260,** 816–819.
44. Strand, M., Prolla, T. A., Liskay, R. M., and Petes, T. D. (1993) Destabilization of tracts of simple repetitive DNA in yeast by mutations affecting DNA mismatch repair. *Nature* **365,** 274–276.
45. Kunkel, T. A. (1993) Slippery DNA and diseases. *Nature* **365,** 207–208.
46. Wooster, R., Cleton-Jansen, A-M., Collins, N., Mangion, J., Cornelis, R. S., Cooper, C. S., et al. (1994) Instability of short tandem repeats (microsatellites) in human cancers. *Nature Genet.* **6,** 152–156.
47. Hess, P., Aquilina, G., Dogliotti, E., and Bignami, M. (1994) Spontaneous mutations at *aprt* locus in a mammalian cell line defective in mismatch recognition. *Somat. Cell Mol. Genet.* **20,** 409–421.
48. Huang, J., Papadopoulos, N., McKinley, A. J., Farrington, S. M., Curtis, L. J., Wyllie, A. H., et al. (1996) *APC* mutations in colorectal tumors with mismatch repair deficiency. *Proc. Natl. Acad. Sci. USA* **93,** 9049–9054.
49. Markowitz, S., Wang, J., Myeroff, L., Parsons, R. E., Sun, L., Lutterbaugh, J., et al. (1995) Inactivation of the type II TGF-ß receptor in colon cancer cells with microsatellite instability. *Science* **268,** 1336–1338.
50. Rampino, N., Yamamoto, H., Ionov, Y., Li, Y., Sawai, H., Reed, J. C., et al. (1997) Somatic frameshift mutations in the *BAX* gene in colon cancers of the microsatellite mutator phenotype. *Science* **275,** 967–969.
51. Fishel, R., Lescoe, M. K., Rao, M. R. S., Copeland, N. G., Jenkins, N. A., Garber, J., et al. (1993) The human mutator gene homolog *MSH2* and its association with hereditary nonpolyposis colon cancer. *Cell* **75,** 1027–1038.
52. Papadopoulos, N., Nicolaides, N. C., Wei, Y-F., Ruben, S. M., Carter, K. C., Rosen, C. A., et al. (1994) Mutations of a *mutL* homolog in hereditary colon cancer. *Science* **263,** 1625–1629.
53. Leach, F. S., Nicolaides, N. C., Papadopoulos, N., Liu, B., Jen, J., Parsons, R., et al. (1993) Mutations of a *mutS* homolog in hereditary nonpolyposis colorectal cancer. *Cell* **75,** 1215–1225.
54. Nicolaides, N. C., Papadopoulos, N., Liu, B., Wei, Y.-F., Carter, K. C., Ruben, S. M., et al. (1994) Mutations of two *PMS* homologues in hereditary nonpolyposis colon cancer. *Nature* **371,** 75–80.
55. Liu, B., Nicolaides, N. C., Markowitz, S., Willson, J. K. V., Parsons, R. E., Jen, J., et al. (1995) Mismatch repair gene defects in sporadic colorectal cancers with microsatellite instability. *Nature Genet.* **9,** 48–55.
56. Baker, S. M., Plug, A. W., Prolla, T. A., Bronner, C. E., Harris, A. C., Yao, X., et al. (1996) Involvement of mouse *MLH1* in DNA mismatch repair and meiotic crossing over. *Nature Genet.* **13,** 336–342.
57. Han, H.J., Yanagisawa, A., Kato, Y., Park, J-G., and Nakamura, Y. (1993) Genetic instability in pancreatic cancer and poorly differentiated type of gastric cancer. *Cancer Res.* **53,** 5087–5089.
58. Risinger, J. I., Berchuck, A., Kohler, M. F., Watson, P., Lynch, H. T., and Boyd, J. (1993) Genetic instability of microsatellites in endometrial carcinoma. *Cancer Res.* **53,** 5100–5103.

59. Merlo, A., Mabry, M., Gabrielson, E., Vollmer, R., Baylin, S. B., and Sidransky, D. (1994) Frequent microsatellite instability in primary small cell lung cancer. *Cancer Res.* **54,** 2098–2101.
60. Wooster, R., Cleton-Jansen, A.-M., Collins, N., Mangion, J., Cornelis, R. S., Cooper, C. S., et al. (1994) Instability of short tandem repeats (microsatellites) in human cancers. *Nature Genet.* **6,** 152–156.
61. King, B. L., Carcangiu, M. L., Carter, D., Kiechle, M., Pfisterer, J., Pfleiderer, A., et al. (1995) Microsatellite instability in ovarian neoplasmas. *Br. J. Cancer* **72,** 376–382.
62. de Wind, N., Dekker, M., Berns, A., Radman, M., and te Riele, H. (1995) Inactivation of the mouse *Msh2* gene results in mismatch repair deficiency, methylation tolerance, hyper-recombination, and predisposition to cancer. *Cell* **82,** 321–330.
63. Reitmair, A. H., Schmits, R., Ewel, A., Bapat, B., Redston, M., Mitri, A., et al. (1995) *MSH2* deficient mice are viable and susceptible to lymphoid tumours. *Nature Genet.* **11,** 64–70.
64. Baker, S. M., Bronner C. E., Zhang, L., Plug, A. W., Robatzek, M., Warren, G., et al. (1995) Male mice defective in the DNA mismatch repair gene *PMS2* exhibit abnormal chromosome synapsis in meiosis. *Cell* **82,** 309–319.
65. Edelmann, W., Yang, K., Umar, A., Heyer, J., Lau, K., Fan, K., et al. (1997) Mutation in the mismatch repair gene Msh6 causes cancer susceptibility. *Cell* **91,** 467–477.
66. Griffin, S., Branch, P., Xu, Y.-Z., and Karran, P. (1994) DNA mismatch binding and incision at modified guanine bases by extracts of mammalian cells: implications for tolerance to DNA methylation damage. *Biochemistry* **33,** 4787–4793.
67. Kat, A., Thilly, W. G., Fang, W.-H., Longley, M. J., Li, G-M., and Modrich, P. (1993) An alkylation-tolerant, mutator human cell line is deficient in strand-specific mismatch repair. *Proc. Natl. Acad. Sci. USA* **90,** 6424–6428.
68. Swann, P. F., Waters, T. R., Moulton, D. C., Xu, Y-Z., Zheng, Q., Edwards, M., et al. (1996) Role of postreplicative DNA mismatch repair in the cytotoxic action of thioguanine. *Science* **273,** 1109–1111.
69. Waters, T. R. and Swann, P. F. (1997) Cytotoxic mechanism of 6-thioguanine: hMutSα, the human mismatch binding heterodimer, binds to DNA containing S^6-methylthioguanine. *Biochemistry* **36,** 2501–2506.
70. Fram, R. J., Cusick, P. S., Wilson, J. M., and Marinus, M. G. (1985) Mismatch repair of *cis*-diamminedichloroplatinum(II)-induced DNA damage. *Mol. Pharmacol.* **28,** 51–55.
71. Boyer, J. C., Umar, A., Risinger, J. I., Lipford, J. R., Kane, M., Yin, S., et al. (1995) Microsatellite instability, mismatch repair deficiency, and genetic defects in human cancer cell lines. *Cancer Res.* **55,** 6063–6070.
72. Koi, M., Umar, A., Chauhan, D. P., Cherian, S. P., Carethers, J. M., Kunkel, T. A., et al. (1994) Human chromosome 3 corrects mismatch repair deficiency and microsatellite instability and reduces *N*-methyl-*N'*-nitro-*N*-nitrosoguanidine tolerance in colon tumor cells with homozygous *hMLH1* mutation. *Cancer Res.* **54,** 4308–4312.
73. Umar, A., Koi, M., Risinger, J. I., Glaab, W. E., Tindall, K. R., Kolodner, R. D., et al. (1997) Correction of hypermutability, *N*-methyl-*N'*-nitro-*N*-nitrosoguanidine resistance, and defective DNA mismatch repair by introducing chromosome 2 into human tumor cells with mutations in *MSH2* and *MSH6*. *Cancer Res.* **57,** 3949–3955.
74. Fink, D., Nebel, S., Aebi, S., Zheng, H., Cenni, B., Nehmé, A., et al. (1996) The role of DNA mismatch repair in platinum drug resistance. *Cancer Res.* **56,** 4881–4886.
75. Fink, D., Nebel, S., Aebi, S., Nehmé, A., and Howell, S. B. (1997) Loss of DNA mismatch repair due to knockout of MSH2 or PMS2 results in resistance to cisplatin and carboplatin. *Int. J. Oncol.* **11,** 539–542.
76. Aebi, S., Fink, D., Gordon, R., Kim, H. K., Zheng, H., Fink, J. L., et al. (1997) Resistance to cytotoxic drugs in DNA mismatch repair-deficient cells. *Clin. Cancer Res.* **3,** 1763–1767.
77. Rode, P., Kupiec, N., Teicher, B., Emi, Y., and Bubley, G. (1996) The effect of a homozy-

gous *hMLH1* mutation on antitumor alkylating agent sensitivity. *Proc. Am. Assoc. Cancer Res.* **37,** 380.
78. Zamble, D. B. and Lippard, S. J. (1995) Cisplatin and DNA repair in cancer chemotherapy. *Trends Biochem. Sci.* **20,** 435–439.
79. Naredi, P., Heath, D. D., Enns, R. E., and Howell, S. B. (1995) Cross-resistance between cisplatin, antimony potassium tartrate, and arsenite in human tumor cells. *J. Clin. Invest.* **95,** 1193–1198.
80. Aebi, S., Kurdi-Haidar, B., Gordon, R., Cenni, B., Zheng, H., Fink, D., et al. (1996) Loss of DNA mismatch repair in acquired resistance to cisplatin. *Cancer Res.* **56,** 3087–3090.
81. Anthoney, D. A., McIlwrath, A. J., Gallagher, W. M., Edlin, A. R. M., and Brown, R. (1996) Microsatellite instability, apoptosis, and loss of p53 function in drug-resistant tumor cells. *Cancer Res.* **56,** 1374–1381.
82. Drummond, J. T., Anthoney, A., Brown, R., and Modrich, P. (1996) Cisplatin and Adriamycin resistance are associated with MutLα and mismatch repair deficiency in an ovarian tumor cell line. *J. Biol. Chem.* **271,** 19645–19648.
83. Mello, J. A., Acharya, S., Fishel, R., and Essigmann, J. M. (1996) The mismatch-repair protein hMSH2 binds selectively to DNA adducts of the anticancer drug cisplatin. *Chem. Biol.* **3,** 579–589.
84. Duckett, D. R., Drummond, J. T., Murchie, A. I. H., Reardon, J. T., Sancar, A., Lilley, D. M. J., et al. (1996) Human MutSα recognizes damaged DNA base pairs containing O^6-methylguanine, O^4-methylthymine, or the cisplatin-d(GpG) adduct. *Proc. Natl. Acad. Sci. USA* **93,** 6443–6447.
85. Yamada, M., O'Regan, E., Brown, R., and Karran, P. (1997) Selective recognition of a cisplatin-DNA adduct by human mismatch repair proteins. *Nucleic Acids Res.* **25,** 491–495.
86. Mu, D., Tursun, M., Duckett, D. R., Drummond, J. T., Modrich, P., and Sancar, A. (1997) Recognition and repair of compound DNA lesions (base damage and mismatch) by human mismatch repair and excision repair systems. *Mol. Cell Biol.* **17,** 760–769.
87. Nehmé, A., Baskaran, R., Aebi, S., Fink, D., Nebel, S., Cenni, B., et al. (1997) Differential induction of c-Jun NH_2-terminal kinase and c-Abl kinase in DNA mismatch repair-proficient and -deficient cells exposed to cisplatin. *Cancer Res.* **57,** 3253–3257.
88. Carethers, J. M., Hawn, M. T., Chauhan, D. P., Luce, M. C., Marra, G., Koi, M., et al. (1996) Competency in mismatch repair prohibits clonal expansion of cancer cells treated with *N*-methyl-*N'*-nitro-*N*-nitrosoguanidine. *J. Clin. Invest.* **98,** 199–206.
89. Hawn, M. T., Umar, A., Carethers, J. M., Marra, G., Kunkel, T. A., Boland, C. R., et al. (1995) Evidence for a connection between the mismatch repair system and the G_2 cell cycle checkpoint. *Cancer Res.* **55,** 3721–3725.
90. Brown, R., Hirst, G. L., Gallagher, W. M., McIlwrath, A. J., Margison, G. P., van der Zee, A. G. J., et al. (1997) hMLH1 expression and cellular responses of ovarian tumour cells to treatment with cytotoxic anticancer agents. *Oncogene* **15,** 45–52.
91. Risinger, J. I., Umar, A., Boyd, J., Berchuck, A., Kunkel, T. A., and Barrett, J. C. (1996) Mutation of *MSH3* in endometrial cancer and evidence for its functional role in heteroduplex repair. *Nature Genet.* **14,** 102–105.
92. Fink, D., Zheng, H., Nebel, S., Norris, P. S., Aebi, S., Lin, T-P., et al. (1997) *In vitro* and *in vivo* resistance to cisplatin in cells that have lost DNA mismatch repair. *Cancer Res.* **57,** 1841–1845.
93. Richards, B., Zhang, H., Phear, G., and Meuth, M. (1997) Conditional mutator phenotypes in hMSH2-deficient tumor cell lines. *Science* **277,** 1523–1526.
94. Branch, P., Aquilina, G., Bignami, M., and Karran, P. (1993) Defective mismatch binding and a mutator phenotype in cells tolerant to DNA damage. *Nature* **362,** 652–654.
95. Fink, D., Nebel, S., Norris, P. S., Baergen, R. N., Wilczynski, S. P., Costa, M. J., et al. (1998) Enrichment for DNA mismatch repair-deficient cells during treatment with cisplatin. *Int. J. Cancer* **77,** 741–746.

96. Fink, D., Nebel, S., Norris, P. S., Aebi, S., Kim, H. K., Haas, M., et al. (1998) The effect of different chemotherapeutic agents on the enrichment of DNA mismatch repair-deficient tumour cells. *Br. J. Cancer* **77,** 703–708.
97. de las Alas, M. M., Aebi, S., Fink, D., Howell, S. B., and Los, G. (1997) Loss of DNA mismatch repair: effects on the rate of mutation to drug resistance. *J. Natl. Cancer Inst.* **89,** 1537–1541.
98. Kinzler, K. W. and Vogelstein, B. (1996) Lessons from hereditary colorectal cancer. *Cell* **87,** 159–170.
99. Skipper, H. E., Schabel, F. M., and Lloyd, H. H. (1978) Experimental therapeutics and kinetics: selection and overgrowth of specifically and permanently drug-resistant tumor cells. *Semin. Hematol.* **15,** 207–219.
100. Tomlinson, I. P. M., Novelli, M. R., and Bodmer, W. F. (1996) The mutation rate and cancer. *Proc. Natl. Acad. Sci. USA* **93,** 14800–14803.
101. Loeb, L. A. (1994) Microsatellite instability: marker of a mutator phenotype in cancer. *Cancer Res.* **54,** 5059–5063.
102. Ben-Yehuda, D., Krichevsky, S., Caspi, O., Rund, D., Polliack, A., Abeliovich, D., et al. (1996) Microsatellite instability and p53 mutations in therapy-related leukemia suggest mutator phenotype. *Blood* **88,** 4296–4303.
103. Fujita, M., Enomoto, T., Yoshino, K., Nomura, T., Buzard, G. S., Inoue, M. and Okudaira, Y. (1995) Microsatellite instability and alterations in the *hMSH2* gene in human ovarian cancer. *Int. J. Cancer* **64,** 361–366.
104. Fink, D., Nebel, S., Aebi, S., Zheng, H., Kim, H. K., Christen, R. D. and Howell, S. B. (1997) Expression of the DNA mismatch repair proteins hMLH1 and hPMS2 in normal human tissues. *Br. J. Cancer* **76,** 890–893.
105. Thibodeau, S. N., French, A. J., Roche, P. C., Cunningham, J. M., Tester, D. J., Lindor, N. M., Moslein, G., Baker, S. M., Liskay, R. M., Burgart, L. J., Honchel, R. and Halling, K. C. (1996) Altered expression of hMSH2 and hMLH1 in tumors with microsatellite instability and genetic alterations in mismatch repair genes. *Cancer Res.* **56,** 4836–4840.
106. Lim, P. C., Tester, D., Cliby, W., Ziesmer, S. C., Roche, P. C., Hartmann, L., Thibodeau, S. N., Podratz, K. C. and Jenkins, R. B. (1996) Absence of mutations in DNA mismatch repair genes in sporadic endometrial tumors with microsatellite instability. *Clin. Cancer Res.* **2,** 1907–1911.
107. Fink, D., Aebi, S. and Howell, S. B. (1998) The role of DNA mismatch repair in drug resistance. *Clin. Cancer Res.* **4,** 1–6.

III CLINICAL ANTITUMOR ACTIVITY AND TOXICOLOGY OF PLATINUM DRUGS

8 Clinical Experience with Cisplatin and Carboplatin

Martin S. Highley and A. Hilary Calvert

CONTENTS

1. INTRODUCTION

Malignant disease is a major cause of mortality, killing approximately 25% of individuals in the Western world. The most common cancers are those originating in the lung, breast, colon, and rectum *(1)*. Improvements in curability and survival are dependent on advances in early detection, surgery, radiotherapy, and chemotherapy, but once widespread metastatic disease has become established chemotherapy is a central component of management. The era of chemotherapy commenced in the late 1940s and 1950s with the clinical introduction of the classical alkylating agents (e.g., nitrogen mustard, cyclophosphamide and melphalan), and antimetabolites [e.g., methotrexate and 5-fluorouracil (5-FU)], with a marked improvement in the treatment of lymphomas and leukemias. The next major advance was the appearance of cisplatin in 1972. Over the last 25 years the use of cisplatin and its less toxic analog carboplatin has influenced the chemotherapeutic management of many common solid tumors. As a result, metastatic germ cell tumors are now curable (Fig. 1), and the outlook for patients with ovarian cancer and certain childhood tumors has improved significantly. However, less impact has been made on

From: *Platinum-Based Drugs in Cancer Therapy*
Edited by: L. R. Kelland and N. Farrell © Humana Press Inc., Totowa, NJ

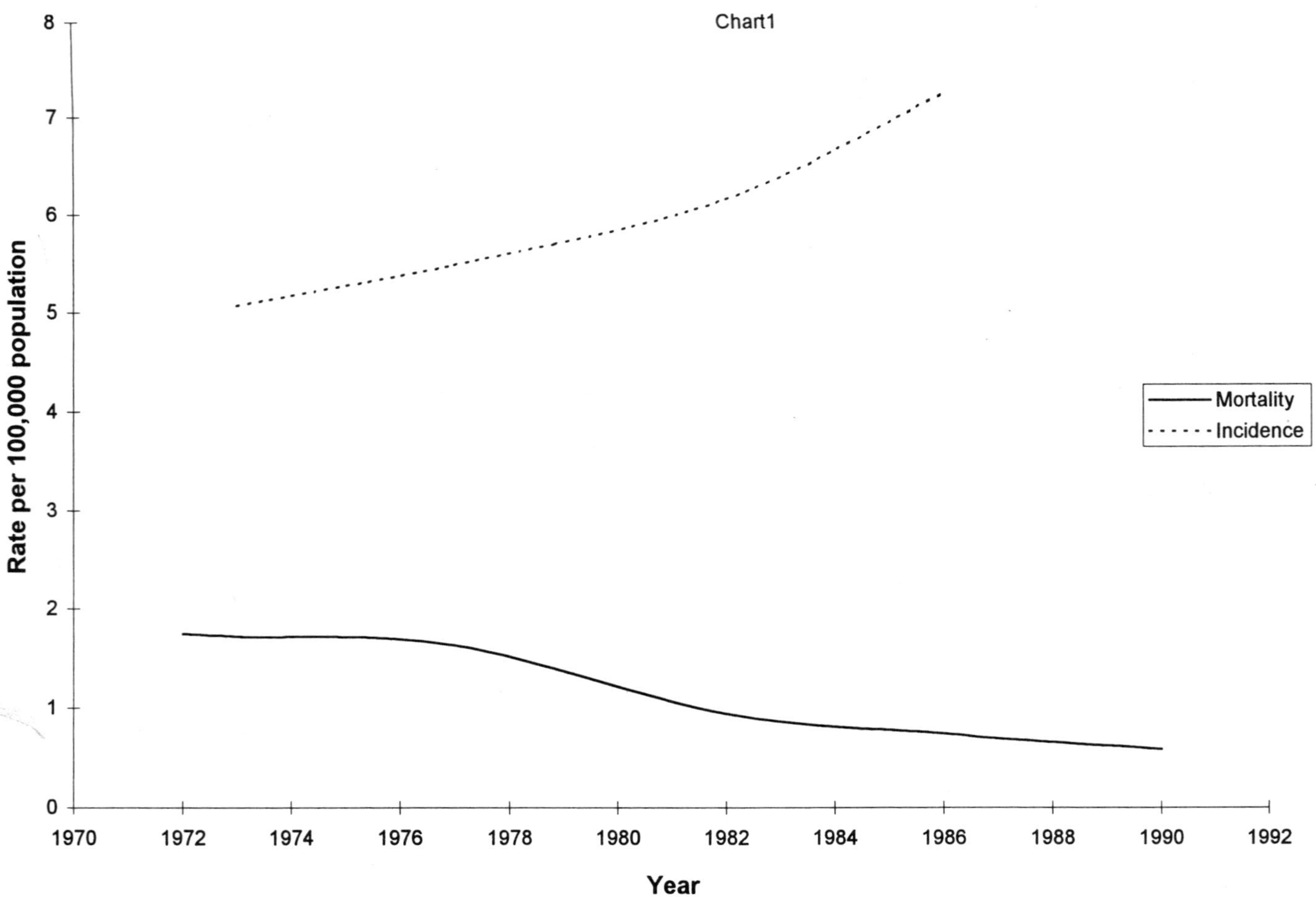

Fig. 1. Mortality and incidence of testicular cancer in England and Wales (ages 15–34 years, per 100,000 population).

other numerically more important tumors. This chapter discusses the clinical use of cisplatin and carboplatin, their toxicities, and their effects on different tumor types.

2. CISPLATIN TO CARBOPLATIN: A CHANGING TOXICITY PROFILE

The optimum use of cisplatin was at first hindered by dose-limiting nephrotoxicity. This was later minimized by hydration before and after, with or without mannitol, but even with standard doses the glomerular filtration rate (GFR) can decrease by 25% or more, a deterioration that may not be reversible and that may lead to an increased risk of hypertension. The need for rigorous hydration often restricts the use of cisplatin to in-patients. Cisplatin also causes a cumulative peripheral neuropathy, which although mainly sensory in nature can lead to motor impairment, presumably due to proprioceptive loss. Ototoxicity, in the form of tinnitus or high tone hearing loss as a result of destruction of the hair cells of the cochlea, is an additional problem. Persistent hypomagnesemia and hypocalcemia also occur and are more common in children. Other side effects remain troublesome, particularly severe nausea and vomiting, although their incidence and severity has been much reduced by the introduction of the 5-hydroxytriptamine$_3$ (5-HT$_3$) antagonists such as ondansetron. The relatively mild nature of the myelosuppression of cisplatin given at conventional doses is an advantage. In children, who are often cured with cisplatin-containing regimens, hearing and renal impairment can be a significant lifelong burden.

Soon after the introduction of cisplatin, the search was on for second-generation platinum derivatives with a more acceptable toxicity profile, and in 1988 carboplatin became routinely available. In cisplatin, a central platinum atom is surrounded by two chloride atoms and two ammonia molecules; in carboplatin the two chloride atoms are replaced by the 1,1-cyclobutanedicarboxylate moiety. To be effective, cisplatin must be activated by hydrolysis and loss of the chlorine atoms to produce a positive ion, which is highly electrophilic and capable of interacting with DNA. In carboplatin, the platinum atom is located in a six-membered ring, resulting in a lower rate of activation. Differences in the rate of activation lead to differences in toxicity; the more reactive cisplatin is more toxic than the less reactive carboplatin. Therefore, for clinical purposes, there is a window of reactivity for platinum complexes, currently represented by cisplatin and carboplatin. A compound more reactive than cisplatin will be unduly toxic; one less reactive than carboplatin would probably require such a high-dose that its use would be prevented by pharmaceutical considerations.

Carboplatin is associated with little or no renal toxicity so there is no need for hydration, facilitating its use in the out-patient setting. Peripheral neurotoxicity is rare, and nausea and vomiting are reduced compared with cisplatin. The incidence of hearing loss and tinnitus is lower than with cisplatin, although younger children, those with brain tumors, and those who have received cranial irradiation are more susceptible than other individuals. Ototoxicity in children has been reported to be moderate for 56% of patients receiving cisplatin and severe for 25%; among those receiving carboplatin, moderate and severe ototoxicity develop in 13% and 3%, respectively *(2)*. Carboplatin causes less hypomagnesemia and hypocalcemia than cisplatin, but more myelosuppression, particularly thrombocytopenia, which is dose limiting and usually manifests about 14 d after treatment. More severe thrombocytopenia and granulocytopenia occur in patients with a diminished GFR. Both cisplatin and carboplatin can cause allergic reactions, most often in the form of facial flushing, erythema, and pruritus. These usually occur during a rechallenge with platinum compounds, sometimes years after the initial exposure. Fertility after cisplatin or carboplatin administration has mainly been studied following the treatment of testicular cancers. At cumulative doses of more than 400 mg/m^2 cisplatin, irreversible impairment of gonadal function is likely. There is a significantly higher chance of recovery for carboplatin-treated patients, compared with those who receive cisplatin.

In clinical practice, peripheral neuropathy, ototoxicity, and renal impairment are usually reversible up to a certain point, and dosages are therefore modified if changes develop in baseline GFRs, or audiograms, or if there is progressive clinical peripheral neuropathy. Experience with cisplatin has defined the tumor types most appropriate for platinum therapy, and carboplatin has tended to establish itself as a substitute for cisplatin, usually as a result of a more favorable toxicity profile.

3. THE IMPORTANCE OF PHARMACOKINETICS

Carboplatin is less protein bound than cisplatin and is primarily eliminated by renal excretion, entirely through glomerular filtration. The maximum concentration of free drug in the plasma (C_{max}), clearance of free drug, and the area under the free drug plasma concentration-time curve (AUC) are important pharmacokinetic parameters of carboplatin and cisplatin. The AUC of carboplatin permits the prediction of thrombocytopenia, although the exact relationship alters with successive cycles on account of cumulative bone marrow toxicity. Calculating doses to produce moderate to severe myelosuppression aids dose optimization. The simpler pharmacokinetics of carboplatin permitted Calvert et al. *(3)* to derive a relationship among dose, AUC, and GFR (Eq. [1], the Calvert formula), showing that the dose of carboplatin can be optimally and individually determined from the GFR.

$$\text{dose of carboplatin (mg)} = \text{target AUC (GFR + 25)}. \quad [1]$$

Further evidence of this principle is provided by retrospective studies. Jodrell et al. *(4)* compared the Calvert-derived AUC for the initial cycle of single-agent carboplatin and subsequent myelosuppression in 450 untreated and 578 previously treated patients with ovarian cancer. There was a significant correlation between calculated AUC and thrombocytopenia and leukopenia. Once AUC was accounted for, the only other pretreatment factors affecting toxicity were performance status and pretreatment with other cytotoxic agents. There was also a relationship between calculated AUC and antitumor response rate, although the response rate tended to reach a plateau at AUCs exceeding about 5 mg/mL × min. A similar relationship exists within the pediatric population, and the GFR has also been used to estimate the dose of carboplatin necessary to obtain an AUC of 4–6 for children with malignant germ cell tumors *(5)*.

The dose of carboplatin can therefore be considered in terms of the AUC, which is a measure of carboplatin exposure. The introduction of the AUC as a dosing unit was a novel concept, an improvement on dosing by surface area, allowing the reduction of toxicity. The determination of carboplatin doses using AUC methods has now been almost universally accepted. Ideally the GFR, uncorrected for surface area, is determined using ^{51}Cr-labeled ethylenediamine tetraacetic acid (EDTA) clearance. However other methods of estimating GFR, such as the Cockcroft and Gault formula (Eq. [2]) *(6)*, or 24-h creatinine clearance assessments (Eq. [3]) can also be used, but are less accurate when dealing with individuals with very low or very high GFRs.

$$\mathrm{GFR} = C\,(140 - \mathrm{A})\,W/P \qquad [2]$$

where C = constant (1.23 in males and 1.05 in females), A = age (years), W = weight (kg), and P = serum creatinine (μ*M/L)*.

$$\mathrm{GFR} = UV/P \qquad [3]$$

where V = volume of urine produced in 24 h, U = concentration of creatinine in urine, and P = serum creatinine.

In early work with carboplatin, 400 mg/m^2 was regarded as the standard dose, based on surface area. With the development of AUC-derived dosing, an AUC of 7 repeated once every 4 weeks is now common practice when carboplatin is administered as a single agent, and an AUC of 5 is used in combination regimens. AUCs of 4–6 are usually employed in patients who have been moderately or heavily pretreated, or when a 3-weekly regimen is given. The standard dose of cisplatin as a single agent is 75 or 100 mg/m^2 given every 3 weeks.

The use of infusional therapy has increased steadily since 1983, as it has become evident that continuous exposure of tissues to chemotherapeutic agents leads to altered properties. Most work has been performed with 5-FU, but both cisplatin and carboplatin have been administered by prolonged continuous intravenous infusion. However an improvement in the therapeutic index has usually not been observed, and dose-limiting toxicities are not changed. Smit et al. *(7)* gave a 21-d infusion of carboplatin with a maximum tolerated dose of 30 mg/m^2/d, and 6 weeks between treatments. The major toxicities were myelosuppression and decreased GFRs.

4. THE USE OF CISPLATIN AND CARBOPLATIN IN DIFFERENT TUMOR TYPES

4.1. Germ Cell Tumors

4.1.1. Teratoma

Before 1975, teratoma patients with bulky abdominal lymphadenopathy or advanced metastatic disease were rarely cured. Einhorn and Donohue *(8)* were the first to use cisplatin, in combination with vinblastine and bleomycin (PVB), in malignant teratoma, with astounding success. The routine use of cisplatin-based combination regimens, frequently BEP (Table 1), now commonly leads to a cure.

In assessing the activity of treatment regimens, the terms complete response and partial response are used. A complete response (CR) is defined as the complete disappearance of all objective evidence of disease (physical or radiologic), lasting at least 1 month. A partial response (PR) is defined as a decrease in the sum of the product of perpendicular diameters of measurable lesions of at least 50%, lasting at least 1 month. Duration of response and survival are other important indicators of activity.

The Medical Research Council (MRC) and the European Organisation for Research and Treatment of Cancer (EORTC) have investigated the use of carboplatin, etoposide, and bleomycin in good-prognosis teratoma patients *(9)*. In all, 598 patients were randomized to receive four cycles of BEP or CEB (carboplatin AUC 5 in place of the cisplatin); 94.4% of patients treated with BEP had a complete response compared with 87.3% in the carboplatin arm (p = 0.009). More treatment failures were seen in the carboplatin-treated patients, and it was concluded that combination chemotherapy based on carboplatin was inferior to that based on cisplatin. Interestingly, a study of a group of patients treated with this regimen showed a very strong correlation between relapse rate and retrospectively calculated AUC, with virtually all the relapses occurring in patients who had received an AUC of less than 5, suggesting that inadequate carboplatin dosage may be an important factor in these trials *(10)*. Bleomycin can cause problems with lung toxicity and the cisplatin plus etoposide (EP) combination has also been investigated. A randomized study comparing EP with etoposide plus carboplatin (EC) has also favored the cisplatin combination, although carboplatin doses were based on surface area *(11)*. Event-free and relapse-free survival were inferior for patients given EC, and myelosuppression was more severe, possibly because many patients receiving carboplatin had a calculated AUC greater than 5.

4.1.2. Seminoma

Combination regimens containing cisplatin are also very effective against metastatic seminoma *(12)*, although the high radiosensitivity of this condition and frequent solitary regional spread has resulted in less experience with plat-

Table 1
Examples of Common Treatment Regimens Containing Cisplatin or Carboplatin

Malignancy	*Regimen*
Teratoma and seminoma	**BEP** Bleomycin 30 U d 2 Etoposide 120 mg/m^2 d 1–3 Cisplatin 50 mg/m^2 d 1–2 Every 3 weeks, for 4 cycles
Ovarian carcinoma	Cisplatin 75 mg/m^2 d 1 + Taxol 135 mg/m^2 d 1 or Carboplatin AUC 5 d 1 + Taxol 175 mg/m^2 d 1 Every 3 weeks, for 6 cycles
SCLC	Carboplatin AUC 5 d 1 + Etoposide 100 mg/m^2 d 1–3 Every 3 weeks, for 6 cycles
NSCLC	**MIC** Mitomycin C 6 mg/m^2 d 1 Ifosfamide 3 g/m^2 d 1 Cisplatin 50 mg/m^2 d 1 Every 3 weeks, for 4–6 cycles
Head and neck cancer	Cisplatin 100 mg/m^2 d 1 5-FU infusion 1000 mg/m^2/d, d 1–4 Every 3 weeks, for 6 cycles
Transitional cell carcinoma of the bladder/urinary tract	**MVAC** Methotrexate 30 mg/m^2 d 1, 15, and 22 Vinblastine 3 mg/m^2 d 2, 15, and 22 Adriamycin 30 mg/m^2 d 2 Cisplatin 70 mg/m^2 d 2 Every 4 weeks, for 4–6 cycles
Cervical carcinoma	**BIP** Bleomycin 30 mg d 1 Ifosfamide 5 g/m^2 d 2 Cisplatin 50 mg/m^2 d 2 Every 3 weeks, for 4–6 cycles
Gastric carcinoma	**ECF** Epirubicin 50 mg/m^2 Cisplatin 60 mg/m^2 5-FU 200 mg/m^2/d by continuous infusion Every 3 weeks, for 6–8 cycles

inum-based treatment than in teratoma. However, with large-volume retroperitoneal disease, radiotherapy can lead to a higher recurrence rate and an increased risk of renal damage. Platinum-based combination chemotherapy is now used in patients with abdominal masses more than 5 cm in diameter, supradiaphragmatic node metastases, or extranodal metastases. A variety of cisplatin-based combinations, e.g., BEP, EP, and PVB, have a high success rate, with 70–90% of patients achieving prolonged progression-free survival. There is as yet no evidence to suggest that carboplatin is inferior to cisplatin in the treatment of seminoma, unlike the situation in teratoma. The substitution of carboplatin is of major importance since the cure rate is high, the treated population is young, and the severity of some side effects is worsened by their chronicity, the full effect of which has yet to be expressed. Single-agent carboplatin is also effective in the adjuvant treatment of stage I seminoma. Oliver et al. *(13)* treated 78 patients with one or two cycles of carboplatin and experienced only one relapse after a median follow-up of 44 months; and the MRC is currently comparing adjuvant carboplatin with radiotherapy in a Phase III trial.

4.2. Ovarian cancer

There has been a significant increase in the 5-year survival rate from ovarian cancer over the last 25 years, and the introduction of cisplatin in advanced disease has been a contributory factor. Despite this improvement, however, most patients with advanced epithelial ovarian cancer still die of their disease; the 5-year survival rate for patients with stage III disease remains between 15 and 30%, and fewer than 5% of patients with stage IV disease live for 5 years. A metaanalysis of 8139 patients in 45 trials, performed by the Advanced Ovarian Cancer Trialists Group, investigated the effectiveness of platinum compounds as single agents or as components of combination chemotherapy in advanced disease *(14)*. Although firm conclusions concerning the most effective forms of treatment for advanced ovarian cancer were not reached, the results suggested that in terms of survival, immediate platinum-based treatment was superior to nonplatinum regimens, platinum in combination was better than single-agent platinum when used in the same dose, and cisplatin and carboplatin were equally effective. Platinum-based therapy is now regarded as standard treatment and is also used in the adjuvant setting.

To improve survival, studies of the effect of platinum dose intensity have been conducted in advanced ovarian cancer. In vitro studies suggest that a 10-fold increase in dose is required to influence response and survival *(15)*. Dose-response relationships have usually been demonstrated in randomized trials *(16,17)*, although their overall significance remains in some doubt. Kaye et al. *(16)* investigated six cycles of cyclophosphamide 750 mg/m^2 with either high-dose (100 mg/m^2) or low-dose (50 mg/m^2) cisplatin. Survival benefit was evident after 2 years for the high-dose arm, but after 4 years of follow-up the difference was much less marked, whereas neurotoxicity was more persistent after higher cisplatin doses. A survival advantage for an intense high-dose regimen (120 mg/m^2 vs 60 mg/m^2, every 3–4 weeks) was also observed in a smaller randomized trial *(18)*. In contrast, McGuire et al. *(19)* compared eight doses of cisplatin 50 mg/m^2 plus cyclophosphamide 500 mg/m^2 with four doses of cisplatin 100 mg/m^2 plus cyclophosphamide 1000 mg/m^2, (the same total dose of both drugs), with no significant difference in response or survival. Perhaps the total dose of cisplatin given over 18–24 weeks is more important for survival than the average weekly cisplatin dose intensity.

Retrospectively calculated increases in carboplatin AUC values are associated with significant improvements in overall objective response rates *(4)*. Calvert et al. *(20)* determined the maximum tolerated AUC of carboplatin given every 2 weeks for 4 courses. Recombinant human granulocyte colony-stimulating factor was used to support the leukocyte count, and platelet transfusions were given as necessary. They demonstrated that the AUC intensity of carboplatin administration can be approximately doubled compared with standard treatment (400 mg/m^2 every 4 weeks or AUC 7 every 4 weeks) with an acceptable level of toxicity. However, the incidence of thrombocytopenia, very low up to an AUC of 7 every 2 weeks, increased abruptly for higher AUCs. It was suggested that a further increase in AUC might be possible by using a more effective method of platelet support. A prospective investigation using an AUC of 12 every 4 weeks compared with an AUC of 6 every 4 weeks *(21)* showed that there was little difference in disease-free or overall survival although the administered dose intensity of the high-dose arm was only 30% higher than that of the control arm, owing to toxicity causing dose delays. A further study compared an AUC of 4 with an AUC of 8 in 222 patients and did not demonstrate any difference in the outcome between the two groups *(22)*.

Prior response to cisplatin therapy influences the likelihood of a secondary response to carboplatin. Studies suggest significant cross-resistance between cisplatin and carboplatin in patients with ovarian cancer and response rates of less than 5% in disease resistant to cisplatin. Gore et al. *(23)* studied 54 patients following remission with cisplatin or carboplatin. On relapse they were given the same agent or the alternative platinum compound; no differences in response rate or survival were observed. However, the progression-free interval dictated response to second-line treatment. If relapse occurred less than 18 months after initial treatment, the response rate was 17%, compared with 53% if relapse occurred later, when a doubling of median survival following second-line therapy was also observed.

Combination regimens containing cisplatin in advanced disease are associated with overall responses of 60–80% and CRs of around 50%. Cisplatin with cyclophosphamide was initially the standard combination treatment for advanced ovarian cancer, but comparative studies of cisplatin 100 mg/m^2 + cyclophosphamide 600 mg/m^2 *(24)* or cisplatin 75 mg/m^2 + cyclophosphamide 600 mg/m^2 *(25)* vs carboplatin 300 mg/m^2 + cyclophosphamide 600 mg/m^2 have shown that the combination of carboplatin and cyclophosphamide is equivalent. The importance of not climbing the shoulder of the dose-response curve is seen in the results of a clinical trial comparing carboplatin plus cyclophosphamide with cisplatin plus cyclophosphamide in previously untreated patients with primarily suboptimal stage III or IV ovarian cancer *(26)*. Using a low carboplatin dose of 150 mg/m^2 every 3 weeks, carboplatin plus cyclophosphamide was associated with a lower progression-free interval and decreased survival compared with cisplatin plus cyclophosphamide. The second International Collaborative Ovarian Neoplasm study (ICON 2) compared cyclophosphamide (500 mg/m^2) plus Adriamycin (50 mg/m^2) plus cisplatin (50 mg/m^2) (CAP) with single-agent carboplatin (AUC 5) in 1526 patients with previously untreated ovarian cancer *(27)*. The results showed a median survival of 33 months and a 2-year survival of 60% for both groups. There was no evidence that CAP or carboplatin were more or less effective in different subgroups defined by age, stage, residual disease, differentiation, histology, or center. CAP was more toxic, causing more alopecia, leukopenia, and nausea but less thrombocytopenia. These results suggested that there was no advantage of CAP compared with single-agent carboplatin.

In contrast to combinations of platinum drugs with anthracyclines or alkylating agents, trials examining combinations with paclitaxel have been more consistent in demonstrating an improvement in outcome. A randomized comparison of cisplatin 75 mg/m^2 plus cyclophosphamide 600 mg/m^2 compared with cisplatin 75 mg/m^2 plus paclitaxel 135 mg/m^2 given over 24 h, showed significantly improved response rates, progression-free survival (13 vs 18 months), and overall survival (24 vs 38 months) *(28)*. This result has been confirmed in an independent study of similar design except that paclitaxel was infused over 3 h *(29)*. A further comparison of cisplatin and carboplatin, both given in combination with paclitaxel, has shown that the two treatments are equally effective, but that the carboplatin arm is significantly less toxic *(30)*. It is also of interest that the combination of carboplatin and paclitaxel seems to be associated with less thrombocytopenia than the use of single-agent carboplatin, suggesting that the paclitaxel has a protective effect on carboplatin-induced thrombocytopenia *(31)*. These results have focused interest on the combination of carboplatin and paclitaxel, which is currently the most widely used regimen for the treatment of ovarian cancer, and is also extremely popular in other histologies.

Both cisplatin and carboplatin can be given intraperitoneally. Responses are uncommon in patients with tumor nodules greater than 0.5–1 cm, and even when residual disease is of small volume they are unlikely unless a PR to initial systemic therapy containing platinum is obtained; one-third of such systemically sensitive patients enter a CR following salvage intraperitoneal cisplatin or carboplatin treatment. A retrospective analysis of patients with microscopic disease achieving a surgically documented CR with cisplatin or carboplatin therapy showed no overall difference, but lower rates were seen in patients with small-volume macroscopic disease (maximum tumor diameter less than 0.5 cm) treated with carboplatin *(32)*. A recent randomized study comparing intraperitoneal cisplatin with intravenous cisplatin, given with cyclophosphamide in chemotherapy naive patients with stage III ovarian cancer, found a longer median survival in the intraperitoneal cisplatin group (49 vs 41 months) *(33)*. This advantage was not influenced by the extent of residual disease.

4.3. Pediatric Malignancies

Cisplatin is used in more than half of children suffering from malignant disease and is a valuable component of front-line therapy for intracranial tumors, neuroblastoma, sarcomas, retinoblastomas, germ cell tumors and hepatoblastoma. It has also been used in salvage regimens for these tumors and for other common pediatric malignancies such as Hodgkin's lymphoma, non-Hodgkin's lymphoma and Wilms' tumor. Neuroblastoma, Wilms' tumor, rhabdomyosarcoma, and Ewing's sarcoma have shown some sensitivity to carboplatin. A 50% single-agent response rate to carboplatin in Wilms tumor is similar to those seen with older nonplatinum regimens. Primary osteosarcomas are most common in children and young adults, and cisplatin produces regression in 15–20% of patients with metastatic osteosarcoma. Carboplatin seems to have less activity than cisplatin in this condition, possibly because patients treated with carboplatin have usually received prior cisplatin. Platinum compounds have not found a place in the first-line treatment of leukemias, but activity to single-agent carboplatin has been seen in adult patients with relapsed or refractory acute non-lymphocytic leukemia, with response rates of 29% and 44% *(34,35)*. A median duration of response of greater than 6 months has been reported, with three CRs persisting for longer than 12 months *(34)*.

Carboplatin penetrates the blood-brain barrier more readily than cisplatin, with cerebrospinal fluid to plasma ultrafiltrate AUC ratios of approximately 30%, and single-agent carboplatin has activity in pediatric brain tumors, particularly medulloblastoma and ependymoma. In a summary of Phase II data, Gaynon *(36)* described response rates of 30% for medulloblastoma, 18% for ependymoma, 6% for brainstem glioma, 7% for low-grade astrocytoma, and 5% for high-grade astrocytoma. One trial found a PR rate of 73% for astrocytoma, but the tumor grade was not stated. For cisplatin, response rates of 44, 0, and 11% were seen in medulloblastoma, brainstem glioma, and malignant astrocytoma, respectively. A number of children achieve a prolonged period of stable disease following carboplatin, but whether this is a true effect of carboplatin or the natural history of a subset of children with more slowly growing malignancies is uncertain.

4.4. Lung Cancer

4.4.1. Small Cell Lung Cancer

Small cell lung cancer (SCLC) metastasizes early during development but is a highly chemosensitive tumor. Although good responses and improvements in survival are often seen, relapse can occur soon after stopping chemotherapy. Only 3% of patients achieve a cure, and these may represent a particular biologic subgroup. In those with limited stage disease, (tumor confined to one hemithorax with or without ipsilateral supraclavicular lymphadenopathy or a pleural effusion), chemotherapy is given with radiotherapy. Chemotherapeutic agents may enhance the activity of radiotherapy at the primary site by radiosensitization or additional direct cytotoxicity, and both carboplatin and cisplatin are radiosensitizers.

It became apparent during the 1980s that cisplatin was one of the most active chemotherapeutic agents in all types of lung cancer. Cisplatin and carboplatin have a similar spectrum of activity, but the lower toxicity of the latter has led to its increasing usage. In 1985 Smith et al. *(37)* described the use of single-agent carboplatin in previously untreated patients with SCLC, with a response rate of 60%. Subsequent Phase I and II trials confirmed CRs in approximately 10–30% of previously untreated patients, with an overall response rate of approximately 40–70%. Corresponding figures in patients who have received prior chemotherapy are approximately 5 and 20%, respectively.

The binary combination of platinum compound and etoposide is a widely used regimen in SCLC. Carboplatin plus etoposide is associated with CR rates of between 30 and 40%, overall response rates of 80%, and median survivals of 9–15 months in patients with limited disease, whereas in those with extensive disease lower CR rates of 9–13%, overall response rates of approximately 70%, and median survivals of 8–9 months are usual. One study compared etoposide 300 mg/m^2 on d 1–3 plus cisplatin 50 mg/m^2 on d 1–2 with etoposide 300 mg/m^2 on d 1–3 plus carboplatin 300 mg/m^2 on d 1, given every three weeks, with no difference in efficacy *(38)*.

In an attempt to improve these figures, dose intensity has been increased, but cure rates have not improved. In nonrandomized trials objective response rates are better, but toxicity is worse, and there is no survival benefit. More intensive combination chemotherapy has been investigated, and Smith et al. *(39)* have reported a 94% overall response rate, with 72% CRs, in patients with limited disease using the carboplatin plus etoposide plus ifosfamide combination. Toxicity was substantial and improvement in survival only modest. High-dose carboplatin (800–1600 mg/m^2) has been used successfully without the need for bone marrow support, but again significant toxicity resulted *(40)*.

4.4.2. Non-Small Cell Lung Cancer

In contrast to SCLC, non-small cell lung cancer (NSCLC) often remains localized to its primary site and the surgical approach, in the early stage of the disease process, offers the best chance of cure. Surgery is appropriate in stages I–IIIA. In stage IIIA disease metastases are present in ipsilateral mediastinal and/or subcarinal lymph nodes. Stage IIIB NSCLC involves contralateral mediastinal or hilar nodes, or scalene or supraclavicular nodes, or invades central structures in the chest, and management is less well defined. The role of neoadjuvant therapy in stage III disease—attempting to reduce tumor burden, thereby making the patient operable—has been of considerable interest in recent years. Those with stage IV disease and distant metastases are managed with chemotherapy, although NSCLC is less chemosensitive than SCLC. Radiotherapy is important in stage III disease and also in the palliative setting.

Cisplatin-based regimens have proved important in most stages of NSCLC. Survival has been improved when cisplatin is given postoperatively to those with stage II or IIIA disease, with radiotherapy in stage IIIB disease, or alone in stage IV disease. Cisplatin is one of the most active agents in NSCLC with an overall response rate of about 20%, which is increased with doses higher than 100 mg/m^2. Studies of carboplatin have recorded a 10% response rate, lower than that achieved with cisplatin, but suboptimal dosing may be a factor. In trials evaluating carboplatin combinations in advanced NSCLC, response rates range from 9–38% and median survival from 17–38 weeks. These results are similar to those obtained with regimens not containing carboplatin. A prospective, randomized Phase III trial compared etoposide (100 mg/m^2 d 1–3) plus cisplatin (120 mg/m^2 d 1) with etoposide plus carboplatin (325 mg/m^2 d 1); response rate (27 vs 16%, $p = 0.07$) and median survival (30 vs 27 weeks) were similar *(41)*. The carboplatin combination was better tolerated. Many Phase II trials have suggested that three-drug regimens are more effective than two-drug regimens, but this has not been confirmed in the Phase III setting.

The Non-Small Cell Lung Cancer Collaborative Group has performed a metaanalysis of 9387 patients from 52 randomized trials to evaluate the effect of chemotherapy on survival *(42)*. They found that cisplatin-containing regimens favored chemotherapy, significantly so when used with radical radiotherapy and supportive care.

More recently it has been shown that various combinations of cisplatin or carboplatin, in particular the combination of cisplatin and paclitaxel, but also combinations with gemcitabine, docetaxel, navelbine, and irinotecan can also prolong survival in NSCLC (reviewed in ref. *43*). Carboplatin in combination with paclitaxel has been reported to have response rates in the region of 30–60% *(44)*, although a preliminary report of a randomized trial comparing this combination with the more conventional cisplatin/etoposide regimen does not currently show a difference in survival *(45)*.

Combined chemoradiotherapy in locally advanced NSCLC has increased in importance over the last few years. Survival benefit may result from control of local disease from radiotherapy, or metastatic disease from chemotherapy. Several studies have suggested that chemotherapy followed by thoracic irradiation is superior to radiotherapy alone, in terms of both survival and the development of distant metastases. The administration of cisplatin immediately before radiotherapy appears to maximize radiation enhancement, particularly when multiple fractions of radiation are given. In one study patients received either vinblastine plus cisplatin followed by radiotherapy, or radiotherapy alone *(46)*. Those in the chemotherapy group had a median survival of 14 months, compared with 10 months for those given radiotherapy alone. In a comparison of radiotherapy with radiotherapy plus cisplatin, given either weekly or daily, to inoperable patients, survival was significantly improved in the radiotherapy plus daily cisplatin group (1-, 2-, and 3- year survivals of 54, 26 and 16%, respectively) compared with the radiotherapy-only group (respective survivals of 46, 13, and 2%) *(47)*. The survival benefit of daily combined treatment resulted from improved control of local disease. Less work has been performed investigating carboplatin plus radiotherapy combinations, but an early study suggested a response rate of 33% in stage III inoperable disease using concurrent carboplatin and radiotherapy *(48)*.

The neoadjuvant approach has also been assessed. Rosell et al. *(49)* performed a randomized trial comparing preoperative chemotherapy plus surgery with surgery alone in patients with stage IIIA disease. Chemotherapy comprised three cycles of the MIC regimen (See Table 1). All patients received mediastinal irradiation after surgery. Although only 60 patients were included, the median survival was 26 months in patients given chemotherapy before surgery, compared with 8 months in patients treated with surgery alone ($p < 0.001$). The median disease-free survival was also significantly different; 20 months with chemotherapy compared with 5 months without.

4.5. Head and Neck Cancer

It became apparent in the mid 1970s that cisplatin was a highly effective drug in the treatment of squamous cell carcinoma of the head and neck. The influence of platinum compounds is substantial, and cisplatin and carboplatin are now among the most commonly used single agents in the palliation of recurrent disease. The addition of 5-FU has increased response rates but not survival. Chemoradiotherapy incorporating cisplatin-based regimens have been investigated since the early 1980s.

Most chemoradiotherapy studies have employed cisplatin with 5-FU, and it is accepted that cisplatin and infusional 5-FU (Table 1) is the safest and most active combination. Cisplatin does not produce mucositis and is one of the better radiopotentiators and sensitizers. Studies indicate a higher clinical CR rate, extended duration of disease-free survival, and possibly improved overall survival, for patients treated with chemoradiotherapy rather than radiotherapy alone. There is no survival difference giving cisplatin and then 5-FU sequentially, rather than simultaneously, but improved regional control is seen with simultaneous administration in stage III disease. Merlano et al. *(50)* compared alternating courses of chemotherapy (cisplatin plus 5-FU) and radiotherapy with radiotherapy alone, in patients with unresectable disease, finding better local control and disease-free survival, and unusually, a survival advantage for the combined treatment approach. A comparison of radiotherapy alone with radiotherapy and cisplatin 20 mg/m^2/week showed a significantly higher overall response rate in patients receiving cisplatin (73 vs 59%), but there was no difference in CR rate or survival *(51)*. A higher dose of cisplatin, 100 mg/m^2 every 3 weeks, given during radiotherapy has produced a CR rate of 71% *(52)*.

Cisplatin and 5-FU has also been used as adjuvant therapy. In one study patients with resected stage III or IV squamous cell carcinoma of the oral cavity, oropharynx, hypopharynx, or larynx and negative margins of resection, were given immediate radiotherapy or three cycles of adjuvant cisplatin plus 5-FU followed by radiotherapy *(53)*. No difference in disease-free or overall survival was observed, but the development of distant metastases was less likely following chemotherapy.

The activity of carboplatin is comparable to that of cisplatin in patients with recurrent and metastatic head and neck tumors. Nutritional support is vital in head and neck cancer patients, and the less severe nausea and vomiting with carboplatin is an important factor. Carboplatin with concomitant radiotherapy has been evaluated. Fractionating the carboplatin dose is less myelosuppressive than bolus dosing. A study of 103 patients with advanced head and neck carcinoma treated with radiotherapy plus carboplatin 60–70 mg/m^2/d, d 1–5 and 29–33, showed 1- and 2-year survival rates of 77 and 53%, respectively *(54)*. Phase I studies with carboplatin and simultaneous radiotherapy have produced results comparable to those reported with cisplatin and cisplatin plus 5-FU regimens and radiotherapy.

Cisplatin plus 5-FU, carboplatin plus 5-FU, and cisplatin plus 5-FU plus leucovorin (PFL) are commonly used in the neoadjuvant setting. The overall response rates (approximately 80%) and CR rates (approximately 35%) are similar, but there is considerable variation in toxicity; carboplatin plus 5-FU is tolerated the most easily, and PFL is the most toxic. The use of neoadjuvant cisplatin plus 5-FU infusion and radiotherapy allows laryngeal preservation in two-thirds of treated patients. Although there is a higher rate of local recurrence compared with laryngectomy and postoperative radiotherapy, there is a lower rate of distant metastases.

4.6. Bladder Cancer

Cisplatin and carboplatin are two of the most effective single agents in the treatment of bladder cancer, and they form the basis of most combination chemotherapy regimens. Cisplatin is associated with a response rate of 17–40%, but toxicity is a problem, particularly nephrotoxicity, which can be aggravated by ureteric obstruction. The results of single-agent carboplatin in bladder cancer have been variable. In one study 25 patients with locally advanced or metastatic urothelial cancer were treated with 400–450 mg/m^2 carboplatin every four weeks, producing two CRs *(55)*, whereas other trials have generated negative results.

Combination chemotherapy is regarded as more effective than single-agent treatment, and such combinations should contain a platinum analog. However, MVAC (see Table 1) is the only combination protocol that has been shown to be superior to single-agent cisplatin. In one study, 39% of patients given MVAC responded, with a median survival of 12.5 months *(56)*; corresponding figures for cisplatin alone were 12% and 8.2 months. The binary combinations of cisplatin and methotrexate, and cisplatin and Adriamycin, are no better than cisplatin alone. Cisplatin is preferred, as the evidence of equivalence with carboplatin is not as strong as with other tumors. A randomized study comparing MVEC (methotrexate, vinblastine, epirubicin, and cisplatin) with M-VEC (methotrexate, vinblastine, epirubicin, and carboplatin) yielded an overall response rate of 71% in the cisplatin arm compared with 41% in the carboplatin-treated patients *(57)*. Unfortunately, the toxicities of the MVAC regimen are considerable, and the MVMJ regimen, substituting the less cardiotoxic mitoxantrone for Adriamycin and carboplatin for cisplatin, has been used successfully *(58)*. For a more detailed discussion of randomized trials comparing cisplatin with carboplatin in bladder, germ cell, ovarian, lung, and head and neck malignancies, the reader is referred to a recent review of the literature *(59)*.

4.7. Cervical Cancer

Platinum compounds have been investigated extensively as single agents in cervical cancer, and with treatment every three weeks there is a slight advantage with cisplatin doses of 100 mg/m^2 compared with 50 mg/m^2. However, despite consistent activity in phase II trials, response rates have not exceeded 30–40%. Furthermore, the duration of response and survival following single-agent therapy are relatively brief at 6–9 months, except in a small subset (less than 10%) of patients who achieve a CR. The combination of bleomycin, ifosfamide, and cisplatin (BIP) (Table 1) has become popular, with overall response rates of up to 69%, although combination chemotherapy has not yet been shown to be superior to single-agent therapy in a randomized trial. The addition of 5-FU to cisplatin has not resulted in a higher response rate or longer response duration or longer survival compared with cisplatin alone. A 32% response rate has been seen with doxorubicin and cisplatin.

4.7. Breast cancer

Metastatic breast cancer remains a common disease, with an incidence of approximately 22,000 cases per year in the United Kingdom. Standard regimens often produce a remission, but patients with widespread metastatic disease are rarely cured. Single-agent cisplatin, used first line in metastatic breast cancer, has shown activity with overall responses of about 50%, and a median duration of response of 4–5 months. Phase III trials of cisplatin-containing regimens, testing against standard regimens, have sometimes shown increased overall response rates, but no increase in overall survival. Coupled with the inconvenience of administration, the greater toxicity of cisplatin-containing schedules ensured continued unpopularity. Unfortunately, carboplatin does not seem to possess the same activity and as first-line single-agent therapy yields response rates of the order of 20%. There is few data regarding carboplatin dose-response relationships in breast cancer, and perhaps higher doses are needed to match the results seen with cisplatin. Both cisplatin and carboplatin have been employed in regimens of high-dose chemotherapy and autologous bone marrow transplantation in metastatic breast cancer.

4.8. Gastrointestinal Tract Cancer

Carcinomas in the upper, middle, and most of the lower esophagus are squamous in origin and are treated similarly to head and neck squamous cell carcinomas. Hence cisplatin and carboplatin, in combination with 5-FU infusions, form the basis of most chemotherapy treatments. Chemoradiotherapy is important in downstaging the disease before operation and in the treatment of local residual disease.

Gastric carcinomas are adenocarcinomas, and for treatment purposes these include adenocarcinomas arising in the lower esophagus from Barrett's epithelium. Cisplatin and carboplatin have activity as single agents in gastric carcinoma, with response rates of approximately 20 and 5%, respectively. However, combination regimens have been more successful. ECF (Table 1) has proved useful, with response rates approaching 70%, and a doubling of median survival from around 20 to 40 weeks. Cisplatin has been successfully replaced by carboplatin in this regimen.

5-FU remains the cornerstone of treatment for colorectal carcinoma, and the combination of cisplatin and 5-FU has not been shown to be superior to 5-FU alone. Anal carcinomas are of squamous origin, and 5-FU with cisplatin is commonly used in association with radiotherapy.

4.9. Adenocarcinoma of Unknown Primary Site

Poorly differentiated carcinoma (PDC), poorly differentiated adenocarcinoma (PDA), and the more common well-differentiated adenocarcinoma of unknown primary site can present chemotherapeutic problems. Patients with PDC and PDA are considered as a separate group as some are very sensitive to cisplatin-containing regimens. Initial reports describing this sensitivity related mainly to patients with clinical features suggestive of extragonadal germ cell tumors [i.e., young men, mediastinal or retroperitoneal tumors, elevated human chorionic gonadotropin (HCG) or α-fetoprotein (AFP)]. Further evidence of this responsiveness has since emerged. In one study, 220 patients with PDC and PDA of unknown primary site were prospectively evaluated and treated with cisplatin-based chemotherapy *(60)*. The CR rate was 26%, and the PR rate was 36%. The median survival was 12 months and the 12-year actuarial survival 16%.

4.10. Other Solid Tumors

Cisplatin and carboplatin have been used in salvage regimens for lymphomas. Malignant melanoma and prostate cancer respond poorly to chemotherapy, but platinum compounds compare favorably with other cytotoxic agents in these conditions.

5. USE OF PLATINUM COMPOUNDS IN HIGH-DOSE CHEMOTHERAPY WITH AUTOLOGOUS STEM CELL SUPPORT

5.1. High-Dose Treatment

High-dose chemotherapy with autologous stem cell support is now used routinely in the treatment of lymphomas, and less often in the management of patients with teratoma, or breast and ovarian carcinomas. The dose-limiting toxicity of bone marrow suppression, important when chemotherapy is administered conventionally, can be circumvented by the use of stem cells. For the process to be successful, the disease must be very chemosensitive, as in the case of lymphoma and teratoma, or moderately chemosensitive and of low volume as in the adjuvant treatment of breast and ovarian carcinomas. The collection and reinfusion of stem cells has largely replaced the previous technique of harvesting bone marrow. Chemotherapy is initially given as a stem cell mobilizing agent, in conjunction with granulocyte colony-stimulating factor, following which the number of stem cells in the circulation increases, allowing their collection and storage. High-dose chemotherapy, at doses that obliterate the marrow, is then administered followed by reinfusion of the stem cells into the circulation. The stem cells repopulate the marrow spaces with bone marrow recovery. Cyclophosphamide and etoposide are the most widely used mobilizing agents. The dose-response relationships of cisplatin and carboplatin are important factors supporting their inclusion in high-dose chemotherapy regimens. However, cisplatin is a poor candidate on account of associated neurotoxicity and nephrotoxicity. In contrast, the dose-limiting toxicities of carboplatin, thrombocytopenia, and leukopenia can be successfully managed, allowing the use of this agent in the high-dose setting. High-dose carboplatin has been used to treat teratoma, ovarian carcinoma, and breast cancer but is less useful in lymphoma. The chemosensitivity of SCLC implies that this disease should be amenable to high-dose treatment, but such approaches have been disappointing, with no prolongation of survival.

5.2. High-Dose Treatment for Teratoma

The cure rate of patients with multiple relapses of germ cell cancer treated with high-dose chemotherapy is 15–20%, even though a good initial response can often be obtained. High-dose treatment has been used following multiple relapses of teratoma, as primary salvage therapy, i.e., in patients with recurrence or first relapse and, more recently, as primary therapy. Studies of high-dose carboplatin in primary salvage therapy have frequently been performed in patients pretreated with cisplatin. Further conventional therapy (mainly BEP) is given to induce remission followed by consolidation using high-dose carboplatin, usually with etoposide, with or without cyclophosphamide or ifosfamide, and with stem cell support. Up to 50% can achieve a CR with 2-year survivals of up to 50%. High-dose carboplatin and etoposide in patients with cisplatin-refractory germ cell tumors has produced 24% CR and 21% PR rates, with a median survival of 7.6 months *(61)*. High-dose chemotherapy has been used as part of first-line treatment in selected patients with germ cell cancer *(62)*. Conventional platinum-based chemotherapy is administered, and those patients with a slow fall in serum HCG or AFP after two or three treatment cycles are given high-dose carboplatin and etoposide with autologous bone marrow support. A randomized phase III study is currently in progress comparing four cycles of BEP with two cycles of BEP plus two cycles of high-dose therapy containing carboplatin, etoposide, and cyclophosphamide, in the first-line treatment of very poor risk patients.

5.3. High-Dose Treatment for Ovarian Cancer

Current evidence suggests that increasing the dose intensity of cisplatin to 25 mg/m^2/week, or carboplatin to an AUC of 4/week, provides therapeutic advantage, but beyond these doses no further benefit is bestowed, only increasing toxicity. Whether a second higher threshold exists is not known, but its possibility provides the rationale for the investigation of high-dose platinum regimens in ovarian cancer. This approach remains experimental and confined to clinical trials. To date, results are not superior to those achieved with standard approaches. A pilot Phase II study of three cycles of high-dose paclitaxel plus carboplatin, with one of high-dose melphalan, each followed by peripheral stem cell support, in previously untreated patients, generated a 34% pathologic CR rate. Gastrointestinal toxicity and neuropathy were seen in 76 and 62% of patients, respectively *(63)*.

5.4. High-Dose Treatment for Breast Cancer

Carboplatin is commonly used in high-dose regimens with stem cell support *(64)*, and for some patients with high-risk early-stage or metastatic disease such regimens can result in extended disease-free survival. Adjuvant therapy may be most worthwhile, as micrometastatic disease unresponsive to standard doxorubicin-based adjuvant chemotherapy may be destroyed by high-dose chemotherapy.

6. CONCLUSIONS AND FUTURE CLINICAL DIRECTIONS

Cisplatin and carboplatin have influenced the practice of medical oncology immensely over the last 25 years. They have been extensively investigated and are established in the treatment of many tumor types. Carboplatin can replace cisplatin in some—but not all—situations, and carboplatin is currently the only platinum agent that can be used in high-dose strategies. Current research is focusing on several areas. Efforts are being made to develop methods of ameliorating side effects, particularly the nonhematologic effects of cisplatin. An example of such an approach is the use of glutathione, a tripeptide thiol. This has been shown in randomized studies to protect against cisplatin-induced neuropathy. For example, Cascinu et al. *(65)* showed that 89% of patients in a placebo arm developed neurotoxicity, compared with 17% of those given glutathione. The introduction of new growth factors such as thrombopoeitin may allow the use of higher platinum dosages. Second, new platinum derivatives with different toxicity profiles and spectra of activity are under investigation, and progress may be made in the treatment of tumors not currently regarded as platinum sensitive. Third, the combination of platinum compounds with newer agents, such as the taxanes, topoisomerase 1 inhibitors, gemcitabine, raltitrexed, and navelbine is currently under way and seems likely to reveal new active combinations.

REFERENCES

1. Office for National Statistics. (1997). *The Health of Adult Britain 1841–1994*. Office for National Statistics, London, Vol. 2, Chapter 17, pp. 30–59.
2. Gaynon, P. S., Ettinger, L. J., Baum, E. S., et al. (1990) Carboplatin in childhood brain tumours: a Childrens Cancer Study group phase II trial. *Cancer* **66,** 2465–2469
3. Calvert, A. H., Newell, D. R., Gumbrell, L. A., et al. (1989) Carboplatin dosage: prospective evaluation of a simple formula based on renal function. *J. Clin. Oncol.* **7,** 1748–1756.
4. Jodrell, D. I., Egorin, M. J., Canetta, R. M., et al. (1992) Relationships between carboplatin exposure and tumor response and toxicity in patients with ovarian cancer. *J. Clin. Oncol.* **10,** 520–528.
5. Pinkerton, C. R., Broadbent, V., Horwich, A., et al. (1990) "JEB"—a carboplatin based regimen for malignant germ cell tumours in children. *Br. J. Cancer* **62,** 257–262.
6. Cockcroft, D. W. and Gault, M. H. (1976) Prediction of creatinine clearance from serum creatinine. *Nephron* **16,** 31–41.
7. Smit, E. F., Willemse, P. H. B., Sleijfer, D. T. et al. (1991) Continuous infusion carboplatin on a 21-day schedule: a phase I and pharmacokinetic study. *J. Clin. Oncol.* **9,** 100–110.
8. Einhorn, L. H. and Donohue, J. D. (1977) Cis-diamminedichloroplatinum, vinblastine, and bleomycin combination chemotherapy in disseminated testicular cancer. *Ann. Intern. Med.* **87,** 293–298.
9. Horwich, A., Sleijfer, D. T., Fossa, S. D., Kaye, S. B., Oliver, R. T. D., Cullen, M. H., et al. (1997) Randomised trial of bleomycin, etoposide, and cisplatin compared with bleomycin, etoposide, and carboplatin in good-prognosis metastatic nonseminomatous germ cell cancer: a multiinstitutional Medical Research Council/European Organisation for Research and Treatment of Cancer trial. *J. Clin. Oncol.* **15,** 1844–1852.

10. Childs W. J., Nicholls J., Horwich A. (1992) The optimisation of carboplatin dose in carboplatin, etoposide and bleomycin combination chemotherapy for good prognosis metastatic nonseminomatous germ cell tumours of the testis. *Ann. Oncol.* **3,** 291–296.
11. Bajorin, D. F., Sarosdy, M. F., Pfister, D. G., Mazumdar, M., Motzer, R. J., Scher, H. I., et al. (1993) Randomised trial of etoposide and cisplatin versus etoposide and carboplatin in patients with good-risk germ cell tumors: a multiinstitutional study. *J. Clin. Oncol.* **11,** 598–606.
12. Peckham, M. J., Horwich, A., and Hendry, W. F. (1985) Advanced seminoma: treatment with cis-platinum based combination chemotherapy or carboplatin (JM8). *Br. J. Cancer* **52,** 7–13.
13. Oliver, R. T., Edmonds, P. M., Ong, J. Y., et al. (1994) Pilot studies of 2 and 1 course carboplatin as adjuvant for stage I seminoma: should it be tested in a randomised trial against radiotherapy? *Int. J. Radiat. Oncol. Biol. Phys.* **29,** 3–8.
14. Advanced Ovarian Trialists Group. (1991) Chemotherapy in advanced ovarian cancer: an overview of randomised clinical trials. *BMJ* **303,** 884–893.
15. Calvert, A. H., Newell, D. R., Gore, M. E. (1992) Future directions with carboplatin: can therapeutic monitoring, high-dose administration, and hematologic support with growth factors expand the spectrum compared with cisplatin? *Semin. Oncol.* **19 (Suppl 2),** 155–163.
16. Kaye, S. B., Paul, J., Cassidy, J., Lewis, C. R., Duncan, I. D., Gordon, H. K., et al. (1996) Mature results of a randomised trial of two doses of cisplatin for the treatment of ovarian cancer. *J. Clin. Oncol.* **14,** 2113–2119.
17. Murphy, D., Crowther, D., Renninson, J., et al. (1993) A randomised dose intensity study in ovarian carcinoma comparing chemotherapy given at four week intervals for six cycles with half dose chemotherapy given for twelve cycles. *Ann. Oncol.* **4,** 377–383.
18. Ngan, H. Y., Choo, Y. C., Cheung, M., et al. (1989) A randomised trial of high-dose vs low dose cisplatin combined with cyclophosphamide in the treatment of advanced ovarian cancer. *Chemotherapy* **35,** 221–227.
19. McGuire, W. P., Hoskins, W. J., Brady, M. F., et al. (1995) Assessment of dose intensive therapy in suboptimally debulked ovarian cancer: a Gynaecologic Oncology Group study. *J. Clin. Oncol.* **13,** 1589–1599.
20. Calvert, A. H., Lind, M. J., Ghazal-Aswad, S., Gumbrell, L., Millward, M. J., Bailey, N. P., et al. (1994) Carboplatin and granulocyte colony-stimulating factor as first-line treatment for epithelial ovarian cancer: a phase I dose-intensity escalation study. *Semin. Oncol.* **21. (Suppl 12)** 1–6.
21. Gore, M., Mainwaring, P., A'Hern, R., MacFarlane, V., Slevin, M., Harper, P. et al. (1998) Randomized trial of dose-intensity with single-agent carboplatin in patients with epithelial ovarian cancer. *J. Clin. Oncol.* **16,** 2426–2434.
22. Jakobsen, A., Bertelsen, K., Andersen, J. E., Havsteen, H., Jakobsen, P., Moeller, K. A., et al. (1997) Dose-effect study of carboplatin in ovarian cancer: a Danish Ovarian Cancer Group study. *J. Clin. Oncol.* **15** 193–198.
23. Gore, M. E., Fryatt, I., Wiltshaw, E., Dawson, T. (1990) Treatment of relapsed carcinoma of the ovary with cisplatin or carboplatin following initial treatment with these compounds. *Gynecol. Oncol.* **36,** 207–211.
24. Alberts, D. S., Green, S., Hannigan, E.V., et al. (1992) Improved therapeutic index of carboplatin plus cyclophosphamide versus cisplatin plus cyclophosphamide: Final report by the Southwest Oncology Group of a phase III randomised trial in stages III and IV ovarian cancer. *J. Clin. Oncol.* **10,** 706–717.
25. Swenerton, K., Jeffrey, J., Stuart, G., et al. (1992) Cisplatin-cyclophosphamide versus carboplatin-cyclophosphamide in advanced ovarian cancer: a randomised phase III study of the National Cancer Institute of Canada Clinical Trials Group. *J. Clin. Oncol.* **10,** 718–726.
26. Edmonson, J. H., McCormack, G. W., Wieand, H. S., et al. (1989) Cyclophosphamide-cisplatin versus cyclophosphamide-carboplatin in stage III-IV ovarian carcinoma: a comparison of equally myelosuppressive regimens. *J. Natl. Cancer Inst.* **81,** 1500–1504.

27. Parmar, M. K. B., Torri, V., Bonaventura, A., Bonazzi, C., Colombo, N., Delaloye, J.-F., et al. (1998) ICON 2: randomised trial of single-agent carboplatin against three-drug combination of CAP (cyclophosphamide, doxorubicin, and cisplatin) in women with ovarian cancer. *Lancet.* **352,** 1571–1576.
28. McGuire, W. P., Hoskins, W. J., Brady, M. F., Kugera, P.C., Partridge, E. E., Look, K. Y., et al. (1996). Cyclophosphamide and cisplatin compared with paclitaxel and cisplatin in stage III and stage IV ovarian cancer. *N. Engl. J. Med.* **334,** 1–6.
29. Stuart, G., Bertelsen, K., Mangioni, C., Trope, C., James, K., Cassidy, J., et al. (1998) Updated analysis shows a highly significant improved overall survival (OS) for cisplatin-paclitaxel as first line treatment of advanced ovarian cancer: mature results of the EORTC-GCCG, NOCOVA, NCIC CTG and Scottish Intergroup Trial. *Proc. AACR* **34,** Abstract no 1394.
30. du Bois, A., Richter, B., Warm, M., Costa, S., Bauknecht, T., Lück, H. J., et al. (1998) Cisplatin/paclitaxel vs carboplatin/paclitaxel as 1st-line treatment in ovarian cancer. *Proc. ASCO* **34,** Abstract no 1395.
31. Calvert, A. H. (1997) A review of the pharmacokinetics and pharmacodynamics of combination carboplatin/paclitaxel. *Semin. Oncol.* **24,** S2-85–S2-90.
32. Markman, M., Reichman, B., Hakes, T., et al. (1993) Evidence supporting the superiority of intraperitoneal cisplatin compared to intraperitoneal carboplatin for salvage therapy of small volume residual ovarian cancer. *Gynecol. Oncol.* **50,** 100–104.
33. Alberts, D. S., Liu, P. Y., Hannigan, E. V., O'Toole, R., Williams, S. D., Young, J. A., et. al. (1996) Intraperitoneal cisplatin plus intravenous cyclophosphamide versus intravenous cisplatin plus intravenous cyclophosphamide for stage III ovarian cancer. *N. Engl. J. Med.* **335,** 1950–1955.
34. Martinez, J. A., Martin, G., Sanz, G. F., et al. (1991) A phase II trial of carboplatin infusion in high-risk acute nonlymphoblastic leukemia. *J. Clin. Oncol.* **9,** 39–43.
35. Meyers, F. J., Welborn, J., Lewis, J. P., et al. (1989) Infusion carboplatin treatment of relapsed and refractory acute leukaemia: evidence of efficacy with minimal extramedullary toxicity at intermediate doses. *J. Clin. Oncol.* **7,** 173–178.
36. Gaynon, P. S. (1994) Carboplatin in pediatric malignancies. *Semin. Oncol.* **21 (Suppl 12),** 65–76.
37. Smith, I. E., Harland, S. J., Robinson, B. A., et al. (1985) Carboplatin: a very active new cisplatin analogue in the treatment of small cell lung cancer. *Cancer Treat. Rep.* **69,** 43–46.
38. Skarlos, D. V., Samantas, E., Kosmidis, P., Fountzilas, G., Angelidou, M., Palamidas, P., et al. (1994) Randomised comparison of etoposide-cisplatin vs. etoposide-carboplatin and irradiation in small-cell lung cancer. A Hellenic Co-operative Oncology Group Study. *Ann. Oncol.* **5,** 601–607.
39. Smith, I. E., Perrin, T. J., Ashley, S. A., Woodiwiss, J., Forgeson, G. V., Yarnold, J. R., et al. (1990) Carboplatin, etoposide, and ifosfamide as intensive chemotherapy for small-cell lung cancer. *J. Clin. Oncol.* **8,** 899–905.
40. Gore, M. E., Calvert, A. H., Smith, I. E. (1987) High-dose carboplatin in the treatment of lung cancer and mesothelioma: a phase I dose escalation study. *Eur. J. Cancer Clin. Oncol.* **23,** 1391–1397.
41. Klastersky, J., Sculier, J. P., Lacroix, H. et al. (1990) A randomised study comparing cisplatin or carboplatin plus etoposide in patients with advanced non-small lung cancer: European Organisation for Research and Treatment of Cancer protocol 07861. *J. Clin. Oncol.* **8,** 1556–1562.
42. Non-Small Cell Lung Cancer Collaborative Group. (1995) Chemotherapy in non-small cell lung cancer: a meta-analysis using updated data on individual patients from 52 randomised clinical trials. *BMJ* **311,** 899–909.
43. Bunn, P. A. Jr., and Kelly K. (1998) New chemotherapeutic agents prolong survival and im-

prove quality of life in non-small cell lung cancer: a review of the literature and future directions. *Clin. Cancer Res.* **4,** 1087–1100.

44. Bunn, P. A. Jr. (1996) The North American experience with paclitaxel combined with cisplatin or carboplatin in lung cancer. *Sem. Oncol.* **23 (Suppl 16)**, 18–25.
45. Belani, C. P., Natale, R. B., Lee, J. S., Socinski, M., Robert, F., Waterhouse, D., et al. (1998) Randomized phase III trial comparing cisplatin/etoposide versus carboplatin/paclitaxel in advanced and metastatic non-small cell lung cancer (NSCLC). *Proc ASCO* **34,** abstract no 1751.
46. Dillman, R. O., Seagren, S. L., Propert, K. J., et al. (1990) A randomised trial of induction chemotherapy and high-dose radiation therapy in stage III non-small cell lung cancer. *N. Engl. J. Med.* **323,** 940–945.
47. Schaake-Koning, C., Van Den Bogaert, W., Dalesio, O., et al. (1992) Effects of concomitant cisplatin and radiotherapy on inoperable non-small-cell lung cancer. *N. Engl. J. Med.* **326,** 524–530.
48. Belani, C. P. and Aisner, J. (1994) Combined chemotherapy and radiation in locally advanced non-small cell lung cancer. *Semin. Oncol.* **21 (Suppl 6),** 79–90.
49. Rosell, R., Gomez-Codina, J., Camps, C., Maestre, J., Padille, J., Canto, A., et al. (1994) A randomised trial comparing preoperative chemotherapy plus surgery with surgery alone in patients with non-small-cell lung cancer. *N. Eng. J. Med.* **330,** 153–158.
50. Merlano, M., Vitale, V., Rosso, R., et al. (1992) Treatment of advanced squamous cell carcinoma of the head and neck with alternating chemotherapy and radiotherapy. *N. Engl. J. Med.* **327,** 1115–1121.
51. Haselow, R. E., Warshaw, M. G., Okin, M. M., et al. (1990) Radiation alone versus radiation plus weekly low-dose cis-platinum in unresectable cancer of the head and neck, in *Head and Neck Cancer,* vol 2, (Fee, W. E., Jr., Goepfert, H., Johns, M. E., et al., eds.), Decker, Toronto, pp. 279–281.
52. Marcial, V. A., Pajak, T. F., Mohiuddin, M., et al. (1990) Concomitant cisplatin chemotherapy and radiotherapy in advanced mucosal squamous cell carcinoma of the head and neck. *Cancer* **66,** 1861–1868.
53. Laramore, G. E., Scott, C. B., Al-Sarraf, M., et al. (1992) Adjuvant chemotherapy for resectable squamous cell carcinoma of the head and neck: report on Intergroup Study 0034. *Int. J. Radiat. Oncol. Biol. Phys.* **23,** 705–713.
54. Zamboglou, N., Schnabel, T., Kolotas, C., et al. (1994) Carboplatin and radiotherapy in the treatment of head and neck cancer: six years' experience. *Sem. Oncol.* **21 (Suppl 12),** 45–53.
55. Raabe, N. K., Fossa, S. D., and Paro G. (1989) Phase II study of carboplatin in locally advanced and metastatic transitional cell carcinoma of the urinary bladder. *Br. J. Urol.* **64,** 604–607.
56. Loehrer, P. J., Einhorn, L. H., Elson, P. J. et al., (1992) A randomised comparison of cisplatin alone or in combination with methotrexate, vinblastine, and doxorubicin in patients with metastatic urothelial carcinoma: a cooperative group study. *J. Clin. Oncol.* **10,** 1066–1073.
57. Petrioli, R., Frediani, B., Manganelli, A., Barbanti, G., De Capua, B., De Lauretis, A., et al. (1996) Comparison between a cisplatin-containing regimen and a carboplatin containing regimen for recurrent or metastatic bladder cancer patients. A randomised phase II study. *Cancer* **77,** 344–351.
58. Waxman, J., and Wasan, H. (1994) Platinum based chemotherapy for bladder cancer. *Semin. Oncol.* **21 (Suppl 12),** 54–60.
59. Lokich, J. and Anderson, N. (1998) Carboplatin versus cisplatin in solid tumors: an analysis of the literature. *Ann. Oncol.* **9,** 13–21.
60. Hainsworth, J. D., Johnson, D. H., Greco, F. A. (1992) Cisplatin-based combination chemotherapy in the treatment of poorly differentiated carcinoma and poorly differentiated adenocarcinoma of unknown primary site: results of a 12-year experience. *J. Clin. Oncol.* **10,** 912–922.

61. Nichols, C. R., Andersen, J., Lazarus, H. M., et al. (1992) High-dose carboplatin and etoposide with autologous bone marrow transplantation in refractory germ cell cancer: an Eastern Co-operative Oncology Group study. *J. Clin. Oncol.* **10,** 558–563.
62. Motzer, R., Gulati, S., Crown, J., et al. (1992) High-dose chemotherapy and autologous bone marrow rescue for patients with refractory germ cell tumors: early intervention is better tolerated. *Cancer* **69,** 550–556.
63. Aghajanian, C., Fennelly, D., Shapiro, F., et al. (1998) Phase II study of "dose-dense" high-dose chemotherapy treatment with peripheral-blood progenitor-cell support as primary treatment for patients with advanced ovarian cancer. *J. Clin. Oncol.* **16,** 1852–1860.
64. Crown, J., Kritz, A., Vahdat, L., et al. (1993) Rapid administration of multiple cycles of high-dose myelosuppressive chemotherapy in patients with metastatic breast cancer. *J. Clin. Oncol.* **11,** 1144–1149.
65. Cascinu, S., Cordella, L., Del Ferro, E., Fronzoni, M., and Catalano, G., (1995) Neuroprotective effect of reduced glutathione on cisplatin-based chemotherapy in advanced gastric cancer: a randomised double-blind placebo-controlled trial. *J. Clin. Oncol.* **13,** 26–32.

9 Clinical Experience

Platinum and Taxanes

Michelle Vaughan, Francisco Sapunar, and Martin Gore

CONTENTS

1. INTRODUCTION

The platinum drugs are widely used in cancer therapy. In recent years they have been successfully combined with the taxanes, especially for the treatment of patients with cancers of the ovary, lung, breast, and head and neck. This chapter presents some of the evidence on the use of platinum and taxane regimens in these malignancies.

2. OVARIAN CANCER

Ovarian carcinoma is the sixth most common malignancy in women and is the leading cause of death from gynecologic malignancy in the Western world *(53)*. The earliest stages of this disease can be treated by surgery alone, with excellent results *(37)*; however, as the signs and symptoms of this malignancy are nonspecific, the most patients (75%) present when the disease has spread beyond the ovary and is consequently rarely curable. The standard treatment for ovarian cancer is surgical debulking followed by chemotherapy.

2.1. The Platinum Drugs

There are a number of cytotoxic agents with well-defined activity in ovarian cancer; of these, the platinum drugs are accepted as the most effective single

From: *Platinum-Based Drugs in Cancer Therapy*
Edited by: L. R. Kelland and N. Farrell © Humana Press Inc., Totowa, NJ

agents in this disease *(2)*. Despite their widespread use, several unanswered questions remain concerning platinum administration.

2.1.1. Combination vs Single Agent

In the 1980s and early 1990s most centers used platinum therapy for ovarian cancer, but there was debate as to whether the addition of other chemotherapeutic agents to single-agent cisplatin or carboplatin conferred significant benefit. A metaanalysis of six trials by the Advanced Ovarian Cancer Trialists Group (AOCTG) involving 925 patients suggested that platinum combination therapy achieved superior survival over single-agent platinum *(2)*, with a risk ratio of 0.85 [confidence interval (CI) 0.72–1.0] and the benefit just reaching statistical significance ($p = 0.03$). It has, however, been difficult to demonstrate this advantage in individual randomized trials. In 1992 the Gruppo Interregionale Cooperativo Oncologico Ginecologia published the long-term results of a three-arm study comparing single-agent cisplatin, cisplatin, and cyclophosphamide, and the combination of cisplatin, cyclophosphamide, and Adriamycin (CAP) *(25)*. In all, 565 patients were randomized between 1980 and 1985; the median survivals of the three groups were not significantly different at 19, 20, and 23 months, respectively. Similarly, the 7-year overall survival figures did not differ significantly among the three groups (9.6, 14.5, and 17.2%, respectively), although Cox's model did show borderline significance for the difference between single-agent cisplatin and CAP.

Two recent publications have added further data to this debate. First, the recently published results of a trial designed to compare optimal dose carboplatin with the CAP regimen showed no difference between the two arms. Second, the AOCTG have updated their 1991 analysis and have only been able to show a statistically significant benefit for combination therapy when a subset of trials are considered.

Despite the absence of compelling evidence from randomized trials, many clinicians favor the use of combination chemotherapy in young, fit, and optimally debulked patients, while acknowledging that the absolute survival benefit is likely to be small, perhaps in the region of 3% at 5 years *(53)*.

2.1.2. Carboplatin vs Cisplatin

A further controversy has involved the relative merits of using cisplatin or carboplatin. There is no controversy over their toxicity profiles, carboplatin being better tolerated, but there have been many discussions concerning their relative efficacy. The AOCTG metaanalysis looked at 11 trials involving over 2000 patients comparing cisplatin and carboplatin either alone or in combination. No study suggested any superiority for either agent, and the metaanalysis has reflected this, overall relative risk being 1.05 (95% CI 0.94–1.18).

As suggested, the toxicity profiles of the two drugs are quite different, with more severe neurotoxicity, nephrotoxicity, ototoxicity, nausea, and vomiting in patients treated with cisplatin, and more myelotoxicity in carboplatin-treated patients. The significantly more favorable therapeutic index of carboplatin leads many clinicians to choose this agent over cisplatin. It is worthwhile noting, however, that all the trials involving carboplatin in the metaanalysis administered the drug according to surface area, not renal clearance, as is currently recommended. *(10)*; whether this would make a difference is not known. A minority of experts in the field remain to be convinced of the equivalence in efficacy between cisplatin and carboplatin, citing inadequate patient numbers, inadequate carboplatin doses, crossover, and a dearth of long-term follow-up to adequately exclude a benefit for cisplatin *(55)*. They remain uncomfortable with its use in good-prognosis patients with the prospect of long-term survival or even cure. However, all are agreed that for patients with a poor prognosis, carboplatin is the drug of choice.

2.1.3. Length of Treatment/Dose Intensity

As in other malignancies, the issue of optimal dosing of platinum has been investigated in ovarian cancer. Two randomized prospective trials of longer vs shorter treatment periods using combination chemotherapy have failed to provide any evidence that more than six cycles of platinum-based treatment improves survival *(5,26)*.

Early Phase II trials suggested that a dose-response relationship existed with the platinum drugs. However, only 2 of the 11 randomized trials examining this issue have suggested any advantage, and they were among the smallest studies *(4,39)*. None of the trials of platinum dose intensity increased it by more than a factor of 2 because it is not possible to intensify cisplatin doses beyond this. The trials using carboplatin have also not increased the dose by more than this factor, and it remains to be seen whether using carboplatin at higher doses is beneficial. It is impossible to draw any conclusions from the published high-dose trials because although there are 40 reports detailing treatment in over 600 patients, 27 different regimens had been employed and no randomized data exist *(32)*.

2.2. The Taxanes

2.2.1. Introduction

The crude extract of the bark of the Pacific yew *Taxus brevifolia* was first discovered to have cytotoxic properties in the1960s. In 1971, the active constituent paclitaxel was isolated, and it was the first of a new class of antimicrotubule agents, the taxanes *(56)*. Poor water solubility of the isolate, however, meant that it was 10 years before Phase I trials were under way *(13)*. Paclitaxel and the semisynthetic analog docetaxel are the two compounds in the class in current clinical use. Both agents act by stabilizing microtubules and inhibiting depolymerization (and therefore mitosis). Docetaxel treatment results in higher intracellular concentration and has a higher affinity for microtubules and therefore greater potency than paclitaxel *(18,31)*. Docetaxel is also derived from the more renewable resource of the needles of the European yew *Taxus baccata*. Both agents are given by iv infusion and metabolized in the liver, with most inactive metabolites being excreted in the bile.

2.2.2. Taxanes in Relapsed Disease

The first clinical trials of paclitaxel were performed in patients with recurrent disease. Initial studies showed there was a degree of lack of cross-resistance between platinum and paclitaxel with response rates of 16–37% in patients who had failed platinum. Median response durations were 5–10 months, and median survivals of 8–16 months were achieved in this poor-prognosis patient group *(15,16,23,50,52)*.

The differences in response rates seen in the early studies are likely to be due to the heterogeneity of taxane dosing and patient characteristics. For instance, it is clear that patients who relapse over 1 year after the first platinum-based treatment have a good chance of a second response to a further platinum treatment *(21,34)*; the response lessening the shorter the time interval between successive treatments. This relationship also appears to apply to responses seen in Phase II trials of new drugs *(6)*.

More recently a multivariate analysis of 744 patients in four studies looking at agents including paclitaxel, docetaxel, and epirubicin as second- and third-line treatment did not find time from last treatment a significant independent predictor of response to chemotherapy when the time interval was analyzed as a continuous variable *(16)*. The authors suggested that the time interval itself was not the critical variable for response, rather that this was a surrogate for other variables, such as tumor size and biology. In a subsequent publication in abstract form, the group analyzed the same patient database for predictors of overall survival (OS) and time to progression (TTP). They reported that a short time since last chemotherapy did predict for TTP and OS *(54)*, which may mean that factors predicting for OS and TTP are not the same as those predicting for response to chemotherapy.

There is less experience with docetaxel than paclitaxel in patients with cancer of the ovary. Four Phase II trials of docetaxel, including 340 patients with advanced ovarian cancer, have been recently reviewed. The overall response rate was 30%, with response durations ranging between 4 and 17 months. The authors concluded that docetaxel and paclitaxel have similar activity in ovarian cancer *(29)*.

2.2.3. Toxicity

Hypersensitivity reactions complicated treatment in the initial studies of paclitaxel in up to 16% of patients *(44)*. This was thought to be due to the "cremophor EL" vehicle, a polyoxyethylated castor oil used to improve paclitaxel's aqueous insolubility. This complication was reduced by an increased infusion duration and premedication with steroids, antihistamines, and H2 antagonists. The current rate of severe hypersensitivity is now less than 1%, and rapid infusion with appropriate premedication is safe *(40)*.

The dose-limiting toxicity of paclitaxel is neutropenia, with a maximum tolerated dose of 200–250 mg/m^2 in most studies *(20)*. Neuropathy is the next most significant dose-limiting toxicity; it is dose dependant and cumulative but usually reversible *(44)*. Alopecia also occurs in most patients (approximately 90%), and myalgia/arthralgia may also occur in a minority of patients, but it is manageable.

The docetaxel toxicity profile differs somewhat in that fatigue and diarrhea occur more commonly, whereas neuropathy is less frequent and less severe *(11)*. There is also the unique side effect of fluid retention, characterized by peripheral edema and/or pleural effusions. This is cumulative, occurring in approximately 50% of patients after four cycles at 100 mg/m^2 and is probably related to a direct effect on small blood vessels. The onset of the edema can be delayed by the use of glucocorticoids, and the condition is slowly reversible on stopping therapy. *(12,29,49)*.

2.2.4. Dosing and Scheduling

A particular difficulty with paclitaxel administration is that its pharmacokinetics follow nonlinear kinetics, with saturable distribution, metabolism, and elimination *(19)*. This leads to unpredictability in both toxicity and efficacy with changes in dose and rate of administration. Docetaxel, on the other hand, follows linear pharmacokinetics; thus its toxicity and efficacy are not as schedule dependent.

In 1994 Eisenhauer and colleagues *(16)* examined the issue of both schedule and dose of paclitaxel in recurrent carcinoma of the ovary in a large, randomized European-Canadian trial. The 187 patients treated with a 3-h infusion given with premedication of glucocorticoids and H1 and H2 antagonists suffered no more allergic reactions than the 204 patients receiving the same prophylactic regimen and paclitaxel infusion over 24 h. There was also no statistically significant difference in lower incidence of fever and grade 4 neutropenia. Changes in quality of life scores were no different between the two groups, and there were no significant differences in response rates or overall survival. Subsequent pharmacokinetic and clinical studies have suggested that shortening the infusion time to 1 h is safe *(24)*, and this has now been adopted as standard in many institutions.

Cumulative data suggest there may be a dose-response relationship for paclitaxel, with response rates increasing from 19% in patients treated with 135 mg/m^2 to 46% in those given 250 mg/m^2 *(22)*. In the randomized European-Canadian study, response rates with 175 mg/m^2 were higher than with 135 mg/m^2 (20 vs 15%), but this did not reach significance ($p = 0.2$). However, a significant disease-free survival advantage was seen with the higher dose (4.4 months vs 3.2 months, $p = 0.02$).

Weekly administration of paclitaxel has more recently been investigated with a resulting increase in dose intensity and reducing toxicity. The schedule appears to be well tolerated and although the numbers are very small, encouraging response rates in heavily pretreated patients have been reported *(1)*.

2.3. Platinum/Taxane Combinations

2.3.1. Cisplatin and Paclitaxel

Once it was established that the taxanes offered impressive single-agent activity in recurrent ovarian cancer, trials of paclitaxel in combination with platinum agents as first-line treatment began. The first Phase I trial of the combination of paclitaxel and cisplatin *(43)*, found that the sequence of 24-h paclitaxel followed by cisplatin was tolerable. This schedule was therefore chosen for the first prospective randomized trial comparing cisplatin and paclitaxel with the standard treatment of cisplatin and cyclophosphamide performed by the Gynecologic Oncology Group (GOG) 111 trial *(35)*. This landmark trial was undertaken in 386 previously untreated patients with suboptimally debulked stage III and IV disease and good performance status. Patients were treated with cisplatin 75 mg/m^2 and paclitaxel 135 mg/m^2 over 24 h, or cisplatin 75 mg/m^2 and cyclophosphamide 750 mg/m^2. Significant differences in favor of the cisplatin/paclitaxel combination were seen for response rate (73 vs 60%, $p = 0.01$), progression-free survival (18 vs 13 months, $p < 0.001$), and overall survival (38 versus 24 months, $p < 0.001$). Neutropenia, febrile neutropenia, alopecia, and peripheral neuropathy were all significantly greater in the group receiving cisplatin and paclitaxel; however, the differences in toxicity between the arms of the trial were modest, and the combination of cisplatin/paclitaxel was regarded as well tolerated.

These findings have been recently confirmed in an Intergroup study using the same control treatment as in GOG-111 but also including earlier stage and optimally debulked patients, with the shorter schedule of paclitaxel 175 mg/m^2 over 3 h as opposed to 135 mg/m^2 over 24 h, as in GOG 111. This trial also demonstrated an advantage to cisplatin/paclitaxel treatment for response rate (77 vs 66%, $p = 0.02$), progression-free survival. (16 vs 12 months $p = 0.0001$), and overall survival (35 vs 25 months, $p < 0.001$) *(46)*. However, significant neurotoxicity was encountered in patients treated with cisplatin/paclitaxel.

A subsequent GOG trial undertaken in suboptimally debulked stage III and IV patients has compared the combination of cisplatin/paclitaxel with each agent individually *(36)*. This study found that response rates were superior with the combination compared with single-agent paclitaxel but not compared with single-agent cisplatin at a dose of 100 mg/m^2. There were fewer dose reductions and treatment delays with a higher percentage of patients completing six cycles of therapy in the paclitaxel/cisplatin arm. The combination treatment yielded similar progression-free survival and overall survival to single-agent

Table 1
Randomized Trials of Cisplatin and Paclitaxel vs Other Platinum Combinations in Advanced Ovarian Cancer[a]

Study	*No.*	*Stage*	*Cisplatin (mg/m^2)*	*Paclitaxel (mg/m^2)*	*Cyclo (mg/m^2)*	*RR (%)*	*DFS (months)*	*OS (months)*
GOG 111, 1996 (*35*)	386	III–IV	75	135/24 h	—	73*	18***	38**
			75	—	750	60	13	24
Intergroup, 1997 (*46*)	680	IIB–IV	75	175/3 h	—		17	
			75		750		12	
GOG 132, 1997 (*36*)	615	III–IV	75	135/24 h	—	72	14	27
			100	—	—	74	16	30
			—	200/24 h	—	46**	11	26

[a]Cyclo, cyclophosphamide; RR, response rate; DFS, disease-free survival; OS, overall survival.
*$p = 0.01$.
**$p < 0.05$.
***$p < 0.001$.

Table 2
Phase I Trials with Carboplatin and Paclitaxel in Ovarian Cancer[a]

			MTD			
Study	*No.*	*Stage*	*Carboplatin (AUC)*	*Paclitaxel mg/m²)*	*RR (%)*	*Median PFs (months)*
Bookman et al., 1996 (*8*)	39	III–IV	7.5	135/24 h 175/3 h	75	15
Huizing et al., 1997 (*28*)	35	III–IV	300 mg/m^2	200/3 h	78	NS
Bolis et al., 1997 (*7*)	27	IIc–IV	300 mg/m^2	150–250 Not achieved	NS	NS
ten Bokkel Huinink et al., 1997) (*49*)	46	III–IV	9	200/3 h	NS	NS

[a]MTD, maximum tolerated dose; AUC, area under the curve; PFS, progression-free survival.

cisplatin, but better progression-free survival than single-agent paclitaxel. Overall survival was not significantly different in all three groups; however, significant crossover occurred in this trial even before progression was documented, and this undoubtedly confounds the results of this study.

The results of the above three studies are summarized in Table 1.

2.3.2. Carboplatin and Paclitaxel

The favorable therapeutic index of carboplatin, especially its relative lack of neurotoxicity coupled with its ease of administration, has prompted many investigators to substitute it for cisplatin in combination with paclitaxel in first-line studies. A number of Phase I trials have explored different doses and schedules of this combination *(7,8,28,45,48)*. These are tabulated in Table 2. Toxicity profiles of the combination have been found to be highly acceptable, with neutropenia being the dose-limiting toxicity in most studies, followed by peripheral neuropathy and thrombocytopenia.

A consistent finding in these preliminary studies is that although neutropenia has been additive as expected, the combination of carboplatin and paclitaxel has caused less thrombocytopenia than anticipated. Counterintuitively, in two Phase I studies with a fixed dose of carboplatin as the dose of paclitaxel increased, platelet nadirs increased *(7,45)*. There is no indication of a pharmacokinetic interaction between the drugs to explain this observation *(28)*, and a direct effect of paclitaxel on megakaryocytes is thought to be the most likely mechanism *(9)*.

There are three Phase III trials that address the issue of cisplatin-carboplatin equivalence in the context of platinum/paclitaxel combination therapy (Table 3) *(14,38,33)*. Interim reports of two of these studies *(14,38)* suggest greater non-

Table 3
Ongoing Randomized Trials of Paclitaxel with Cisplatin or Carboplatin in Advanced Ovarian Cancer

Study	*No.*	*Stage*	*Cisplatin (mg/m^2)*	*Paclitaxel (mg/m^2)*	*Carboplatin (AUC)*
Neijt	159	IIB–IV	75	175/3 h	—
et al., 1997 (*38*)			—	175/3 h	5
DuBois	660	IIB–IV	75	185/3 h	—
et al., 1997 (*14*)			—	185/3 h	6
GOG 58	700	III	75	135/3 h	—
(unpublished)			—	175/3 h	7.5

hematologic toxicity in the cisplatin/paclitaxel arm, but it is still too early to evaluate the efficacy results of these trials. Most investigators feel that for poorer prognosis patients in whom quality of life is a major issue it is reasonable to use carboplatin/paclitaxel. There is, however, controversy over the use of this combination in patients with good-prognosis disease.

3. LUNG CANCER

3.1. Introduction

There has in the past been pessimism over the use of chemotherapy in lung cancer, the leading cause of cancer death worldwide. Most patients present with non-small cell lung cancer (NSCLC), and only a small proportion (approximately 20%) of these patients are suitable for surgical resection *(82)*. An even smaller proportion are actually cured by surgery or radical radiotherapy; hence the high mortality of this disease and the need to find effective medical means of improving quality of life and survival.

The prognosis of this disease has changed little over the past 20 years, with the overall median survival for all stages being 6–8 months and 5-year survival of 10–15%. In most patients with advanced disease, median survival is only 4–6 months *(82)*.

3.2. Platinum Chemotherapy

In those patients with unresectable disease, single-agent chemotherapy achieves response rates of up to 20%. Cisplatin is considered to be the most active single agent. Single-agent chemotherapy, however, rarely induces complete responses, and median survival is not significantly prolonged *(64)*.

Combination platinum chemotherapy is used more often than single-agent treatment. Agents commonly added to cisplatin include mitomycin, the vinca alkaloids, etoposide, and ifosfamide. Response rates range from 30 to 40%, but complete remissions are seen in less than 5% of patients *(64)*. The toxicity of combination chemotherapy in this patient population with advanced disease and often poor performance status must be balanced against the benefits. Many clinicians have been sceptical about the use of chemotherapy in advanced NSCLC, but trials have shown that chemotherapy induces good symptomatic relief and improved functional status over best supportive care *(70,80)*, as well as a reduction in inpatient time and costs of medical care *(76)*.

Two metaanalyses have also shown that cisplatin-based combination regimens are associated with a modest survival benefit *(82,88)*. The largest of these, a study by the Non-Small Cell Lung Cancer Collaborative Group, looked at 52 randomized trials of chemotherapy in NSCLC and included 9387 patients *(82)*. The survival benefit was 10% at 1-year (from 15 to 25%) compared with best supportive care, with lesser benefits when added to surgery or radiotherapy settings (5 and 2%, respectively at 5 years). This gives a 3-month prolongation of overall survival from 4–6 months to 6–12 months. Chemotherapy therefore offers a benefit to a patient's chemotherapy, but its role still depends very much on individual patient circumstances and preferences.

3.3. Taxanes

Results on the use of paclitaxel in NSCLC have been recently summarized *(62)*. As with ovarian cancer, doses and schedules in these studies vary enormously, from 1- to 24-h infusions and weekly to 3-weekly dosing. Results of the 10 trials evaluating paclitaxel in 316 patients show an overall response rate of 27% (range, 10–56%), with median and 1-year survivals of 8.5 months and 41% (range, 22–53%), respectively.

Docetaxel has similar activity; seven trials in previously untreated patients demonstrate response rates of 31% (range, 21–54%) and median survival of 9 months *(62,85)*. Two trials have looked at docetaxel in the difficult area of platinum-refractory and -resistant patients and have demonstrated response rates of 17% and median survival of 9 months, comparing favorably with other second-line regimens, including paclitaxel *(63,71)*. As in other malignancies, myelosupression, especially neutropenia, was the most significant toxicity. Fluid retention was also encountered but was readily treatable with corticosteroids.

3.4. Platinum/Taxane Combinations

Over the last 2–3 years, several Phase I and II trials have examined combinations of paclitaxel with cisplatin or carboplatin. Six trials involving 215 patients have demonstrated the efficacy of the combination of cisplatin and paclitaxel with response rates of 11–55%, (mean, 41%). The results of these trials are presented in Table 4 *(59,72,77,84,87,89)*. As with ovarian cancer, neurotoxicity (and to a lesser extent myelosuppression), are the dose-limiting side effects. More recently, both the Eastern Cooperative Oncology Group (ECOG)

Table 4
Cisplatin and Paclitaxel in Metastatic Lung Cancer

Study	*No.*	*Cisplatin (mg/m^2)*	*Paclitaxel ($mg/m^2/h$)*	*RR (%)*
Rowinsky et al., 1993 (*87*)	40	75	135–250/96	43
von Pawel et al., 1996 (*89*)	67	75	175/3	43
Pirker et al., 1995 (*84*)	20	50 × 2/7	175/3	35
Georgiadis et al., 1995 (*72*)	17	60–80	100–180/96	55
Belli et al., 1995 (*59*)	29	100–120	135–225	28

Table 5
Carboplatin and Paclitaxel in Metastatic Lung Cancer

Study	*No.*	*Carboplatin (AUC mg/m^2)*	*Paclitaxel ($mg/m^2/h$)*	*RR (%)*
Langer et al., 1995 (*79*)	108	7.5	135–200/3–24	50
De Vore et al., 1996 (*68*)	51	6 or 300 mg/m^2	135–175/3–24	27
Belanir et al., 1996 (*58*)	26	5–11	135–200/24	50
Natale, 1990 (*81*)	49	6	150–250/3	62
Rowinsky et al., 1995 (*86*)	19	7	175–250/3	37
Greco and Hainsworth, 1997 (*74*)	100	6	225/1	38
Kosmidis et al., 1996 (*78*)	21	7	175/3	33
Creaven et al., 1996 (*67*)	26	4–4.5	100–270/1–3	13
Huizing et al., 1997 (*75*)	55	300–400 mg/m^2	100–250/3	11

and the European Organization for Research and Treatment of Cancer (EORTC) have compared cisplatin and paclitaxel with their standard cisplatin/epipodphylotoxin regimens *(60,73)*. In both studies the cisplatin/paclitaxel response rates were superior; 26 vs 12% in the one *(60)* and 44 vs 30% in the other *(73)*. Median survival was significantly improved by 2 months from 7.7 to 9.8 months in the ECOG *(60)*, but not the EORTC *(73)* trial (9.4 vs 9.7 months).

The combination of carboplatin/paclitaxel has been more extensively studied, because of its superior toxicity profile and ease of administration, as outlined earlier. A wide range of doses and regimens have been used: carboplatin AUC 4–7 and paclitaxel 135–250 mg/m^2 in 1–24-h infusions. As with cisplatin/paclitaxel combinations, myelosuppression, and to a lesser extent neuropathy, are the toxicities that limit dose. Response rates are variable (11–62%), but the mean response in all 518 patients in 15 trials is very similar to that seen with the cisplatin/paclitaxel regimen, 39% (Table 5). In addition, two studies have suggested that there may be a dose-response effect with carboplatin/paclitaxel *(62,75)*.

Table 6
Cisplatin and Docetaxel in Metastatic Lung Cancer[a]

Study	*No.*	*Cisplatin (mg/m²)*	*Docetaxel (mg/m²)*	*RR (%)*	*Estimated MOS (months)*
Zalcberg et al., 1995 *(90)*	47	75	75	39	10
Douillard et al., 1995 *(69)*	51	100	75	30	10
Androulakis et al., 1996 *(57)*	53	80	100	48	13
Cole et al., 1995 *(65)*	57	100–175	65–85	51	10.5

[a]MOS, median overall survival.

A smaller number of trials have looked at docetaxel/platinum combinations. This combination appears more attractive than paclitaxel/platinum because of the absence of overlapping neurotoxicity seen with cisplatin and paclitaxel. Four trials in previously untreated advanced-stage patients (Table 6) have demonstrated the effectiveness of the combination of cisplatin and docetaxel given in doses of 75–100 mg/m^2 and 75 mg/m^2, respectively.

In summary, platinum/taxane combinations appear active and well tolerated in advanced lung cancer. Ongoing randomized trials should provide more information about optimal doses and schedules.

4. HEAD AND NECK CANCER

4.1. Introduction

Squamous cell carcinoma (SCC) of the head and neck constitutes a major public health problem, with estimates in 1998 of more than 500,000 new cases worldwide. SCC presents with stage III or IV disease in more than two-thirds of the cases. Standard treatment for head and neck cancer at presentation is surgery and radiotherapy. Despite optimal local therapy, more than half of the cases will ultimately develop local recurrence, and 30% or more will subsequently develop metastatic disease *(91)*. The conventional treatment of patients with advanced laryngeal cancer consists of total laryngectomy and postoperative radiation therapy, which results in overall 5-year survival rates ranging from 0 to 50% *(91)*. Chemotherapy is only considered to be standard treatment for recurrent or metastatic disease, with responses in the order of 15–30% using single-agent drugs as methotrexate, cisplatin, carboplatin, 5-fluorouracil (5-FU) and bleomycin. Median response duration is 4–6 months, and survival following chemotherapy is usually only 6–10 months. Neoadjuvant chemotherapy in conjunction with radiotherapy and/or surgery has been shown to produce responses in up to 90% in patients with stage III/IV disease, and there is a complete response rate of about 50%. Neoadjuvant chemotherapy may have a role in conjunction with radiotherapy in patients with laryngeal cancer in an attempt to avoid surgery and to preserve the larynx. The use of neoadjuvant chemotherapy to reduce the incidence or delay the appearance of metastatic disease is less certain.

The use of concomitant chemotherapy and radiotherapy potentiates the cytotoxic effects of radiation by the inhibition of sublethal damage repair, hypoxic cell sensitization, and cell cycle synchronization. Cisplatin given weekly with concomitant radiotherapy has also demonstrated an increase in response rate to conventional radiotherapy in inoperable head and neck squamous cell carcinoma (73 vs 59%) *(92)*, but no disease-free or overall survival advantage was observed. Optimal integration of 5-FU and radiotherapy requires a high dose of 5-FU (800–1000 mg/m^2/d for 5 d) and/or continuous protracted exposure for synergy to occur *(93)*.

The data on incidence and mortality, and the results of our current treatments clearly demonstrate the need for new approaches to the treatment of head and neck SCC. New chemotherapy agents that have been tested include the taxanes, paclitaxel and docetaxel, both with approximately 35% response rates in relapsed disease.

4.2. Platinum Chemotherapy

Patients treated with single-agent cisplatin have shown response rates of 20–30% in relapsed disease, and this has become the mainstay of multidrug therapy. One of the major advances in chemotherapy was the development of the 4-d continuous infusion 5-FU plus cisplatin schedule. Response rates of 60–90% were reported in previously untreated patients, with complete remissions in 30–50% of patients *(94)*. The addition of leucovorin has been shown to increase the cytotoxicity of 5-FU by enhancing the inhibition of thymidilate synthase *(95)*, which has also been used in combination with cisplatin/infusional 5-FU in patients with head and neck cancer (Table 7). High-dose cisplatin has been used in a Phase II study of 59 patients with unresectable locally advanced disease *(96)*. The planned cisplatin dose was 80 mg/m^2 per week, but few patients achieved this dose intensity. The response rate was 59%, with 15% of patients achieving a complete response, similar to that of combination regimens; the pattern of toxicity was different, however, with a higher incidence of ototoxicity and marrow suppression being dose limiting (Table 8).

Current standard treatment for metastatic disease is combination chemotherapy. In 1992 Forastiere et al. *(97)* reported the experience of the SWOG in 277 patients with locally recurrent or metastatic head and neck cancer. At that time methotrexate was considered standard therapy for this group of patients and previous Phase II trials reported similar response rates to those seen with

Table 7
Neoadjuvant Combination Cisplatin, no Taxol in Locally Advanced or Inoperable Head and Neck Cancer[a]

	No.	*Treatment*	*RR (%)*	*CR*	*SV/comments*
Veterans Affairs, 1991 (*100*)	332	Cisplatin/5-FU/DXT	85	31	68%/2 y
		vs			
		Surgery/DXT			62%/2 y
					Less metastatic disease with chemoDXT
Vokes et al., 1992 (*107*)	64	PMB × 2	79	21	Median SV 22 mo
		PFL × 2, then	81	29	Not reached
		Surgery or chemoradiotherapy with FHX-L eow			PMB better for metastatic disease
Adelstein et al., 1993 (*108*)	57	Cisplatin 75 mg/m^2		77	RFS 45%/4 y
		5-FU 1000 mg/m^2/4 d + DXT			OS 49%/4 y
		Evaluation wk 5			
		CR/unresectable = chemoradiotherapy			79% failures are locoregional
		PR/SD/resectable = surgery and chemoDXT			
Shirinian et al., 1994 (*105*)	64	Cisplatin/bleomycin/5-FU	75		71%/2 y
		Cisplatin/5-FU, then			
		DXT or surgery if <PR			
Taylor et al., 1994 (*103*)	214	a. Cisplatin 100 mg/m^2	78	50	Similar
		5-FU 1000 mg/m^2 5 d × 3, then DXT	93	52	

		b. Cisplatin 60 mg/m^2 5-FU 800 mg/m^2/5 d DXT days 1–5 eow × 7			Better regional control with concomitant treatment
Dragovic et al., 1995 (*110*)	34	Cisplatin 60 mg/m^2 5-FU 750 mg/m^2/5 d Radiotherapy 2 Gy bds		82	38%/3 y
Scneider et al., 1995 (*95*)	39	Cisplatin 100 mg/m^2 5-FU 500 nmg/m^2/5 d Leucovorin 200 mg/m^2/5 d	87.9	63.7	
Lefebvre et al., 1996 (*101*)	194	a. Cisplatin 100 mg/m^2; 5-FU 1000 mg/m^2/5 d/3w; if CR then DXT otherwise surgery and DXT vs b. Surgery and DXT	86	54	57%/3 y 43%/3 y 0% patients preserve larynx in chemotherapy arm Mostly hypopharynx patients
Adelstein et al., 1997 (*102*)	100	a. DXT b. Cisplatin 20 mg/m^2/4 d; 5-FU 1000 mg/m^2/4 d/d 1 & 22; DXT Assess at 50 Gy—CR/PR complete DXT, if <PR = surgery		50 70	RFS 3 y 52 vs 67 Mets 21 vs 10% OS similar but with successful organ preservation 35/57%

[a]SV, survival; DXT, deep x-ray therapy; FHX-L, ????; eow, ????; bds, ????.

Table 8
Neoadjuvant Single-Agent Cisplatin in Locally Advanced Head and Neck Cancer

Study	*No.*	*Treatment*	*RR (%)*	*CR*	*SV/comments*
Slotman et al., 1992 (*106*)	53	Cisplatin 20 mg/m^2/4 d/wk 1&4/DXT, surgery	94	75	Median survival 45 mo OS 55%/5 y
Planting et al., 1997 (*96*)	59	Cisplatin 80 mg/m^2/wk × 6, DXT, surgery/ DXT or second-line chemotherapy	59		OS 56 wk PFS 32 wk 9 patients achieved planned dose intensity

cisplatin *(98)*. Patients were randomized to have three weekly cycles of cisplatin/5-FU, four weekly cycles of carboplatin/5-FU, or weekly methotrexate. The response rates were 32, 21, and 10%, respectively, with complete response in 6, 2, and 2% of patients. Taylor et al. *(99)* reported on an alternate-week schedule of cisplatin/5-FU given with radiotherapy in patients with locally advanced or recurrent disease. Fifty-five percent of the patients achieved a complete response with a median survival of 37 months, which compared favorably with a Radiation Therapy Oncology Group (RTOG) study of radiotherapy alone.

Neoadjuvant chemotherapy has been tested in randomized trials of operable patients. In 1992 the Department of Veteran Affairs Laryngeal Cancer Study Group *(100)*. published a study of 332 patients with previously untreated stage III or IV squamous carcinoma of the larynx who were randomly assigned to receive three cycles of cisplatin and infusional 5-FU induction treatment followed either by radiotherapy or laryngectomy and postoperative radiotherapy. There was a response rate of 85% to induction chemotherapy, with 49% of patients achieving complete response. The larynx was preserved in 64% of the patients in the chemotherapy group. Local recurrences were significantly higher in the chemotherapy arm (12 vs 2%, $p = 0.001$), but the surgery arm presented with a significantly higher incidence of metastasis (17 vs 11%, $p = 0.001$). There was no disease-free (53.3 and 55.9%) or overall survival (68% for both groups) difference with a median follow-up of 33 months. These results supported the findings of non-randomized trials that induction chemotherapy followed by definitive radiotherapy is an effective strategy to achieve laryngeal preservation without compromising overall survival or causing increased toxicity.

Another randomized study of neoadjuvant chemotherapy vs surgery in operable patients was reported by the EORTC *(101)*. Two hundred and two patients with histologically proven squamous cell carcinoma of the pyriform sinus or of the hypopharyngeal aspect of the ariepliglotic fold were included in this trial. They were randomized to have surgery and radiotherapy or induction chemotherapy with two or three cycles of cisplatin/infusional 5-FU followed by radiotherapy if in complete response, or salvage surgery if this had not been achieved. The response rate in the chemotherapy arm was 86%, with a complete response rate of 40–50%. The median follow-up was 51 months, and the 3-year overall survival was 43% for the surgical plus radiotherapy arm vs 57% for the chemotherapy plus radiotherapy arm, the disease-free survival was 31 and 43%, respectively, and the median survival 25 and 44 months, respectively. The incidence of metastasis at 3 years again favored the chemotherapy arm, with 40% of the patients who received chemotherapy being metastasis free, compared with 27%. The survival of patients whose surgery is delayed for a trial of chemotherapy does not appear to be compromised, and laryngeal preservation is feasible in a high proportion of patients, with 30% being alive and disease-free at 3 years with a functioning larynx.

Aldestein and coworkers published their results *(102)* on 100 patients with resectable stage II–IV disease who were randomized to have radiotherapy alone or concomitant chemotherapy with cisplatin and infusional 5-FU for 4 d during weeks 1 and 3 of radiotherapy. Salvage surgery was reserved for residual disease after 50 Gy of radiotherapy, or recurrent disease. Relapse Free Survival (RFS) was 52 and 67%, respectively, and the likelihood of developing metastasis 21 and 10%, favoring the chemotherapy-radiotherapy arm. Overall survival with successful primary site preservation was 35 vs 57% ($p = 0.02$), again favoring the chemoradiation arm.

Patients with locally advanced unresectable disease were randomized to induction chemotherapy in a study by Taylor et al. *(103)* on 214 patients who received three cycles of neoadjuvant cisplatin/infusional 5-FU followed by radiotherapy or seven cycles of concomitant chemoradiotherapy for 5 d every other week. Overall response rates were significantly different, favoring the concomitant chemoradiation arm (78 vs 93%, $p = 0.006$) although complete response rates were similar. There were no overall survival differences between the two treatments. A study by Merlano and colleagues *(104)* reported on 157 patients with unresectable stage III–IV disease treated with neoadjuvant cisplatin/infusional 5-FU for 5 d alternating with radiotherapy or radiotherapy alone. They found complete response rates of 42 and 22%, respectively ($p = 0.037$), and a median survival of 16.5 vs 11.7 months ($p < 0.05$) in favor of the combined treatment group.

Nonrandomized studies of induction chemotherapy have been published in patients with resectable disease at the M.D. Anderson Cancer Center (MDACC) *(105)*. Sixty-four patients with untreated, locally advanced resectable head and neck cancer were enrolled into an induction regime of cisplatin/bleomycin/infusional 5-FU or cisplatin/infusional 5-FU. Radiotherapy was given to all patients after the chemotherapy. Surgery was reserved for patients who achieved less than a partial response to chemotherapy or those with recurrent or residual disease after sequential chemoradiotherapy. The overall response rate was similar for both treatments (75%), and the complete response rates after radiotherapy were 88, 83, and 50% for laryngeal, hypopharyngeal, and oropharyngeal cancers, respectively. At a follow-up of 15–54 months, 44% of patients with laryngeal, 28% with hypopharyngeal, and 22% with oropharyngeal cancers were alive and disease free with larynx preservation. The overall 2-year survival rates were 71, 46, and 38%, respectively. The lower rate of disease-free survival in the oropharyngeal group may reflect the fact that disease at this site that requires laryngectomy is generally very advanced, with a high rate of T3, 4 and N3 disease. A study of preoperative cisplatin chemoradiotherapy followed by curative surgery was published by Slotman et al. *(106)* and involved 53 patients with advanced stage II and IV disease. Response rates to chemoradiation were 94%, with 84% of the patients achieving a complete response. Twenty-three percent of the patients did not undergo surgery for a variety of reasons. The follow-up of this study was 8 years, and the median survival for all patients was 45 months. The 5-year actuarial survival rate was 43% for all patients, 55% for patients who had chemoradiotherapy and surgery, and 18% for those who did not undergo surgery.

Vokes and colleagues *(107)* have used induction chemotherapy on inoperable patients in a nonrandomized setting. They administered neoadjuvant chemotherapy to 64 previously untreated patients with locoregionally advanced disease. All patients received two cycles of induction chemotherapy with cisplatin, bleomycin, and methotrexate (PMB) or cisplatin/infusional 5-FU (PFL). This was followed by surgery when possible and/or chemoradiotherapy with 5-FU, hydroxyurea, and leucovorin. The response rate was 79% (21% complete response) for patients receiving PMB and 81% (29% complete response) for PFL. The median survival was 22 months in the PMB group, and the median survival for those treated with PFL has not been reached, with a median follow-up of 35 months. The locoregional recurrence rates were 30 and 26% for patients treated with PMB and PFL, respectively. This equals or exceeds that for patients treated with induction chemotherapy followed by standard radiotherapy in previous studies at the same institution. The improved regional control rate appears to translate into favorable long-term survival for patients in the PFL group. Aldestein and coworkers *(108)* published a phase II study on 57 patients with unresectable stage III and IV disease who were treated with two cycles of cisplatin/infusional 5-FU and concurrent split-course radiotherapy. There was a complete remission rate of 77%, which was markedly better than the 44.5% in the radiotherapy-only control arm of the ECOG study in patients with unresectable disease *(109)*. At 4 years the projected RFS was 45%, and the overall survival was 49%. The author noted that 79% of the recurrences were locoregional.

The addition of chemotherapy to accelerated fractionation radiotherapy together has been reported by Dragovic and colleagues *(110)* in a study of 34 patients with stage IV previously untreated inoperable disease. The rationale behind accelerated radiotherapy is that accelerated tumor repopulation during conventionally fractionated radiotherapy could be an important determinant of local control probability *(111)*. Treatment with cisplatin and continuous infusion 5-FU was given on weeks 1, 3, and 5 together with twice daily radiotherapy, the fractionation being more than 6 h apart. The response rate was high (94%), with 82% patients achieving a complete response. The actuarial 3-year survival at a minimum follow-up of 36 months was 38%. Acute mucosal toxicity was acceptable although greater than expected with standard radiotherapy.

4.3. Taxanes

Paclitaxel may be the most active single chemotherapeutic agent for the treatment of head and neck cancer. Preliminary results show a response rate of 37% for single-agent treatment in newly diagnosed patients and those with relapsed disease *(112)*.

There is also preclinical evidence of radiation enhancement by paclitaxel *(113)*. The underlying mechanism of this interaction is thought to be cell cycle arrest in the G_2/M phase of the cell cycle. In vivo studies with murine mammary carcinoma *(114)* have shown that the greatest enhancement of radiation response is not at the time of maximum mitotic arrest by paclitaxel (9 hs), but 1 d after paclitaxel treatment, indicating that paclitaxel may also potentiate tumor response by mechanisms other than blocking the cell cycle in mitosis. Mucosal toxicity with standard doses of paclitaxel is uncommon, and therefore combining it with radiation therapy may be possible without having to interrupt the radiation schedule *(115,116)*.

Forastiere et al. *(117)* reported an ECOG Phase II study of single-agent paclitaxel in patients with recurrent or locally advanced incurable disease. Thirty patients received 250 mg/m^2 over 24 h with granulocyte colony-stimulating factor, (G-CSF) and courses were given every 3 weeks until progression was documented. The response rate was 40%. Severe granulocytopenia occurred in 91% of the patients, but this was short-lived. The median survival was 9 months, with 33% of the patients alive at 1 year. This is in contrast to the median survival of 6–7 months and 1-year survival of 20–25% usually reported in comparable trials using cisplatin and 5-FU. This study established paclitaxel as an active cytotoxic drug for the treatment of squamous cell carcinoma of the head and neck.

Docetaxel (Taxotere) showed clinical activity in patients with advanced or recurrent SCC of the head and neck, with a response rate of 32% in a report from the EORTC on 39 patients *(118)*. This was recently confirmed in a study by Dreyfuss et al. *(119)* on 31 patients with advanced or recurrent disease who were treated with docetaxel 100 mg/m^2 every 3 weeks. The response rate was 42%, with a complete response rate of 13% and a median duration of response of 5 months.

4.4. Platinum/Taxane Combinations

Some studies have demonstrated that there is synergism between paclitaxel and cisplatin *(120)*. Hitt et al. *(121)* reported a Phase I/II study with escalating doses of paclitaxel and a fixed dose of cisplatin as neoadjuvant treatment in 28 patients with locally advanced inoperable head and neck cancer. Chemotherapy was given for 3 weeks and three cycles with G-CSF for paclitaxel doses over 200 mg/m^2. An overall response rate of 78% was reported. A detailed analysis of the data showed that tumors arising in the larynx or hypopharynx seem to respond better to the paclitaxel/cisplatin regimen than those from the oropharynx, oral cavity, or nasal cavity. No dose-limiting toxicity was encountered at paclitaxel doses of 300 mg/m^2 (Table 9).

The ECOG conducted a Phase III trial *(122)* comparing two doses of paclitaxel (135 or 200 mg/m^2/24 h) plus cisplatin 75 mg/m^2 in 197 patients who failed to go into complete response with a cisplatin/5-FU/leucovorin regime or who had previously untreated locally advanced disease. Objective response rates were similar in the two groups (34%). Median and 1-year survival in the two groups were similar, at 7.2 months and 28%, respectively.

Researchers at the Veterans Administration Medical Center *(123)* designed a pilot study to determine the feasibility of combining 3-h infusional paclitaxel with 5-FU and cisplatin in chemotherapy-naive patients with recurrent or advanced disease. Seventeen patients were treated with paclitaxel at a dose of 135 mg/m^2/3 h together with cisplatin 75 mg/m^2 and infusional 5-FU 1 g/m^2/24 h for 3 d for three courses. The major toxicities were neutropenia and mucositis.

Another group *(124)* treated 23 chemotherapy-naive patients with relapsed and/or metastatic disease, with a continuous infusion of cisplatin and 5-FU for 3 d (20 and 200 mg/m^2/d, respectively), and escalating doses of paclitaxel starting at 100 mg/m^2 with no G-CSF. The overall response rate was 38%, and the maximum tolerated dose of paclitaxel was determined to be at 160 mg/m^2.

The addition of ifosfamide to the paclitaxel/cisplatin combination has been investigated by Shin et al. *(125)* at the MDACC. Fifty-three chemotherapy-naive patients with recurrent or metastatic disease were enrolled. The treatment was paclitaxel 175 mg/m^2, cisplatin 60 mg/m^2, and 3 d of ifosfamide at 1 g/m^2/d. Overall response rate was 58%, with 17% of patients achieving a complete response. The median follow-up was 17.7 months and the median survival 8.8 months. The response rate was almost twice that reported in the literature with standard cisplatin/infusional 5-FU treatment in this setting (Table 10).

Table 9
Neoadjuvant Taxol in Advanced or Inoperable Patients with Head and Neck Cancer[a]

Study	*No.*	*Treatment*	*RR (%)*	*CR (%)*	*SV*
B Dunphy, 1997	36	Escalating Taxol 150–265, mg/m^2 Carboplatin AUC 7.5	61	29	NS MTD 230 mg/m^2 w/o G-CSF 250 mg/m^2 w/G-CSF
E Hitt, et al., 1997 *(121)*	28	Escalating Taxol 175–300 mg/m^2 Cisplatin 75 mg/m^2	78	13/28	60%/3 y No DLT at Taxol 300 Larynx and hypopharynx respond better

[a]DLT, dose-limiting toxicity.

Docetaxel has been used with cisplatin in patients with locally advanced, unresectable, or metastatic disease. The EORTC *(126)* reported on 24 patients treated with docetaxel 100 mg/m^2 and cisplatin 75 mg/m^2 every 3 weeks for two to six courses; 24 were evaluable for response at the time of the report, and a response rate of 78% (CR 11%) was achieved. The main toxicity was neutropenia, and 25% of the patients experienced mild sensory neuropathy. The combination of docetaxel with cisplatin, 5-FU, and leucovorin has also been used as induction treatment in a Phase I/II study by Colevas and colleagues *(127)* in cases with locally advanced disease; patients who responded went on to receive radiotherapy. They treated 23 patients with an overall response rate of 100% (61% complete response). The maximum tolerated dose for docetaxel was established at 60 mg/m^2 with neutropenia being the dose-limiting toxicity; other significant toxicities were mucositis, diarrhea, peripheral neuropathy, and sodium-wasting nephropathy.

4.5. Conclusions

Platinums have been considered the mainstay of multidrug therapy in head and neck cancer. The reported response rate for cisplatin as a single agent is 20–30%. The combination of cisplatin and infusional 5-FU over 4 d has increased the response rate to 60–90% in chemotherapy-naive patients. The landmark study of the Veterans Administration group supported the integration of chemotherapy as induction treatment followed by radiotherapy as a way to preserve the larynx in a proportion of patients without having a detrimental effect on survival. This has been corroborated in two studies that have also used concomitant radiochemotherapy with the suggestion of a further improvement in

Table 10
Relapsed or Metastatic Head and Neck Cancer: Combination Treatment with Taxol

Study	*No.*	*Treatment*	*RR (%)*	*CR (%)*	*SV*
Forastiere, 1995	13	Taxol 170 mg/m^2 Ifosfamide 5 g/m^2	5/11 PR		NS
Husssain et al., 1997 (*123*)	17	Escalating Taxol Cisplatin 75 mg/m^2 5-FU 1000 mg/m^2/4 d	71	2/14	Active
Benasso et al., 1977 (*124*)	23	Escalating Taxol 100–180 mg/m^2 Cisplatin 20 mg/m^2/3 d 5-FU 200 mg/m^2/3 d	38		NS Choose Taxol 160 Ciplatin 25/3 d 5-FU 250/3 d
Forastiere et al., 1998 (*117*)	34	Taxol 250 mg/m^2/3 wk G-CSF	40		33%/1 y
Dong, 1998	53	Taxol 175 mg/m^2 Ifosfamide 1 g/m^2/3 d	58	17	Median 8.8 mo

the results compared with a sequential schedule. The survival of patients whose surgery is delayed for a trial of chemotherapy does not appear to be shortened, and larynx preservation is feasible in 64% of patients.

Taxanes appear to be the most active drugs for the treatment of head and neck cancer, with response rates to single-agent therapy of 40% in newly diagnosed and relapsed patients.

The combination of platinum and taxane appears to be promising, as there is synergism between both drugs; response rates in inoperable patients approach 80%, and one-third of patients with platinum-resistant disease respond to combination platimun-taxane treatment.

5. BREAST CANCER

5.1. Introduction

Breast cancer is the most common cancer in women, affecting approximately 1 in 12 women in the United Kingdom during their lifetime. Like ovarian and lung cancer, once the disease has spread to distant organs it is rarely if ever curable. Unlike these malignancies, however, half of those patients with metastatic breast cancer live over 2 years, and up to 10% will live over 10 years. Significant palliation and survival benefit can be obtained by chemotherapy over a number of years, and careful patient selection and sequencing of successive chemotherapy regimens is important to minimize cumulative toxicity.

Most women present with apparently localized disease; a number of these will be treated with adjuvant regimens of proven efficacy such as cyclophosphamide, methotrexate, and 5-FU (CMF), 5-FU, epirubicin, and cyclophosphamide (FEC) or Adriamycin and cyclophosphamide (AC). Patients representing with metastases can benefit from further chemotherapy, but they are incurable and hence the search for new agents with novel mechanisms of action.

The average response rate to chemotherapy for metastatic disease in chemotherapy-naive patients is about 50% *(152)*, but in previously treated patients it is lower (20–25%) *(167)*.

5.2. Platinum Chemotherapy

Carboplatin and cisplatin are known to be active in the treatment of breast cancer, with single-agent response rates of 25–37% in chemotherapy-naive patients *(155,158)*. The combination of a platinum compound and anthracycline results in response rates of 80–86% in such patients, but responses to second-line treatment are disappointing, with the response rate falling to 41–63%. If no anthracycline is used and the accompanying drugs are alkylating agents or 5-FU, the response is in the order of 8–28% *(143)*. Platinum compounds are not used routinely in first-line therapy, as their toxicity relative to other equally effective agents makes them less attractive in the adjuvant setting. This does, however, make them more useful in the treatment of disease recurrence after adjuvant treatment, as platinum resistance is less likely. Initial studies with cisplatin in the treatment of metastatic disease were obviously done as single-agent trials in heavily pretreated patients. Consequently the response rate was very low, on the order of 9%, and of short duration *(170)*. Analysis of the relation between dose intensity and response showed that no patient who received less than 25 mg/m^2/wk of cisplatin achieved an objective remission, compared with an approximately 25% response rate in those whose dose was higher than 33 mg/m^2/wk. In first-line therapy for metastatic disease, it has been shown that the overall response rate is up to 50%, with most patients achieving a partial response and a median duration of 4–5 months only. Combination studies of cisplatin with doxorubicin, etoposide, or 5-FU have demonstrated higher activity, with response rates of 60–70% *(144,149,154)*. Several randomized trials have compared cisplatin-containing regimens with standard CMF or CAP, some of them showing an advantage for the former in terms of response rates, although no trial has demonstrated superiority with regard to overall survival *(168)*. The combination of cisplatin or carboplatin with epirubicin and infusional 5-FU has been extensively used in patients with metastatic or locally advanced breast cancer at the Royal Marsden Hospital. These combinations have given an overall response rate of 81% (17% complete) in patients with metastatic disease and 56% in patients with locally advanced disease *(140,153)*.

Both cisplatin and carboplatin have been used extensively in the context of high-dose chemotherapy and autologous bone marrow transplantation for metastatic breast cancer. Cisplatin in combination with cyclophosphamide and carmustine showed a response rate of 55%; 14% of patients were long-term survivors (3.3–6.5 years, *(163)*). Cisplatin has properties that make it less than ideal for high-dose chemotherapy because the neuro- and nephrotoxicity become dose limiting. Carboplatin has been used instead of cisplatin in the high-dose setting with similar results *(129)*.

Cisplatin has recently been used in combination with a monoclonal antibody against the growth factor receptor Her2/neu. Overexpression of HER2/neu is associated with a number of other adverse prognostic factors and occurs in 25–30% of patients with breast cancer. The synergistic cytotoxic effect of cisplatin and antibodies against HER2/neu appears to involve a decreased capacity of cells that overexpress HER2/neu to repair cisplatin-induced DNA adducts after being exposed to antibody. The response rate to this combination has recently been reported by Pegram and colleagues *(160)*, to be 24% in 37 patients with extensively pretreated advanced breast cancer showing overexpresion of the gene. This appears to be higher than the 8% reported for cisplatin alone in this context.

5.3. Taxanes

The introduction of the taxanes has been a significant advance in the treatment of advanced breast cancer. Single-agent paclitaxel, using administration schedules that vary from 3 to 24 h and in doses ranging from 175 to 250 mg/m^2, produces overall responses in 29–63% of patients with metastatic disease when given as first-line therapy *(145)*. The antitumor efficacy is lower in more heavily pretreated patients, in whom the response rate falls to 6–47% *(143)*. Randomized trials comparing dose levels and administration schedules of single-agent paclitaxel have shown that 175 mg/m^2 gives a very slightly better response rate than 135 mg/m^2 (29 vs 22%) with similar toxicity profiles for the 3-h or 24-h infusion rate *(157)*. Regression analyses for overall response rate, time to progression, and survival indicated that the results achieved with paclitaxel were independent of previous anthracycline exposure and resistance. The median duration of response in 11 studies ranges from 4 to 9 months *(157)*.

A large multi-institutional randomized trial was reported by Sledge and colleagues *(169)* on 739 patients with recurrent or metastatic breast cancer. Patients received doxorubicin (D), paclitaxel (P), or a combination of both as first-line therapy. Patients receiving single-agent treatment were crossed over to the other agent at time of progression. Granulocytopenia was the main toxicity. There was no increased cardiac toxicity with the combination of D+P compared with D alone. The response rates were 34% for D, 33% for P, and 46% for D+P. Median times to treatment failure were 6.2, 5.9, and 8.0 months, respectively. The authors concluded that single-agent D and P have equivalent therapeutic activity; the combination of D+P results in superior overall response rate and time to treatment failure. Even so, the combination was not superior to sequential single-agent treatment with regard to overall survival.

Alkylating agents have also been successfully combined with paclitaxel. A dose-finding study by Pagani et al. *(159)* and co-workers reported on 80 women with metastatic breast cancer treated with paclitaxel and cyclophosphamide. The overall response rate was 25% for patients with prior chemotherapy and 50% for those without prior chemotherapy for metastatic disease. The recommended doses were 200 mg/m^2 for paclitaxel and 1750 mg/m^2 for cyclophosphamide given every 3 weeks. G-CSF was to be used in pretreated patients.

Paclitaxel, when used as neoadjuvant therapy, has been reported to produce response rates of 61% (9% complete) when given as a single agent (200–300 mg/m^2 every 3 weeks x 4, with G-CSF) *(147)* or up to 74% in combination with anthracyclines *(128)*. Paclitaxel 200 mg/m^2 with doxorubicin 60 mg/m^2 or epirubicin 60–90 mg/m^2 was found to be well tolerated in previously untreated patients, but about 20% of patients experienced significant cardiac toxicity *(148)*.

Docetaxel when administered at 100 mg/m^2 as a 1-h infusion produces response rates of 54–68%. Dosages of 100 and 75 mg/m^2 were evaluated in three European trials of docetaxel as first-line chemotherapy for metastatic disease. The response rate was 52% for the lower dose and 68% for the higher *(145)*. Response rates of 10–57% are seen in more heavily pretreated patients *(143)*. A major concern regarding treatment with docetaxel was fluid retention, with the median cumulative dose to the onset of this complication being 400 mg/m^2 in non-premedicated patients. Recent data demonstrate that the prophylactic use of dexamethasone 8 mg orally twice a day for 5 days starting 24 h before docetaxel infusion can significantly delay the onset and reduce the severity of fluid retention, as can increasing the median cumulative dose of docetaxel to 746 mg/m^2 *(165)*. Several studies evaluating second-line docetaxel in patients with previously treated advanced breast cancer have shown it to be highly active, even among patients with a prior history of anthracycline exposure. In an EORTC study, the response rate was 58% in patients with one prior chemotherapy regimen for stage IV disease *(171)*, 53 and 57% in two single-institution U.S. studies of strictly defined anthracycline-resistant metastatic breast cancer *(164,172)*, and 32% in an EORTC multicenter study of patients with anthracycline-resistant disease *(173)*. Responses were seen in visceral and nonvisceral sites of disease, and the median duration of response ranged from 6 to 7 months.

Several Phase III studies have been reported, comparing the efficacy and safety of docetaxel. Chan and colleagues *(142)* reported a response rate of 47% for docetaxel 100 mg/m^2 as first- or second-line therapy in patients previously exposed to an anthracycline, vs 32% for doxorubicin at 75 mg/m^2. The median time to progression was 29 vs 21 weeks. A study comparing second-line docetaxel 100 mg/m^2 with mitomycin 12 mg/m^2/6 weekly plus vinblastine 6 mg/m^2/3 weekly in anthracycline-pretreated patients, with 100 evaluable patients on each arm, showed a response rate of 28 vs 14% in favor of docetaxel *(156)*.

Two U.S. multicenter phase III studies are evaluating docetaxel 100 mg/m^2 vs docetaxel 75 mg/m^2 or paclitaxel 175 mg/m^2/3 h as first- or second-line treatment in metastatic breast cancer.

The combination of docetaxel with doxorubicin has been reported in patients with advanced breast cancer as first-line therapy for metastatic disease *(146)*. The overall response rate in evaluable patients was 90%. The significant activity of docetaxel as a single agent and in combination has provided the rationale to evaluate its role in neoadjuvant therapy. A study by Gradishar *(151a)* reported on 43 patients with stage III disease who were treated with four cycles of docetaxel (100 mg/m^2 every 3 weeks) followed by surgery and four cycles of adjuvant AC; the response rate was 78%, with 2% of patients achieving a complete response.

5.4. Platinum/Taxane Combinations

The rationale behind combining cisplatin with paclitaxel is that cisplatin is active against metastatic breast cancer but is not a component of standard adjuvant chemotherapy, which means that patients who fail after adjuvant therapy may not have cisplatin-resistant disease. In addition, the toxic effects of both drugs are not overlapping, with the exception of neurotoxicity. Preclinical studies suggest synergism between cisplatin and paclitaxel, and sequence-dependent interactions *(166)*. Seven trials have assessed the combination of paclitaxel and cisplatin in advanced breast cancer (Table 11). These are all small trials with consequently variable response rates (21–88%). This combination has not found widespread favor, as response rates are not significantly better than alternative paclitaxel combinations and in some studies an unacceptable degree of neurotoxicity was encountered *(174)*. The commonest schedule of administration is paclitaxel 200 mg/m^2 as a 24-h infusion plus cisplatin 75 mg/m^2.

The combination of carboplatin and paclitaxel has recently been reported in a Phase II trial in patients receiving first-line chemotherapy for advanced or metastatic disease by the North Central Cancer Treatment Group *(161)*. They administered paclitaxel 200 mg/m^2 as a 3-h infusion followed by carboplatin AUC 6 with cycles repeated every 3 weeks to 53 patients. Seventy percent of them had had prior exposure to doxorubicin, and 56% had visceral-dominant disease. The response rate was 60% and the median time to progression 6.7 months. Median overall survival has not yet been reached.

Table 11
Cisplatin and Paclitaxel in Metastatic Breast Cancer

Study	*No. enrolled/ evaluable*	*Cisplatin (mg/m^2)*	*Paclitaxel ($mg/m^2/h$)*	*RR (%)*	*CR (%)*
Browne et al., 1995 (*141*)	13/14	75	135/24	54	2
Berry, et al., 1995 (*130*)	17/17	75	135/3	88	41
Frazier et al., 1995 (*150*)	34/39	75	200/24	44	12
Wasserheit et al., 1996 (*174*)	41/44	75	200/24	53	6
Gelman et al., 1996 (*151*)	27/29	60	90/3[a]	85	11
Sparano, 1996	14/16	60	90/3[a]	21	0
McCaskill, 1996	25/25	60	90/3[a]	60	12

*Given 2-weekly
[a]Given twice a week.

REFERENCES

Ovarian Cancer

1. Abu-Rustum, N. R., Aghajanian, C., Borakat, R. R., Fenelly, D., Shapiro, F., and Spriggs, D. (1997) Salvage weekly paclitaxel in recurrent ovarian cancer. *Semin. Oncol.* **24(Suppl 15),** S15-62–S15-67.
2. Advanced Ovarian Cancer Trialist Group (1991) Chemotherapy in advanced ovarian cancer: an overview of randomized clinical trials. *BMJ* **303,** 884–893.
3. Alberts, P. S., Green, S. Hannigan, E. V., et al. (1992) Improved therapeutic index of carboplatin plus cyclophosphamide versus cisplatin plus cyclophosphamide: final report by the Southwest Oncology Group of a phase III, randomized trial in stages III and IV ovarian cancer. *J. Clin. Oncol.* **10,** 706–717.
4. Bella, M., Cocconi, G., and Lotticci, R. (1994) Mature results of a prospective randomized trial comparing two different dose-intensity regimens of cisplatin in advanced ovarian carcinoma. *Ann. Oncol.* **5(Suppl 80),** 2.
5. Bertelsen, K., Jakobsen, A., Stroyer, I., et al. (1993) A prospective randomized comparison of 6 and 12 cycles of cyclophosphamide, Adriamycin and cisplatin in advanced epithelial ovarian cancer. A Danish Ovarian Study Group trial (DaCOVA). *Gynecol. Oncol.* **49,** 30–35.
6. Blockledge, G., Lawton, F., Redman, C., and Kelly, K. (1989) Response of patients in phase II studies of chemotherapy in ovarian cancer: implications for patient treatment and the design of phase II trials. *Br. J. Cancer* **59,** 650–653.
7. Bolis, G., Scarfone, G., Villa, A., Acerboni, S., Siliprandi, V., and Guarnerio (1997) A phase I trial with fixed dose carboplatin and escalating doses of paclitaxel in advanced ovarian cancer. *Semin. Oncol.* **24(Suppl 2),** S2-23–S2-25.
8. Bookman, M. A., McGuire, W. P., Kilpatrick, D., et al. (1996) Carboplatin and paclitaxel in ovarian carcinoma: a phase I study of the Gynecologic Oncology Group. *J. Clin. Oncol.* **14,** 1895–1902.

9. Calvert, A. H. (1997) A review of the pharmacokinetics and pharmacodynamics of combination carboplatin/paclitaxel. *Semin. Oncol.* **24(Suppl 2),** S2-85–S2-90.
10. Calvert, A. H., Newell, D. R., Gumbrell, L. A., et al. (1989) Carboplatin dosage: evaluation of a simple formula based on renal function. *J. Clin. Oncol.* **7,** 1748–1756.
11. Capri, G., Tarenzi, E., Fulfaro, F., and Gianni, L. (1996) The role of taxanes in the treatment of breast cancer. *Semin. Oncol.* **23(Suppl 2),** 68–75.
12. Chevallier, B., Fumoleau, P., Kerbrat, P., et al. (1995) Docetaxel is a major cytotoxic drug for the treatment of advanced breast cancer. A phase II trial of the Clinical Screening Cooperative Group of the European Organisation for Research and Treatment of Cancer. *J. Clin. Oncol.* **13,** 314–322.
13. Donehower, R. C., Rowinsky, E. K., Grochow, L. K., et al. (1987) Phase I trial of taxol in patients with advanced cancer. *Cancer Treat. Rep.* **71,** 1–7.
14. du Bois, A., Luck, H., Meier, W., et al. (1997) Carboplatin/paclitaxel versus cisplatin paclitaxel as first line chemotherapy in advanced ovarian cancer: an interim analysis of a randomized phase III trial of the Arbeitsgemeinschaft Gynakologische Onkologie Ovarian Cancer Study Group. *Semin. Oncol.* **24(Suppl 15),** S15-44–S15-52.
15. Einzig, A. I., Wiernik, P. H., Sasloff, J., et al. (1992) Phase II study and long-term follow-up of patients treated with taxol for advanced ovarian adenocarcinoma. *J. Clin. Oncol.* **10,** 1748–1753.
16. Eisenhauer, E. A., ten Bokkel Huinink, W. W., Swenerton, K. D., et al. (1994) European-Canadian randomized trial of paclitaxel in relapsed ovarian cancer: high dose versus low dose and long versus short infusion. *J. Clin. Oncol.* **12,** 2654–2666.
17. Eisenhauer, E. A., Vermokken, J. B., and van Glabbeke, M. (1997) Predictors of response to subsequent chemotherapy in platinum pretreated ovarian cancer: a multivarate analysis of 704 patients. *Ann. Oncol.* **8,** 963–968.
18. Gelmon, K. (1994) The taxoids: paclitaxel and docetaxel. *Lancet* **344,** 1267–1272.
19. Gianni, L., Kearns, C. M., Giani, A., et al. (1995) Nonlinear pharmacokinetics and metabolism of paclitaxel and its pharmacokinetic/pharmacodynamic relationships in humans. *J. Clin. Oncol.* **13,** 180–190.
20. Gore, M. E. (1996) The role of taxanes, in *Ovarian Cancer 4*, Chapman & Hall Medical, London, pp. 143–152
21. Gore, M. E., Fryatt, I., Wiltshaw, E., and Dawson, T. (1990) Treatment of relapsed carcinoma of the ovary with cisplatin or carboplatin following initial treatment with these compounds. *Gynecol. Oncol.* **36,** 207–211.
22. Gore, M. E., Levy, V., Rustin, G., et al. (1995) Paclitaxel (Taxol) in relapsed and refractory ovarian cancer: the UK and Eire experience. *Br. J. Cancer* **72,** 1016–1019.
23. Gore, M. E., Preston, N., and A'Hern, R. P. (1995) Platinum-taxol non-cross resistance in epithetial ovarian cancer. *Br. J. Cancer* **7l,** 1308–1310.
24. Greco, F. A. and Hainsworth, J. D. (1996) Paclitaxel via 1-hour infusion: rationale and pharmocology. *Semin. Oncol.* **23(Suppl 15),** 19–20.
25. Gruppo Interregionale Cooperativo Oncologica Ginecologica (1992) Long term results of a randomized trial comparing cisplatin with cisplatin and cyclophosphamide with cisplatin, cyclophosphamide and Adriamycin in advanced ovarian cancer. *Gynecol. Oncol.* **45,** 115–117.
26. Hakes, T., Hoskins, W., Jones, W., et al. (1992) Randomized prospective trial of 5 versus 10 cycles of cyclophosphamide, doxorubicin and cisplatin in advanced ovarian cancer. *Gynecol. Oncol.* **45,** 284–289.
27. Harper, P. (1997). ICON2 and ICON3 data in previously untreated ovarian cancer: results to date. *Semin. Oncol.* **24(Suppl.15),** S15-23–S15-25.
28. Huizing, M. T., Van Warmerdam, L. J. C., Rosing, H., et al. (1997) Phase I and pharmacologic study of the combination paclitaxel and carboplatin as first-line chemotherapy in stage III and IV ovarian cancer. *J. Clin. Oncol.* **15,** 1953–1964.

29. Kaye, S. B., Piccart M., Aapro, M., Francis, P. and Kavanagh, J. (1997) Phase II trials of docetaxel (Taxotere ®) in advanced ovarian cancer—an updated overview. *Eur. J. Cancer.* **33,** 2167–2170.
30. Kaye, S. D., Lewis, C. R., Paul, J., et al. (1992) Randomised study of two doses of cisplatin with cyclophosphamide in epithelial ovarian cancer. *Lancet* **340,** 329–333.
31. Lavelle, F., Bissery, M. C., Combeau, C., et al. (1995) Preclinical evaluation of docetaxel (Taxotere). *Semin. Oncol.* **22(Suppl 4),** 3–16.
32. Mainwaring, P. N., and Gore, M. E. (1995) The importance of dose and schedule in cancer chemotherapy: epithelial ovarian cancer. *Anticancer Drugs.* **6(Suppl 5),** 29–41.
33. Markman, M. (1997) Current status and future directions of platinum/paditaxel-based chemotherapy of ovarian cancer. *Semin. Oncol.* **24(Suppl 11),** S11-24–S11-27.
34. Markman, M., Rothman, R., Hakes, T., et al. (1991) Second-line platinum therapy in patients with ovarian cancer previously treated with cisplatin. *J. Clin. Oncol.* **9,** 389–393.
35. McGuire, W. P., Hoskins, W. J., Brady, M. F., et al. (1996) Cyclophosphamide and cisplatin compared with paclitaxel and cisplatin in patients with stage III and stage IV ovarian cancer. *N. Engl. J. Med.* **334,** 1–6.
36. Muggia, T. M., Brady, P. S., Braly, M. F., et al. (1997) Phase II of cisplatin (P) or paclitaxel (T), versus their combination in suboptimal stage II and IV epithelial ovarian cancer (EOC): Gynecologic Oncology Group (GOG) study # 132. *Proc. Am. Soc. Clin. Oncol.* **16,** 352a.
37. National Institutes of Health Consensus Development Conference Statement. (1994) Ovarian cancer: screening, treatment, and follow-up. *Gynecol. Oncol.* **55,** S4-14
38. Neijt, J. P., Engelholm, S. A., Witteveen, P. O., et al. (1997) Paclitaxel (175 mg/m^2 over 3 hours) with cisplatin or carboplatin in previously untreated ovarian cancer: an interim analysis. *Semin. Oncol.* **24(Suppl 15),** S15-36–S15-39.
39. Ngan H., Choo Y., Cheung M., et al. (1989) A randomized study of high-dose versus low-dose cisplatin combined with cyclophosphamide in the treatment of advanced ovarian cancer. *Chemotherapy* **35,** 221–227.
40. Olsen, J. K., Sood, A. K., Sorosky, J. I., Anderson, B., and Buller, R. E. (1998) Taxol hypersensitivity: rapid retreatment is safe and cost effective. *Gynec. Oncol.* **68,** 25–28.
41. Ozols, R. F., Thigpen, J. T., Dauplat, J., et al. (1993) Dose Intensity. *Ann. Oncol.* **4(Suppl 4**), S49–S56.
42. Piccart, M. J., Bertelsen, G., Stuart, G., et al. (1997) Is cisplatin-paclitaxel (P-T) the standard in first-line treatment of advanced ovarian cancer (OvCa)? The EORTC-GCCG, NOCOVA, NCI-C and Scottish intergroup experience. *Proc. Am. Soc. Clin. Oncol.* **16,** 352a.
43. Rowinsky, E. K., Gilbert, M. R., McGuire, W. P., et al. (1991) Sequences of Taxol and cisplatin: a phase I and pharmacologic study. *J. Clin. Oncol.* **9,** 1692–1703.
44. Rowinsky, E. K., and Donehower, R. C. (1995). Paclitaxel (Taxol) *N. Engl. J. Med.* **332,** 1004–1014.
45. Siddiqui, N., Boddy, A. V., Thomas, H. D., et al. (1997) A clinical and pharmacokinetic study of the combination of carboplatin and paclitaxel for epithelial ovarian cancer. *Br. J. Cancer* **75,** 287–294.
46. Stuart, G., Bertelsen, K., Mangioni, C., et al. (1998) Updated analysis shows a highly significant improved overall survival (OS) for cisplatin-paclitaxel as first line treatment of advanced ovarian cancer: mature results of the EORTC-GCCG, NOCOVA, NCIC CTG and Scottish intergroup trial. *Proc. Am. Soc. Clin. Oncol.* **17,** 361a.
47. Swenerton, K., Jeffrey, J., Stuart, G., et al. (1992) Cisplatin-cyclophosphamide versus carboplatin-cyclophosphamide in advanced ovarian cancer: a randomized phase III study of the National Cancer Institute of Canada Clinical Trials Group. *J. Clin. Oncol.* **10,** 718–726.
48. ten Bokkel Huinink, W., Veenhof, C., Huizing, M., et al. (1997) Carboplatin and paclitaxel in patients with advanced ovarian cancer: a dose-finding study. *Semin. Oncol.* **24(Suppl 2**), S2–21–S2–33.
49. ten Bokkel Huinink, W. W., Prove, A. M., Piccart, M., et al. (1994) A phase II trial with

docetaxel (Laxotere) in second line treatment with chemotherapy for advanced breast cancer. A study of the EORTC Early Clinical Trials Group. *Ann. Oncol.* **5,** 527–532.
50. Thigpen, T., Blessing, J., Ball, H., et al. (1990) Phase II trial of taxol as second line therapy for ovarian carcinoma: a Gynecologic Oncology Group Study. *Proc. Am. Soc. Clin. Oncol.* **9,** 604.
51. Torri, V. (1997). Randomized study of cyclophosphamide, doxorubicin and cisplatin (CAP) vs single agent carboplatin in ovarian cancer patients requiring chemotherapy: interim results of ICON2. *Proc. Am. Soc. Clin. Oncol.* **15,** 280.
52. Trimble, E. L., Adams, J. P., Vera, D., et al. (1993). Paclitaxel for platinum refractory ovarian cancer: results from the first 1,000 patients registered to National Cancer Institute Treatment Referral Centre 9103. *J. Clin. Oncol.* **11,** 2405–2410.
53. Trope, C. and Kristensen, G. (1997) Current status of chemotherapy in gynaecologic cancer. *Semin. Oncol.* **24(5 Suppl. 15),** S15-1–S15-22.
54. Van Glabbeke, M., Vermorken, J., and Eisenhauer, E. (1997) Predictors of survival (OS) and time to progression (TTP) following second- or third-line treatment in advanced ovarian cancer (OVCA): an analysis of 714 patients (PTS) treated with paclitaxel, docetaxel or high dose epirubicin. *Proc. Am. Soc. Clin. Oncol.* **16,** 354a.
55. Vermorken, J. B., ten Bokkel Huinink, W. W., Eisenhauer, E. A., et al. (1993) Carboplatin versus cisplatin. *Ann. Oncol.* **4(Suppl 4),** S41–S48.
56. Wari, M. C., Taylor, H. L., Wall, M. E., et al. (1971) Plant anti-tumour agents VI. The isolation and structur of Taxol, a novel antileukemic and antitumour agent from *Taxus brevifolia. J. Am. Chem. Soc.* **93,** 2325–2329.

Lung Cancer

57. Androulakis, N., Kourousis, C., Kakolyris, S., et al. (1996) First line treatment of non-small-cell lung cancer with docetaxel and cisplatin. Preliminary results of a phase II study. *Ann. Oncol.* **7(Suppl 5),** 98–99.
58. Belani, C. P., Aisner, J., Hiponia, D., et al. (1995) Paclitaxel and carboplatin with and without filgrastim support in patients with metastatic non-small cell lung cancer. *Semin. Oncol.* **22(Suppl 9),** 7–12.
59. Belli, L., Le Chavalier, T., Gottfried, M., et al. (1995) Phase I-II trial of paclitaxel (Taxol) and cisplatin in previously untreated advanced non-small cell lung cancer. *Proc. Am. Soc. Clin. Oncol.* **14,** 348.
60. Bonomi, P., Kim, C., Kugler, K., and Johnson, D. (1997) Results of a phase III trial comparing Taxol-cisplatin regimens to etoposide-cisplatin in non-small cell lung cancer. *Lung Cancer* **18(Suppl 1),** 10.
61. Bunn, P. A. and Kelly, K. (1995) A phase I study of carboplatin and paclitaxel in non-small cell lung cancer: a University of Colorado Cancer Center Study. *Semin. Oncol.* **22(suppl 9),** 2–6.
62. Bunn, P. A. (1997) Defining the role of paclitaxel in lung cancer. Summary of recent studies and implications for future directions. *Semin. Oncol.* **24(Suppl 12)**, S12-15–S12-62.
63. Burris, H., Eckardt, J., Fields, S., et al. (1993) Phase II trials of taxotere in patients with non small cell lung cancer. *Proc. Am. Soc. Clin. Oncol.* **12,** 335.
64. Carney, D. N. (1996) Chemotherapy in the management of patients with inoperable non-small-cell lung cancer. *Semin. Oncol.* **23(Suppl 16)**, 71–75.
65. Cole, J. T., Galla, R. J., Margues, C. B., et al. (1995) Phase I-II study of cisplatin and docetaxel (Taxotere) in non-small-cell lung cancer (NSCLC). *Proc. Am. Soc. Clin. Oncol.* **14,** 357.
66. Cole, J. T., Galla, R. J., Rittenberg, C. N., et al. (1997) Defining the dose of docetaxel (Taxotere) in combination chemotherapy of non-small-cell lung cancer: preserving efficacy with lower dose regimens. *Proc. Am. Soc. Clin. Oncol.* **16,** 465a.

67. Creaven, P. J., Raghavan, D., Perez, R. P., et al. (1996) Early phase studies with paclitaxel/low-dose carboplatin in patients with solid tumors. *Semin. Oncol.* **23(Suppl 16),** 26–31.
68. De Vore, R. F. III., Jagasia, M., Johnson, D. H. (1997) Paclitaxel by either 1-hour or 24-hour infusion in combination with carboplatin in advanced non-small cell lung cancer. Preliminary results comparing sequential phase II trieals. *Semin. Oncol.* **24(Suppl 12),** S12-27–S12-29.
69. Douillard, F. U., Monnier, A., Ibrahim, N., et al. (1995) Preliminary results of the first phase II trial of docetaxel in combination with cisplatin in patients with metastatic or locally advanced non-small cell lung cancer (NSLLC). *Proc. Am. Soc. Clin. Oncol.* **14,** 351.
70. Ellis, P. A., Smith, I. C., Hardy, J. R., et al. (1995) Symptom relief with MVP (mitomycin C, vinblastine and cisplatin) chemotherapy in advanced non-small-cell lung cancer. *Br. J. Cancer* **71,** 366–370.
71. Fossella, F. V., Lee, J. S., Shin, D. M., et al. (1995) Phase II study of docetaxel for advanced or metastatic platinum refractory non small cell lung cancer. *J. Clin. Oncol.* **13,** 643–651.
72. Georgiadis, M. S., Schuler, B. S., Brown, J. E., et al. (1997) Paclitaxel by 96-hour continuous infusion in combination with cisplatin. A phase I trial in patients with advanced lung cancer. *J. Clin. Oncol.* **15,** 735–743.
73. Giaccone. G., Postmus, P., Debruyne, C., et al., for the EORTC LCCG (1997) Final results of an EORTC phase III study of paclitaxel versus teniposide in combination with cisplatin in advanced NSCLC. *Proc. Am. Soc. Clin. Oncol.* **16,** 460a.
74. Greco F. A., Hainsworth, J. D. (1997) Paclitaxel (1-hour infusion) plus carboplatin in the treatment of advanced non-small cell lung cancer: results of a multicenter phase II trial. *Semin. Oncol.* **24(Suppl 12),** S12-14–S12-17.
75. Huizing, M. T., Giaccone, G., van Wormerdam, L. J. C., et al. (1997) Pharmacokinetics of paclitaxel and carboplatin in a dose-escalating and dose-sequencing study in patients with non-small cell lung cancer.
76. Jaakkimainen, L., Goodwin, P. J., Pater, J., et al. (1990) Counting the costs of chemotherapy in a National Cancer Institute of Canada randomized trial in non-small cell lung cancer. *J. Clin. Oncol.* **8,** 1301–1309.
77. Klastersky, J., Sculier, J. P., European Lung Cancer Working Party (1995) Dose finding study of paclitaxel (Taxol) plus cisplatin in patients with non-small-cell lung cancer. *Lung Cancer* **12,** 117–125.
78. Kosimidis, P., Mylonakis, N., Fountzilas, G., Samantos, C., Athonasiodis, A., and Skarlos, P., (1996) Paclitaxel and Carboplatin in inoperable non-small-cell lung cancer. *Semin. Oncol.* **23(Suppl 16),** 68–70.
79. Langer, C. J., Millenson, M., Rosvold E., et al. (1997) Paclitaxel (1 hour) and carboplatin (area under the concentration-time curve 7.5) in advanced non-small cell lung cancer: A phase II study of the Fox Chase Cancer Center and its network. *Semin. Oncol.* **24(Suppl 12),** S12-81–S12-88.
80. Miller, V. A, Rigas, J. R, Francis, P. A, et al. (1995) Phase II trial of a 75-mg/m2 dose of docetaxel with prednisone premedication for patients with advanced non-small cell lung cancer. *Cancer* **75,** 968–972.
81. Natale, R. B. (1996) Preliminary results of a phase I/II clinical trial of paclitaxel and carboplatin in non-small cell lung cancer. *Semin. Oncol.* **23(Suppl 16),** 51–54.
82. Non-Small Cell Lung Cancer Collaborative Group. (1995) Chemotherapy in non-small cell lung cancer: a meta analysis using updated data on individual patients from 52 randomized clinical trials. *BMJ* **311,** 899–909.
83. Paesmans, M., Sculier, J. P., Libert P., et al. For the European Lung Cancer Working Party (1996) Prognostic factors for survival in advanced non-small cell lung cancer: univariate and multivariate analyses including recursive partitioning and amalgamation algorithms in 1,052 patients. *J. Clin. Oncol.* **13,** 1221–1230.

84. Pirker, R., Kraynik, G., Zochbauer, S., Malarjeri, R., Kneussel, M., and Huber, H. (1995) Paclitaxel/cisplatin in advanced non-small-cell lung cancer (NSCLC). *Ann. Oncol.* **6,** 833–835.
85. Ramanathan, R. K., and Belani, C. P. (1997) Chemotherapy for advanced non-small cell lung cancer: past, present and future *Semin. Oncol.* **24,** 440–454.
86. Rowinsky, E. K., Flood, W. A., Santorius, S. L., et al. (1995) Phase I study of paclitaxel as a 3 hour infusion followed by carboplatin in untreated patients with stage IV non-small cell lung cancer. *Semin. Oncol.* **22(Suppl 9),** 48–54.
87. Rowinsky, E. K., Chaudhry, V., Forastiere, A. A., et al. (1993) Phase I and pharmacologic study of paclitaxel and cisplatin with granulocyte colony-stimulating factor: neuromuscular toxicity is dose-limiting. *J. Clin. Oncol.* **11,** 2010–2020.
88. Souquet, P. J., Chauvin, F., Boissell, J. P., et al. (1993) Polychemotherapy in advanced non-small cell lung cancer: a metaanalysis. *Lancet* **342,** 19–21.
89. von Pawel, J., Wagner, H., Niederle, N., et al. (1996) Phase II study of paclitaxel and cisplatin in patients with non-small-cell lung cancer. *Semin. Oncol.* **23(Suppl 16),** 47–50.
90. Zalcberg, J. R., Bishop, J. F., Millward, M.J., et al. (1995) Interim results of a phase II trial of docetaxel in combination with cisplatin in patients with metastatic or locally advanced non-small cell lung cancer (NSCLC). *Eur. J. Cancer,* **3A(Suppl 5),** 1084.

Head and Neck Cancer

91. Dimery, I. W., Hong, W. K. (1993) Overview of combined modality therapies for head and neck cancer. *J. Natl. Cancer Inst.* **85,** 95–111.
92. Haselow, R. E., Adams, G. S., et al. (1983) Simultaneous cis-platinum (DDP) and radiation therapy (RT) for locally advanced unresectable head and neck cancer. *Proc. ASCO* **2,** 160.
93. Weppelman, B., Wheeler, R. H., et al. (1991) A phase I study of prolonged infusion 5-fluorouracil and concomitant radiation therapy in patients with squamous cell cancer of the head and neck. *Int. J. Radiat. Oncol. Biol. Phys.* **20,** 357–360.
94. Rooney, M., Kish, J., et al. Improved complete response rate and survival in advanced head and neck cancer after three-course induction therapy with 120-hours 5-FU and cisplatin. *Cancer* **55,** 1123–1128.
95. Schneider, M., Etienne, M., et al. (1995) Phase II trial of cisplatin, fluorouracil and pure folinic acid for locally advanced head and neck cancer: a pharmacokinetic and clinical survey. *J. Clin. Oncol.* **13,** 1656–1662.
96. Planting, A., Mulder, P., et al. (1997) Phase II study of weekly high-dose cisplatin for six cycles in patients with locally advanced squamous cell carcinoma of the head and neck. *Eur. J. Cancer* **33,** 61–65.
97. Forastiere, A., Metch, B., et al. (1992) Randomized comparison of cisplatin plus fluorouracil and carboplatin plus fluorouracil versus methotrexate in advanced squamous-cell carcinoma of the head and neck: a Southwest Oncology Group study. *J. Clin. Oncol.* **10,** 1245–1251.
98. Grose, W., Lehane, D., et al. (1985) Comparison of methotrexate and cisplatin for patients with advanced squamous cell carcinoma of the head and neck region: a Southwest Oncology Group study. *Cancer Treat. Rep.* **69,** 577–581.
99. Taylor, S.G. IV., Murthy, A. K., et al. (1989) Combined simultaneous cisplatin/fluorouracil chemotherapy and split course radiation in head and neck cancer. *J. Clin. Oncol.* **7,** 846–856.
100. Department of Veteran Affairs Laryngeal Cancer Study Group (1991) Induction chemotherapy plus radiation compared with surgery plus radiation in patients with advanced laygeal cancer. *N. Engl. J. Med.* **324,** 1685–1690.
101. Lefebvre, J. L., Chevalier, D., et al. (1996) Larynx preservation in pyriform sinus cancer:

preliminary results of a European Organization for Research and Treatment of Cancer phase III trial. *J. Natl. Cancer Inst.* **88,** 890–899.
102. Adelstein, D., Saxton, J., et al. (1997) A phase III randomized trial comparing concurrent chemotherapy and radiotherapy with radiotherapy alone in resectable stage III and IV squamous cell head and neck cancers: preliminary results. *Head Neck* **Oct.** 567–575.
103. Taylor, S., Murthy, A., et al. (1994) Randomized comparison of neoadjuvant cisplatin and fluorouracil infusion followed by radiation versus concomitant treatment in advanced head and neck cancer. *J. Clin. Oncol.* **12,** 385–395.
104. Merlano, M., Vitale, V., et al. (1992) Treatment of advanced squamous-cell carcinoma of the head and neck with alternating chemotherapy and radiotherapy. *N. Engl. J. Med.* **327,** 1115–1121.
105. Shirinian, M., Weber, R., et al. (1994) Laryngeal preservation by induction chemotherapy plus radiotherapy in locally advanced head and neck cancer: the MD Anderson cancer center experience. *Head Neck* **Jan/Feb.** 39–44.
106. Slotman, G., Doolitle, C., et al. (1992) Preoperative combines chemotherapy and radiation therapy plus radical surgery in advanced head and neck cancer. *Cancer* **69,** 2736–2743.
107. Vokes, E., Weichselbaum, R., et al. (1992) Favorable long-term survival following induction chemotherapy with cisplatin, fluorouracil and leucovorin and concomitant chemoradiotherapy for locally advanced head and neck cancer. *J. Natl. Cancer Inst.* **84,** 877–882.
108. Adelstein, D., Kalish, L., et al. (1993) Concurrent radiation therapy and chemotherapy for locally unresectable squamous cell head and neck cancer: an Eastern Cooperative Oncology Group pilot study. *J. Clin. Oncol.* **11,** 2136–2142.
109. Haselow, R., Warshaw, M., et al. (1990) Radiation alone versus radiation with weekly low dose cis-platinum in unresectable cancer of the head and neck. *Head Neck Cancer* **2,** 279–281.
110. Dragovic, J., Doyle, T., et al. (1995) Accelerated fractionation radiotherapy.
111. Trott, K., Kummermehr, J. (1985) What is known about tumour proliferation rates to choose between accelerated fractionation or hyperfractionation? *Radiother. Oncol.* **3,** 1–9.
112. Forastiere, A., (1993) Use of paclitaxel (Taxol) in squamous cell carcinoma of the head and neck. *Semin. Oncol.* **20(Suppl 3),** 55–60.
113. Geard, C., Jones, J., et al. (1994) Radiation and Taxol effects on synchronized human cervical carcinoma cell. *Int. J. Radiat. Oncol. Biol. Phys.* **29,** 565–569.
114. Milas, L., Hunter, N., et al. (1994) Enhancement of tumor radioresponse of a murine mammary carcinoma by paclitaxel. *Cancer Res.* **54,** 3506–3510.
115. Forastiere, A. (1994) Paclitaxel (Taxol) for the treatment of head and neck cancer. *Semin. Oncol.* **21(5 Suppl 8),** 49–52.
116. Vokes, E., Haraf, D., et al. (1995) The role of paclitaxel in the treatment of head and neck cancer. *Semin. Oncol.* **22(5 Suppl 12),** 8–12.
117. Forastiere, A., Shank, D., et al. (1998) Final report of a phase II evaluation of paclitaxel in patients with advanced squamous cell carcinoma of the head and neck. *Cancer* **82,** 2270–2274.
118. Castimel, G., Verweij, J., et al. (1994) Docetaxel (Taxotere): an active drug for the treatment of patients with advanced squamous cell carcinoma of the head and neck. EORTC Early Clinical Trials Group. *Ann. Oncol.* **5,** 533–537.
119. Dreyfuss, A., Clark, J., et al. (1996) Docetaxel: an active drug for squamous cell carcinoma of the head and neck. *J. Clin. Oncol.* **14,** 1672–1678.
120. Parker, R., Dabholkar, M., et al. (1993) Influence of Taxol:cisplatin sequencing on cisplatin-DNA adduct repair in human ovarian cancer cells. *Proc. Am. Assoc. Cancer Res.* **34,** 356 (abstract 2122).
121. Hitt, R., Paz-Ares, L., et al. (1997) Phase I/II study of paclitaxel/cisplatin as first-line therapy for locally advanced head and neck cancer. *Semin. Oncol.* **24(6, Suppl 19)** S19-20–S19-24.

122. Forastiere, A., Leong, T., et al. (1997) A phase III trial of high-dose paclitaxel plus cisplatin plus G-CSF versus low-dose paclitaxel plus cisplatin in patients with advanced squamous cell carcinoma of the head and neck (HNSCC): an Eastern Cooperative Oncology Group trial. *Proc. Am. Soc. Clin. Oncol.* **16,** 1367 (abstract).
123. Hussain, M., Salwen, W., et al. (1997) Paclitaxek. cisplatin, and 5-fluorouracil in patients with advanced or recurrent squamous cell carcinoma of the head and neck: a preliminary report. *Semin. Oncol.* **24(6, Suppl. 19),** S19-43–S19-45.
124. Benasso, M., Numico, G., et al. (1997) Chemotherapy for relapsed head and neck cancer: paclitaxek. cisplatin, and 5-fluorouracil in chemotherapy-naive patients. A dose finding-study. *Semin. Oncol.* **24(6 Suppl 19),** S19-46–S19-50.
125. Shin, D., Glisson, B., et al. (1998) Phase II trial of paclitaxel, ifofamide and cisplatin in patients with recurrent head and neck squamous cell carcinoma. *J. Clin. Oncol.* **16,** 1325–1330.
126. Schoffski, P., Wanders, G., et al. (1996) Docetaxel and cisplatin: a highly active regimen for squamous cell carcinoma of the head and neck. *Proc. ASCO* **15,** abstract 871.
127. Colevas, A., Busse, P., et al. (1998) Induction chemotherapy with docetaxel, cisplatin, fluorouracil, and leucovorin for squamous cell carcinoma of the head and neck: a phase I/II trial. *J. Clin. Oncol.* **16,** 1331–1339.

Breast Cancer

128. Anelli, A., Albuquerque, A. A., Tabacof, J., et al. (1997) High response rate of paclitaxel and doxorubicin as neoadjuvant chemotherapy in locally advanced breast cancer (IIIB)—preliminary results. *Breast Cancer Treat.* **46,** 75 (abstract 313).
129. Antman, K., Elder, J., Elias, A., et al. (1990) High-dose cyclophosphamide, thiotepa and carboplatin intensification with autologous bone marrow support in patients with breast cancer responding to standard dose induction therapy. *Proc. ASCO.* **9,** 10.
130. Berry, J., Ezzat, A., El-Warith A., et al. (1996) Sequential taxol/platin:pilot in metastatic breast cancer. *Proc. Am. Soc. Clin. Oncol.* **15,** abstract 243.
140. Bonnefoi, H., Smith, I. E., O'Brien, M. E., et al. Phase II study of continuous infusional 5-fluorouracil with epirubicin and carboplatin (instead of cisplatin) in patients with metastatic/locally advanced breast cancer (infusional ECarboF): a very active and well-tolerated outpatient regiman. *Br. J. Cancer* **73,** 391–396.
141. Browne, M. J., Kennedy, T., Cummings, F. et al. (1996) Phase II study of sequential taxol and cisplatin for the treatment of metastatic breast cancer. *Proc. Am. Soc. Clin. Oncol.* **15,** abstract 245.
142. Chan, S., Friedrichs, K., Noel, D., et al. (1997) A randomized phase III study of Taxotere versus doxorubicin in patients with metastatic breast cancer who have failed an anthracycline containing regimen. *Proc. ASCO* **16,** 154a.
143. Clemons, M., Leahy, M., Valle, J., et al. (1997) Review of recent trials of chemotherapy for advanced breast cancer: the taxanes. *Eur. J. Cancer* **33,** 2183–2193.
144. Cocconi, G., Bisani, G., De Lisi, V., et al. (1989). Platinum (P) and etoposide (e) as first-line chemotherapy for metastatic breast cancer (MBC). Preliminary results of a prospective randomized trial. *Proc. ASCO* **7,** 13.
145. D'Andrea, G. M., and Seidman, A. D. (1997) Docetaxel and paclitaxel in breast cancer therapy: present status and future prospects. *Semin. Oncol.* **24,** 27–44.
146. Dieras, V. (1997) Docetaxel in combination with doxorubicin: a phase I dose-finding study. *Oncology* **6,** 17.
147. Dittrich, C., Jakesz, R., Grant, G., et al. (1997) Preoperative paclitaxel in the first-line therapy of patients with breast cancer T 3/4, N 0–3, M 0, followed by surgery, CMF, tamoxifen and radiotherapy: Phase II trial. *Proc. ASCO* **16,** 167.
148. Dombernowsky, P., et al. (1996) Paclitaxel and doxorubicin, a highly active combination in the treatment of metastatic breast cancer. *Semin. Oncol.* **23,** 13–18.

149. Fernandez-Hidalgo, O., Gonzalez, F., Gil, A., et al. (1989) 120-hours simultaneous infusion of cisplatin and fluorouracil in metastatic breast cancer. *Am. J. Clin. Oncol.* **12,** 397–401.
150. Frazier, A., Wasserheit, C., Hochster, H. et al. (1995). High rate of peripheral neuropathy may limit paclitaxel and cisplatin combination in women with advanced breast cancer. *Proc. Am. Soc. Clin. Oncol.* **14,** abstract 145.
151. Gelmon, K. A., O'Reilly, S. E., Tolcher-A. W., et al. (1996) Phase I/II trial of biweekly paclitaxel and cisplatin in the treatment of metastatic breast cancer. *J. Clin. Oncol.* **14,** 1185–1191.
151a. Gradisher
152. Honig, S. F. (1996) Treatment of metastatic disease: hormonal therapy and chemotherapy, in *Diseases of the Breast* (Harris, J. R., Lippman, M. C., Morrow, M., et al., eds.), JP Lippincott, Philadelphia, pp. 669–734.
153. Jones, A. L., Smith, I. E., O'Brien, M. E., et al. (1994) Phase II study of continuous infusion fluorouracil with epirubicin and cisplatin in patients with metastatic and locally advanced breast cancer: an active new regimen. *J. Clin. Oncol.* **12,** 1259–1265.
154. Kolaric, K., Vukas, D., and Protebica, V. (1988). Combination cyclophosphamide, Adriamycin and platinum (CAP) versus 5-fluorouracil, Adriamycin and cyclophosphamide as primary treatment in metastatic breast cancer: results of a prospective randomized study. *Tumori* **75,** 132–136.
155. Martin, M., Diaz-Rubio, C., Casedo, A., et al. (1992) Carboplatin: an active drug in metastatic breast cancer. *J. Clin. Oncol.* **10,** 433–437.
156. Nabbholtz, J., Thuerlimann, B., Bezwoda, W., et al. (1977) Taxotere versus mitomycin C + vinblastine in patients with metastatic breast cancer who have failed and anthracycline containing regimen: preliminary results of a randomized phase III study. *Proc. ASCO* **16,** 148a.
157. Nabholtz, J. M. et al. (1996) Multicenter randomized comparative study of two doses of paclitaxel in patients with metastatic breast cancer. *J. Clin. Oncol.* **14,** 1858–1867.
158. O'Brien, M. D., Talbot, D. C., and Smith, I. E. (1993) Carboplatin in the treatment of advanced breast cancer: a phase II study using a pharmacokinetically guided dose schedule. *J. Clin. Oncol.* **11,** 2112–2117.
159. Pagani, O., Sessa, C., Martinelli, G., et al. (1997) Dose-finding study of paclitaxel and cyclophosphamide in advanced breast cancer. *Ann. Oncol.* **8,** 655–661.
160. Pegram, M. D., Lipton, A., Hayes, D., et al. (1998) Phase II study of receptor-enhanced chemosensitivity using recombinanr humanized anti-p185 HER2/neu monoclonal antibody plus cisplatin in patients with HER2/neu overexpressing metastatic breast cancer refractory to chemotherapy treatment. *J. Clin. Oncol.* **16,** 2659–2671.
161. Perez, E., Suman, J., Krook, P., et al. (1988) Phase II study of paclitaxel plus carboplatin as first-line chemotherapy for women with metastatic breast cancer (MBC): a north central cancer treatment group trial. *Proc. ASCO* **17,** 635.
162. Perez, E. A., and Hartman, L. C. (1996) Paclitaxel and carboplatin for advanced breast cancer. *Semin. Oncol.* **23(Suppl 11),** 41–45.
163. Peters, W. P., Shpall, E. J., Jones, R. B., et al. (1990) High-dose combination of cyclophosphamide (CPA), cisplatin (CDDP) and carmustine (BCNU) in bone marrow support as initial treatment for metastatic breast cancer: three-six year follow-up. *Proc. ASCO* **9,** 10.
164. Radvin, P., Burris, H., Cooke, G., et al. (1995) Phase II evaluation of docetaxel in advanced anthracycline-resistant or anthracenedione resistant breast cancer. *J. Clin. Oncol.* **13,** 2879–2885.
165. Radvin, P., Valero, V., Nabholtz, J., et al. (1996) Efficacy of a 5-day corticosteroid premedication in ameliorating Taxotere induced fluid retention. *Proc. ASCO* **15,** 124 (abstract).

166. Rowinsky, E. K., Gilbert, M. R., McGuire, W. P., et al. (1991) Sequences of Taxol and cisplatin: a phase I and pharmacologic study. *J. Clin. Oncol.* **9,** 1692–1703.
167. Seidman, A. D. (1996) Chemotherapy for advanced breast cancer: a current perspective. *Sem. Oncol.* **23(Suppl 2),** 55–59.
168. Sledge, G. W. (1992) Cisplatin and platinum analogues in breast cancer. *Semin. Oncol.* **19,** 78–82.
169. Sledge, G. W., Neuberg, D., Ingle, J., et al. (1997) Phase III trial of doxorubicin (A) vs. paclitaxel vs doxorubicin + paclitaxel (A & T) as first-line therapy for metastatic breast cancer (MBC): An intergroup trial. *Proc. ASCO* **16,** 1.
170. Sledge, G. W., Roth, B. J. (1989) Cisplatin in the management of breast cancer. *Semin. Oncol.* **16,** 110–115.
171. ten Vokkel Huinink, W., Prove, A., Piccart, M., et al. (1994) A phase II trial of docetaxel (Taxotere) in second line treatment with chemotherapy for advanced breast cancer. A study of the EORTC Early Clinical Trials Group. *Ann. Oncol.* **5,** 527.
172. Valero, V., Holmes, F., Walters, R., et al. (1995) Phase II trial of docetaxel: a new highly effective antineoplastic agent in the management of patients with anthracycline-resistant or anthracenedione-resistant breast cancer. *J. Clin. Oncol.* **13,** 2886–2894.
173. Vorobiof, D., Chasen, M., Moeken, R. (1996) Phase II trial of single agent docetaxel in previously treated patients with advanced breast cancer. *Proc. ASCO* **15,** 120 (abstract).
174. Wasserheit, C., Frazein, A., Oratz-R, et al. (1996) Phase II trial of paclitaxel and cisplatin in women with advanced breast cancer: an active regimen with limiting neurotoxicity. *J. Clin. Oncol.* **14,** 1993–1999.

10 Clinical Experience

DACH-Based Platinum Drugs

Peter J. O'Dwyer, James P. Stevenson, and Steven W. Johnson

CONTENTS

1. INTRODUCTION

The discovery of cisplatin as an active antitumor drug some 30 years ago *(1)* led to a search for more active and less toxic analogs even before the full potential of this class had been revealed. In 1972, Connors and colleagues *(2)* published a series of novel platinum structures with antitumor activity and first proposed a role for different substituents. Dr. Connors made the prescient observation that, based on cross-resistance profiles that resembled those of alkylating agents, cisplatin might not be sufficiently different from the compounds then available, the clinical limitations of which were well known. Using measures of therapeutic index (ratio of efficacy to toxicity), he determined that a series of cyclic amine derivatives had particular promise *(2)*.

The 1,2-diaminocyclohexane (DACH) derivatives were selected by Burchenal and colleagues *(3,4)* for preclinical development based on their activity in resistant murine leukemias (Fig. 1). The laboratory of Kidani examined various steric configurations of the DACH derivatives and found that the *trans*-R,R-stereoisomer yielded the optimal therapeutic index in both sarcoma-180 and P388 models. Interestingly, they also predicted that oxalato-DACH derivatives (such as oxaliplatin) would have superior therapeutic indices *(5,6)*.

From: *Platinum-Based Drugs in Cancer Therapy*
Edited by: L. R. Kelland and N. Farrell © Humana Press Inc., Totowa, NJ

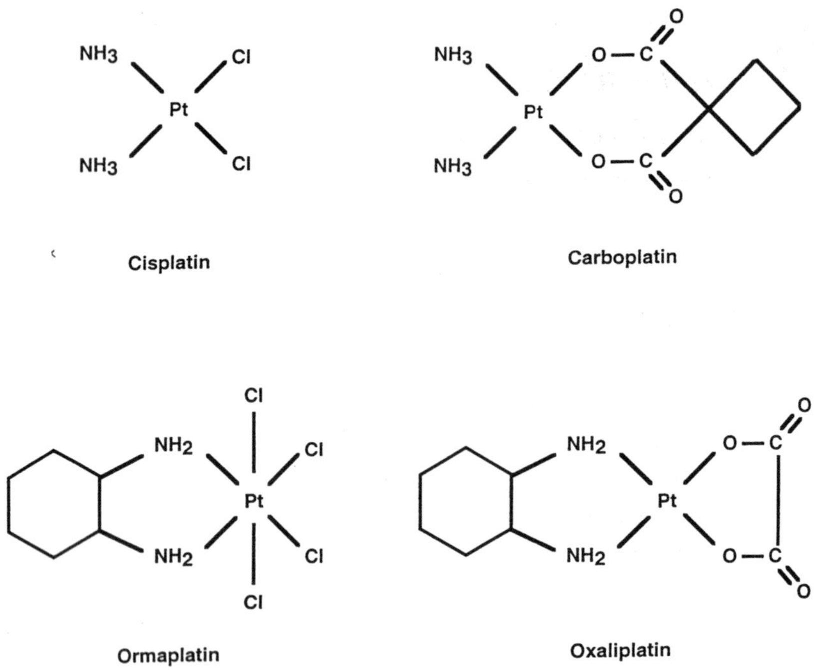

Fig. 1. Structures of platinum complexes.

Two more recent in vitro studies indicated the potential for DACH-based platinum derivatives to exhibit a spectrum of activity different from that of cisplatin and carboplatin. In two cell lines derived from the cisplatin-sensitive A2780 tumor by stepwise exposure to increasing concentrations of cisplatin, DACH-tetrachloro-Pt(IV) (tetraplatin) exhibited substantially less cross-resistance in the resistant lines *(7)*. In a series of ovarian cancer cell lines characterized at the Institute of Cancer Research in the United Kingdom, cisplatin and carboplatin showed a similar pattern of response, whereas that to tetraplatin was entirely different *(8)*. These observations implied different mechanisms of cytotoxicity among the two classes of platinum derivatives, which, as we shall see, has been supported by recent data.

The conclusion was supported further in a study by Rixe and colleagues *(9)* using the 60-cell line tumor screen developed at the National Cancer Institute (NCI). The patterns of sensitivity to individual drugs in these lines are similar for drugs of known similar mechanisms *(10)*. Conversely, it has been shown that the mechanism of an unknown antitumor agent can be predicted (or established to be different) by a comparative analysis against the database of previously studied drugs, using the COMPARE algorithm *(11)*. It was shown that the DACH derivatives tetraplatin and oxaliplatin exhibit quite different profiles from cisplatin and carboplatin in this screen. The potential for their activity in cisplatin-resistant tumors was thereby supported.

In this chapter we will summarize the continuing developments with the DACH derivatives. Clinical trials of these compounds were slow in coming to fruition: tetraplatin (also known as ormaplatin for standard nomenclature) did not reach the clinic until the early nineties, mainly because of difficulties with formulation. Oxaliplatin began to be developed contemporaneously and was shown to have a more tolerable toxicity profile. The promise of this agent in ongoing clinical studies will be illustrated.

2. INTERACTIONS OF DACH COMPOUNDS AND DNA

DNA is believed to be the primary cytotoxic target of the platinum drugs, and in order for this reaction to occur, the parent compounds must become aquated. The biotransformation of oxaliplatin to form a reactive species, 1,2-DACH diaquo platinum(II), is facilitated by HCO_3^- and $H_2PO_4^-$ ions *(12)*. These weak nucleophiles, present in the blood and intracellularly, can displace the oxalate group of oxaliplatin. The resulting intermediates are unstable and are hydrolyzed to the diaquated species. This species may then react with nucleophiles such as the N7 position of guanine to form various types of DNA adducts. These adducts include dG-Pt monoadducts, d(GpG)Pt, d(ApG)Pt, and d(GpNpG)Pt intrastrand crosslinks, and $d(G)_2Pt$ interstrand crosslinks *(13)*. The differences between the adducts formed by oxaliplatin and cisplatin reside primarily in the relative amounts of adducts formed. Oxaliplatin intrastrand adducts form more slowly due to a slower rate of conversion from monoadducts; however, they are formed at similar DNA sequences and regions as cisplatin adducts. Saris et al. *(14)* reported that oxaliplatin forms predominantly d(GpG)Pt and d(ApG)Pt intrastrand crosslinks in vitro and in cultured cells; however, at equitoxic doses oxaliplatin forms fewer DNA adducts compared with cisplatin. This suggests that oxaliplatin lesions are more cytotoxic than those formed by cisplatin *(14,15)*.

Although it is has been demonstrated that cells treated with platinum drugs undergo apoptosis, the basis for the differences in cytotoxicity observed between DACH compounds and other platinum drugs such as cisplatin and carboplatin is unknown. One explanation has been provided recently in a computer modeling study of the d(GpG)Pt adduct formed by oxaliplatin *(16)*. This study revealed that when bound to DNA, cisplatin and oxaliplatin have similar DNA bend, base rotation, and base propeller. The only difference is in the protrusion of the DACH moiety of oxaliplatin into the major groove of DNA, which produces a bulkier adduct than that seen with cisplatin. Therefore it is possible that the bulkier, more hydrophobic adduct formed by oxaliplatin is a more effective inhibitor of DNA synthesis than that of cisplatin. Page and colleagues *(17)* studied the effect of the DACH ligand versus the ethylenediamine ligand on inhibiting the transformation of repair-deficient *Escherichia coli* with platinated plasmid. Platinum adducts with the DACH carrier ligand were significantly more effective than those with the ethylenediamine ligand, suggesting that the DACH ligand is a more efficient inhibitor of replication and transcription.

Another important finding relates to the manner in which cisplatin and DACH platinum DNA adducts are recognized intracellularly. Different types of adducts may be recognized by different proteins or protein complexes, which may ultimately influence cellular responses such as repair, survival, or death. For example, the mismatch repair (MMR) protein complex has been shown to bind to DNA damaged by cisplatin, but not oxaliplatin *(18)*. This may be due to steric hindrance by the DACH ring, preventing the MMR complex from recognizing the lesion. The binding of the MMR complex to cisplatin-damaged DNA has been implicated in cisplatin cytotoxicity. Cells that are defective in MMR may replicate DNA uninterrupted past cisplatin-induced lesions and as a result may not arrest and undergo apoptosis *(19)*. MMR-deficient cells have been reported to be slightly more resistant to cisplatin but not to oxaliplatin *(20,21)*. More work in this area, however, needs to be conducted in order to increase our understanding of how platinum-DNA adduct formation leads to cell death.

3. CLINICAL PHARMACOLOGY OF DACH COMPOUNDS

In general, the pharmacokinetic differences observed between platinum drugs may be attributed to the structure of their leaving groups. Platinum complexes containing leaving groups that are less easily displaced exhibit reduced plasma protein binding, longer plasma half-lives, and higher rates of renal clearance. These features are evident in the pharmacokinetic properties of cisplatin, carboplatin, oxaliplatin, and ormaplatin. Other aspects of platinum drug pharmacokinetics have been thoroughly reviewed elsewhere *(22–25)*.

Following oxaliplatin infusion, platinum accumulates into three compartments: plasma-bound platinum, ultrafilterable platinum, and platinum associated with erythrocytes. Approximately 85% of the total platinum is bound to plasma at 2–5 h post infusion *(26)*. The disappearance of total platinum and ultrafiltrates is biphasic. The half-lives for the initial and terminal phases are 26 min and 38.7 h, respectively, for total platinum and 21 min and 24.2 h, respectively, for ultrafilterable platinum *(25)*. A prolonged retention of platinum is observed in red blood cells, which may be responsible for oxaliplatin toxicity. Unlike cisplatin, which accumulates as both protein-bound and free platinum, total plasma platinum does not accumulate to any significant level following multiple courses of oxaliplatin treatment *(26)*. This may explain why neurotoxicity associated with oxaliplatin therapy is reversible. Oxaliplatin is eliminated predominantly by the kidneys, with more than 50% being excreted in the urine at 48 h. Although the data indicate that cumulative oxaliplatin exposure is the most predictive of neurotoxicity of any pharmacokinetic parameter, investigation of pharmacodynamic correlates will continue to be a focus during its ongoing clinical development.

Oxaliplatin pharmacokinetics do not appear to be altered in combination therapy. This is supported by data from Phase I studies of oxaliplatin/5-fluorouracil (5-FU) and oxaliplatin/irinotecan *(26,27)*. However, Papamichael and colleagues *(28)* recently reported significantly decreased 5-FU area under the curve (AUC) values in patients who received oxaliplatin prior to a 48-h continuous infusion of 5-FU as part of a randomized study. The authors hypothesized that oxaliplatin increased 5-FU anabolism; the exact mechanism for this potential interaction is unclear.

We found the pharmacokinetic profile of ormaplatin to be essentially similar to that of other platinum derivatives in our Phase I study of d 1 and 8 administration over 30 min *(29)*. Plasma platinum concentration vs time curves declined biexponentially and best fit a three-compartment model. We detected a prolonged $t_{1/2}\gamma$ of 109 h and relatively low total clearance of 9.4 mL/min/m^2 in patient plasma, indicative of platinum binding to plasma proteins. Approximately 60% of platinum was protein bound at the end of infusion, with approximately one-half remaining irreversibly bound at 48 h. The AUCs of plasma and ultrafilterable platinum increased linearly with dose (r^2 = 0.707 for plasma, and 0.765 for ultrafiltrate). We found no pharmacodynamic relationship between platinum AUC or clearance values and the development of the peripheral neurotoxicity that became dose limiting in our trial. Interestingly, mean urinary excretion of platinum following ormaplatin dosing was only 10%, which is low in comparison with that seen with other platinum agents. The low urinary excretion of ormaplatin coupled with the relatively large volume of distribution of ultrafilterable platinum (range, 158–279 L/m^2) we observed is indicative of greater lipophilicity and the potential for accumulation in neural tissue.

4. TOXIC PROFILE DIFFERENT FROM CISPLATIN AND CARBOPLATIN

Much like their COMPARE profile, initial clinical experiences with the DACH compounds revealed a novel toxicity pattern distinct from that of other platinum analogs (Table 1). Malonato-platinum was one of the first DACH analogs to enter the clinic in the 1970s. Gastrointestinal toxicities in the form of nausea and vomiting were the principal side effects in Phase I studies, and activity was observed in leukemias, less so in solid tumors *(30)*. The poor solubility of malonato-platinum cut short its development; however, the late 1980s

Table 1
Toxicity Profiles of Cisplatin, Carboplatin, and DACH Analogs

	Cisplatin	*Carboplatin*	*Oxaliplatin*	*Ormaplatin*
Myelosuppression		•		
Nephrotoxicity	•			
Neurotoxicity	•		•	•
Ototoxicity	•			
Nausea/vomiting	•	•	•	•

and early 1990s saw the long-awaited appearance of ormaplatin in the clinic. The ormaplatin experience was also rather short, as will be described. In the interim, investigators in France began a methodical evaluation of oxaliplatin, the one DACH analog that appears to have fulfilled its early promise.

As was seen with malonato-platinum, the early report by Mathe and colleagues *(31)* suggested that nausea and vomiting were the predominant side effects associated with oxaliplatin administration. However, they escalated to a predetermined dose of 45 mg/m^2 every 3 weeks, but a true maximum tolerated dose (MTD) was not reached. No nephrotoxicity or hematologic toxicity was observed at these doses; interestingly, four tumor responses were reported.

The report by Extra et al. *(32)* in 1990 shed light on the clinically relevant toxicities of oxaliplatin, as they reached a true MTD of 200 mg/m^2 when given as a 6-h infusion every 4 weeks. Again, nausea and vomiting were common, with grade 3/4 episodes occurring in over half of the 44 patients treated. This was observed even at the initial dose level of 45 mg/m^2 and did not appear to be dose related; antiemetic pretreatment instituted at doses higher than 90 mg/m^2 allowed further dose escalation. Grade 1/2 diarrhea occurred in 24% of treatment courses. Myelosuppression was mild (generally grade 1/2 thrombocytopenia that was dose related), and no nephrotoxicity was encountered, even though aggressive hydration was not employed. No alopecia or ototoxicity occurred. Neurotoxicity became apparent at doses of 135 mg/m^2 and was dose limiting at 200 mg/m^2. The onset, time-course, and characteristics of the neurologic side effects were very dissimilar from those produced by cisplatin and are described below.

4.1. Neurotoxicity

The substantial Phase I and II clinical experience with oxaliplatin has indicated that it consistently produces acute, transient neurologic toxicity in most patients treated at the recommended Phase II dose of 130–135 mg/m^2 as a 2-h infusion every 3 weeks. The symptomatology produced is generally mild and consists of a peripheral sensory neuropathy characterized by paresthesias and cold-induced dysesthesias in a stocking-glove and perioral distribution, frequently occurring near the end of or shortly after drug infusion and lasting for less than 1 week. Electromyograms performed in six patients treated on the Extra et al. *(32)* study revealed an axonal sensory neuropathy, but nerve conduction velocities were unchanged, and peripheral nerve biopsies revealed decreased myelinization and replacement with collagen pockets. The neurologic effects appear to be cumulative in that they become more pronounced and of greater duration with successive cycles; however, unlike those with cisplatin, they are reversible with drug cessation. In their review of 682 patient experiences, Brienza et al. *(33)* reported that 82% of patients who experienced more than grade 2 neurotoxicity had their symptoms regress within 4–6 months. Laryngopharyngeal spasm and cold dysesthesias have also been reported but are not associated with significant respiratory symptoms and can be prevented by prolonging the infusion duration.

4.2. Ormaplatin (Tetraplatin)

Ormaplatin became the next DACH compound to undergo clinical investigation in the early 1990s. Several administration schedules were studied, including a single short infusion every 28 d, d 1 and 8 every 28 d, and a daily × 5 infusion monthly *(29,34–36)*. Neurotoxicity in the form of delayed peripheral sensory neuropathy became prohibitive at low cumulative doses, including all five patients who received total doses of more than 165 mg/m^2 on the daily × 5 schedule reported by O'Rourke et al. *(34)*, and its further development was abandoned. The functional impairment experienced by some of the affected patients was so severe that they went from being ambulatory to wheelchair bound. A unique characteristic of the disabling neurologic effects was that they progressively worsened even after drug cessation and did not appear to be related to prior platinum exposure.

We performed nerve conduction studies on all patients treated with more than 45 mg/m^2 in our trial of the d 1, 8 schedule and detected decreased amplitudes and prolonged latency times in two of three patients who experienced grade 3 symptoms, consistent with axonal damage and subsequent demyelinization. This is not unlike the nerve conduction patterns associated with cisplatin-induced neuropathy. It should be noted that whereas mild nausea and vomiting were also associated with ormaplatin dosing, no significant nephrotoxicity, myelosuppression, or ototoxicity was observed, similar to other DACH analogs.

4.3. Chronomodulation

Chronobiology and the impact of circadian rhythms on the pharmacokinetics and toxicities of cancer chemotherapy was actively investigated by Levi and Hrushesky *(37,38)* at the University of Minnesota in the 1970s. The continued study of this field at the Institut du Cancer in Villejuif, coupled with the nearly exclusive French development of oxaliplatin during the 1980s led to the initial investigation of oxaliplatin using chronomodulated delivery. Caussanel and Levi *(39)* randomly assigned 25 patients to receive oxaliplatin as a continuous intravenous infusion over 5 d every 3 weeks at a flat rate or a chronomodulated rate, with peak drug delivery in the chronomodulated arm occurring at 4 PM. The initial dose administered over 5 d in each arm was 125 mg/m^2, and doses were escalated by 25 mg/m^2/course as tolerated. Doses up to 200 mg/m^2/course were tolerated by 36% of patients with chronomodulated delivery, whereas no patient who received a constant infusion could be escalated to this level. Nausea and vomiting were nearly twice as common with the flat infusion rate, and grade 2 or greater neutropenia occurred in 19% of treatment courses on this arm and only 2% with circadian delivery. The greatest difference observed was in the incidence of neurotoxicity, which was 10 times greater in the patients who received a constant infusion (28% of courses vs 2%, $p < 0.001$). It is of note that all tumor responses (2 partial and 1 minor) occurred with chronomodulated delivery. The authors concluded that oxaliplatin could be administered at greater dose intensity and was significantly less toxic as a continuous infusion with circadian variation. Phase II and III trials of this schedule were then investigated.

5. OXALIPLATIN: ACTIVE IN COLON CANCER

The rather striking activity displayed by oxaliplatin against colon carcinoma cell lines and preclinical evidence of synergism with 5-FU, irinotecan, and other thymidylate synthase (TS) inhibitors led to a rather substantial development effort in colorectal cancer, a malignancy with limited chemotherapeutic options. Single-agent studies in untreated and 5-FU-refractory patients have been reported, as well as various combination trials in similar populations (Tables 2 and 3).

5.1. Single-Agent Studies

Oxaliplatin displayed significant activity when given as a 2-h infusion every 3 weeks to previously untreated colorectal cancer patients in two separate Phase II studies. Diaz-Rubio and colleagues *(40)* in Madrid treated 25 patients with measurable disease and observed a 20% partial response rate, with 32% of patients maintaining stable disease. The median overall survival was 14.5 months, and no patients experienced grade 3/4 toxicity. In a larger study of 39 patients, Becouarn et al. *(41)* reported a response rate of 24% (41% stable disease); 74% of patients were alive at 1 year, and median overall survival was approximately 13 months. These studies confirmed the preclinical effectiveness of oxaliplatin in colon cancer and established it to be at least comparably active to the standard treatment options 5-FU and irinotecan.

Oxaliplatin trials in 5-FU-pretreated colorectal cancer patients displayed a consistent response rate of 10%, indicating detectable activity in this heterogeneous population. Two studies of the 2-h infusion at the recommended Phase II

Table 2
Oxaliplatin Phase II Results in Colorectal Cancer[a]

Author	*Regimen*	*No.*	*RR (%)*	*MS (mo)*	*Comments*
Diaz-Rubio et al. (*40*)	L-OHP 130 mg/m^2 q 3 wk	25	20	14.5	Previously untreated patients
Becouarn et al. (*41*)	L-OHP 130 mg/m^2 q 3 wk	38	24	13.2	Previously untreated patients
Machover et al. (*42*)	L-OHP 130 mg/m^2 q 3 wk	58	11	8.2	Previously treated patients
Diaz-Rubio et al. (*40*)	L-OHP 130 mg/m^2 q 3 wk	51	10	NR	Previously treated patients
Levi et al. (*43*)	L-OHP 175 mg/m^2/course CHR × 5d q3 wk	29	10	9	Previously treated patients
Levi et al. (*44*)	L-OHP 125 mg/m^2/course 5-FU 3500 mg/m^2/course LV 1500 mg/m^2/course All by 5 d, CHR q 3 wk	93	58	15	Pretreated and untreated patients; RR and MS similar in both groups
Bertheault-Cvitkovic et al. (*46*)	L-OHP 100 mg/m^2/course 5-FU 2800 mg/m^2/course LV 1200 mg/m^2/course All by 4 d, CHR q 2 wk	50	48 (3 CRs)	17.8	RR 40% in 37 previously treated patients; 5-FU escalated to median of 3200 mg/m^2
Levi et al. (*45*)	L-OHP 100 mg/m^2/course 5-FU 2800 mg/m^2/course LV 1200 mg/m^2/course All by 4 d, CHR q 2 wk	90	67 (3 CRs)	19	Previously untreated patients
de Gramont et al. (*51*)	L-OHP 100 mg/m^2 q 2 wk 5-FU 3 g/m^2 48 h CI q 2 wk LV 500 mg/m^2 daily × 2	46	46 (1 CR)	17	Previously treated patients
Gerard et al. (*53*)	L-OHP 130 mg/m^2 q3 wk 5-FU 2.6 g/m^2 24 h CI q wk LV 500 mg/m^2 prior to 5-FU	37	28	10	Previously treated patients
Buechele et al. (*54*)	L-OHP 60 mg/m^2 q wk 5-FU 2.6 g/m^2 24 hr CI q wk LV 500 mg/m^2 prior to 5-FU	14	7	NR	Patients progressed on prior 24-h CI 5-FU; only 14/38 patients evaluable

[a]RR, response rate; CR, complete response; MS, median survival; NR, not reported; CHR, chronomodulated infusion; CI, continuous infusion.

Table 3
Randomized Studies of Oxaliplatin in Colorectal Cancer[a]

Author	*Regimen*	*No.*	*RR (%)*	*MS (mo)*	*Comments*
Giacchetti et al. (*48*)	L-OHP 125 mg/m^2 q 3 wk 5-FU 3500 mg/m^2 5 d CHR LV 1500 mg/m^2 5 d CHR	100	53	NR	$p < 0.001$ for RR; PFS 3 mo greater in L-OHP arm ($p = 0.19$)
	5-FU 3500 mg/m^2 5 d CHR LV 1500 mg/m^2 5 d CHR	100	16	NR	
Levi et al. (*45*)	L-OHP 100 mg/m^2 5 d CHR 5-FU 3000 mg/m^2 5 d CHR LV 1500 mg/m^2 5 d CHR	45	53	23	$p = 0.03$ for MS; results may have been affected by L-OHP inactivation by 5-FU in CI arm
	L-OHP 100 mg/m^2 5 d CI 5-FU 3000 mg/m^2 5 d CI LV 1500 mg/m^2 5 d CI	47	32	19	
Levi et al. (*49*)	L-OHP 100 mg/m^2 5 d CHR 5-FU 3000 mg/m^2 5 d CHR LV 1500 mg/m^2 5 d CHR	93	51	15.9	$p = 0.003$ for response; GI and neurotoxicity significantly less in CHR arm
	L-OHP 100 mg/m^2 5 d CI 5-FU 3000 mg/m^2 5 d CI LV 1500 mg/m^2 5 d CI	93	29	16.9	
de Gramont et al. (*52*)	L-OHP 85 mg/m^2 q 2 wk 5-FU 2 g/m^2 48 h CI q 2 wk LV 200 mg/m^2 daily × 2	210	57	NR	Interim analysis of first 200 patients; $p < 0.05$ for response
	5-FU 2 g/m^2 48 h CI q 2 wk LV 200 mg/m^2 daily × 2	210	26	NR	

[a]RR, response rate; CR, complete response; MS, median survival; CHR, chronomodulated infusion; CI, continuous infusion; NR, not reported.

dose of 130 mg/m^2 have been reported *(42)*. Machover et al. *(42)* treated 58 patients (57% had received two prior chemotherapy regimens) and in addition to the responses observed a 42% stable disease rate and median overall survival of 8.2 months, with survival in responders ranging from 9 to 18.5 months. Overall survival was not as striking in the study of Diaz-Rubio et al. *(40)* of 51 patients, 31% of whom maintained stable disease, with survival in the five responders ranging from 4 to 12 months. The investigation of 5-d chronomodulated oxaliplatin infusion by Levi and colleagues *(43)* produced similar results in 29 evaluable patients, with a median overall survival of 9 months.

5.2. Combination Trials

Most combination studies have incorporated 5-FU and leucovorin (LV) at varying schedules of administration, given their known activity in colorectal cancer and synergism displayed with oxaliplatin in vitro. Again, French investigators almost exclusively conducted early combination trials, and as a result the 5-FU schedules tested were the biweekly 48-h infusion developed by de Gramont and the 5-d chronomodulated infusion used by the group in Villejuif.

The first experience of Levi and colleagues *(44)* with combined oxaliplatin (125 mg/m^2) and 5-FU (3500 mg/m^2)/LV (1500 mg/m^2) chronomodulated infusion over 5 d every 3 weeks yielded an overall response rate of 58% (5% complete response) and median survival of 15 months in 93 colorectal cancer patients, of whom one-half had received no prior therapy. Response and survival rates were similar regardless of prior treatment status. Response rates of 40–67% and median survival times of 17–19 months were reported in two separate studies of intensified chronomodulated delivery of the combination over 4 d every 2 weeks *(45,46)*. Superior results occurred in the multicenter study of Levi et al. of 90 untreated patients *(45)*. Only one randomized study to date has addressed the relative contribution of oxaliplatin to the efficacy of chronomodulated combination oxaliplatin/5-FU/LV *(47)*. Giachetti et al. *(48)* treated 400 patients with the combination or 5-FU/LV chronotherapy alone and noted greater response rates in the oxaliplatin/5-FU/LV arm but no differences in median survival. Crossover effects have been hypothesized as contributing to the observed survival equivalence.

Two separate reports by Levi et al. *(49,50)* describe randomized data comparing chronomodulated oxaliplatin/5-FU/LV over 5 d every 3 weeks with the same combination given as a constant infusion. The initial trial enrolled 92 patients; a higher response rate and 4-month survival advantage (23 vs 19 months $p = 0.03$) were noted in the chronomodulated arm; however, this study was terminated early when it became evident that the basic pH of the 5-FU solution could inactivate oxaliplatin in the catheters of those receiving constant-rate infusions. In the subsequent study, patients had double-lumen catheters placed, and a total of 186 patients were randomized. Although a significantly higher response rate was noted in the chronotherapy group (51% vs 29%, $p = 0.003$), median survival times (15.9 months vs 16.9 months, $p = 0.46$) and 3-year survival rates (22% vs 21%) were similar in both groups. The incidence of grade 3/4 mucositis and peripheral neuropathy was significantly greater with constant-rate infusion.

The more widely accepted biweekly regimen of 48-h high-dose 5-FU (3–4 g/m^2) infusion developed by de Gramont et al. *(51)* in Paris has also been combined with oxaliplatin in Phase II/III trials. This group administered oxaliplatin 100 mg/m^2 prior to each dose of 5-FU/LV and observed a 46% response rate (one complete response) and median survival of 17 months in 46 previously treated colorectal cancer patients *(51)*. Of note is that half of the responses occurred in patients who had previously progressed while receiving the 48-h 5-FU regimen alone, confirming oxaliplatin's preclinical evidence of synergy with and lack of cross-resistance to 5-FU. The results of a European multicenter randomized trial of the de Gramont regimen with and without oxaliplatin (85 mg/m^2 over 2 h on d 1) every 2 weeks in 420 untreated patients were recently reported *(52)*. A doubling of the response rate (57% vs 26%, $p < 0.05$) was observed with the combination, and the progression-free survival rate was nearly 3 months longer in the oxaliplatin-treated patients (39.6 vs 27.8 weeks). Neurotoxicity, gastrointestinal toxicity, and neutropenia were greater with combination therapy but tolerable overall. The European Organization for Research and Treatment of Cancer (EORTC) is presently comparing the biweekly oxaliplatin/48-h 5-FU regimen with the intensified chronomodulated combination (96-h infusion every 2 weeks) in a large randomized study of untreated metastatic colorectal cancer patients (Table 4). Welcome data regarding the overall value of chronotherapy in this setting is anticipated as a result.

Limited data regarding oxaliplatin combined with more commonly used 5-FU regimens in colon cancer are available. Oxaliplatin has demonstrable activity when administered every 3 weeks (130 mg/m^2) or weekly (60 mg/m^2) prior to 24 h high-dose 5-FU/LV (2.6 g/m^2 over 24-h) in previously treated patients *(53,54)*. A large (800 patients) multicenter Phase II trial evaluating the addition of oxaliplatin to four different 5-FU regimens following progression on the same (daily bolus x 5 "Mayo," weekly bolus with LV, weekly high-dose infusion, prolonged continuous intravenous infusion) has recently completed accrual in the United States. Randomized studies in advanced disease will follow in the United States, and Phase III adjuvant colorectal trials are planned in Europe.

Recent combination studies have focused on other active agents in colorectal cancer, including irinotecan and the TS inhibitor tomudex. Demonstrable in vitro synergy and lack of overlapping toxicities make the oxaliplatin/irinotecan combination appealing *(55)*, and Phase I trials of the every 2- and 3-week schedule of both drugs indicate activity in 5-FU-pretreated patients, with no reported pharmacokinetic interaction *(56)*. Fizazi and colleagues *(57)* were able

Table 4
Ongoing Randomized Trials of Oxaliplatin in Colorectal Cancer[a]

Study	*Regimen*
EORTC 5963	L-OHP 100 mg/m^2/course 5-FU 2800 mg/m^2/course LV 1200 mg/m^2/course All by 4 d, CHR q 2 wk vs L-OHP 100 mg/m^2 q 2 wk 5-FU 3 g/m^2 48 h CI q 2 wk LV 500 mg/m^2 daily × 2
de Gramont et al (*52*)	L-OHP 100 mg/m^2 q 2 wk 5-FU 3 g/m^2 48 h CI q 2 wk LV 500 mg/m^2 daily × 2 vs Irinotecan 200 mg/m^2 q 2 wk 5-FU 3 g/m^2 48 h CI q 2 wk LV 500 mg/m^2 daily × 2

[a]CHR, chronomodulated infusion; CI, continuous infusion.

to administer full doses of tomudex and oxaliplatin every 3 weeks in their Phase I study. Stomatitis, asthenia, and amaurosis fugax became dose limiting at a tomudex dose of 3.5 mg/m^2 and oxaliplatin 130 mg/m^2. An ongoing Phase III trial in France randomizes untreated metastatic colorectal cancer patients to either oxaliplatin or irinotecan plus the de Gramont 48-hour 5-FU regimen.

This bulk of evidence establishes oxaliplatin as the third agent, in addition to 5-FU and irinotecan, with significant activity in colorectal cancer, and its value is becoming universally accepted. Acceptance was slowed by its limited geographic development in the clinic, but emerging data from all of Europe and the United States provide confirmatory evidence. The responses seen in 5-FU-refractory patients have led to the present investigations of oxaliplatin as front-line therapy for patients with this common malignancy, and its optimal use in combination continues to be defined.

6. DEVELOPMENT OF OXALIPLATIN IN OTHER TUMORS

Oxaliplatin exhibited low levels of cross-resistance against A2780 ovarian cancer cell lines selected for cisplatin resistance, and ovarian cancer has thus become the other large therapeutic focus in its clinical development. Activity in platinum-refractory patients has been observed, and oxaliplatin will probably become an important addition to the chemotherapeutic options available to the gynecologic oncologist.

Chollet et al. *(58)* and Dieras et al. *(59)* have reported two separate Phase II studies of single-agent oxaliplatin in women with platinum-pretreated ovarian cancers. In the Chollet et al. *(58)* study, 31 evaluable patients, most of whom were platinum refractory, received oxaliplatin 100–130 mg/m^2 as a short infusion; a 29% overall response rate was observed (including 3 of 18 platinum-refractory patients), and median survival time was 12 months. Dieras et al. *(59)* investigated a similar schedule and observed a similar response rate of 30%; whereas only 1 of 13 platinum-refractory patients had a radiographic response, four others maintained disease stability and had a more than 50% decline in serum CA 125 level.

These promising results have led to further randomized and combination trials. Misset and colleagues *(60)* reported their randomized results in 1998 comparing the combination of oxaliplatin and cyclophosphamide with the cisplatin/cyclophosphamide regimen, which was the standard initial therapy for untreated patients at the time of study initiation. Results from this multicenter study of 182 patients indicated no significant differences in response rate and median survival time, whereas patients in the oxaliplatin arm experienced significantly less grade 3/4 hematologic toxicity, nausea/vomiting, and neurotoxicity. The emergence of paclitaxel and its incorporation into front-line therapy with cisplatin or carboplatin has led investigators to study the oxaliplatin/paclitaxel combination. Kalla et al. *(61)* found that full doses of both drugs could be delivered to platinum-pretreated patients every 3 weeks, with no additive or unexpected toxicity; 9 of 18 evaluable patients manifested responses, and median survival was greater than 13 months. The interesting combination of full-dose oxaliplatin and cisplatin has been studied in 25 pretreated ovarian cancer patients by Soulie et al. *(62)*, and responses were evident in both platinum-refractory and -sensitive patients. Hematologic and neurologic toxicity were more pronounced with both drugs; the characteristics of the neuropathy were similar to that seen with oxaliplatin as it was reversible with treatment cessation. Epirubicin/ifosfamide and paclitaxel have been added to the platinum combination in separate studies, and these approaches seem feasible and active *(63,64)*. The carboplatin/oxaliplatin combination is also being investigated *(65)*.

The results of a randomized study recently completed by the EORTC comparing single-agent paclitaxel or oxaliplatin in pretreated patients are awaited. U.S. trials in ovarian cancer are expected to begin soon.

The data on oxaliplatin activity in other tumor types are scant but exist nevertheless. Monnet and colleagues *(66,67)* detected a 13% response rate to single-agent oxaliplatin in untreated non-small cell lung cancer, and this same group observed responses in 6 of 15 patients treated on their Phase I/II combination trial with weekly vinorelbine. Responses have also been reported in anthracycline-resistant breast cancer (3/14 patients) and relapsed non-Hodgkin's lymphoma (9/22 patients) *(68,69)*. The data in lymphoma are interesting in that the median response duration was 14 months and all responders had low-grade or intermediate-grade disease, yet curiously no other data have been obtained in this disease. No responses were observed in another small study of 14 patients with malignant astrocytomas *(70)*.

ACKNOWLEDGMENTS

This work was supported by the NIH, DHHS, grant CA 16520.

REFERENCES

1. Rosenberg, B. (1985) Fundamental studies with cisplatin. *Cancer* **55,** 2303–2316.
2. Connors, T. A., Jones, M., Ross, W. C. J., Braddock, P. D., Khokhar, A. R., and Tobe, M. J. (1972) New platinum complexes with anti-tumor activity. *Chem. Biol. Interac.* **5,** 415–424.
3. Burchenal, J. H., Kalaker, K., Dew, K., and Lokyst, L. (1979) Rationale for development of platinum analogs. *Cancer Treat. Rep.* **63,** 1493.
4. Burchenal, J. H., Irani, G., Kern, K., Lokys, L., and Turkevich, J. (1980) 1,2-Diaminocyclohexane platinum derivatives of potential clinical value. *Rec. Res. Cancer Res.* **74,** 146.
5. Kidani, Y. and Inagaki, K. (1978) Antitumor activity of 1,2-diaminocyclohexane-platinum complexes against sarcoma-180 ascites form. *J. Med. Chem.* **21,** 1315–1318.
6. Noji, M., Okamoto, K., and Kidani, Y. (1981) Relation of conformation to antitumor activity of platinum (II) complexes of 1,2-cyclohexanediamine and 2-(aminomethyl)cyclohexylamine isomers against leukemia P388. *J. Med. Chem.* **24,** 508–515.
7. Behrens, B. C., Hamilton, T. C., Masuda, H., Grotzinger, K. R., Whang-Peng, J., Louie, K., Knutsen, T., McKoy, W. M., Young, R. C., and Ozols, R. F. (1987) Characterization of a cis-diamminedichloroplatinum (II)-resistant human ovarian cancer cell line and its use in evaluation of platinum analogues. *Cancer Res.* **47,** 414–418.
8. Hills, C. A., Kelland, L. R., Abel, G., Siracky, J., Wilson, A. P., and Harrap, K. R. (1988) Biological properties of ten human ovarian carcinoma cell lines, calibration in vitro against four platinum complexes. *Br. J. Cancer* **59,** 527–534.
9. Rixe, O., Ortuzar, W., Alvarez, M., Parker, R., Reed, E., Paull, K. D., and Fojo, T. (1996) Oxaliplatin, traplatin, cisplatin, and carboplatin, spectrum of activity in drug-resistant cell lines and in the cell lines of the National Cancer Institute's Anticancer Drug Screen Panel. *Biochem. Pharmacol.* **52,** 1855–1865.
10. van Osdol, W. W., Myers, T. G., Paull, K. D., Kohn, K. W., and Weinstein, J. N. (1994) Use of the Kohonen self-organizing map to study the mechanisms of action of chemotherapeutic agents. *J. Natl. Cancer Inst.* **86,** 1853–1859.
11. Paull, K. D., Shomaker, R. H., Hodes, L., Monks, A., Scudiero, D. A., Rubinstein, L., et al. (1989) Display and analysis of patterns of differential activity of drugs against human tumor cell lines: development of mean graph and COMPARE algorithim. *J. Natl. Cancer Inst.* **81,** 1088–1092.
12. Mauldin, S. K., Plescia, M., Richard, F. A., Wyrick, S. D., Voyksner, R. D., and Chaney, S. G. (1998) Displacement of the bidentate malonate ligand from (d,l-*trans*-1,2-diaminocyclohexane)malonatoplatinum(II) by physiologically important compounds in vitro. *Biochem. Pharmacol.* **37,** 3321–3333.
13. Jennerwein, M. M., Eastman, A., Khokhar, A. (1989) Characterization of adducts produced in DNA by isomeric 1,2-diaminocyclohexaneplatinum(II) complexes. *Chem. Biol. Interact.* **70,** 39–49.
14. Saris, C. P., van de Vaart, P. J., Rietbroek, R. C., Blommaert, F. A. (1996) In vitro formation

of DNA adducts by cisplatin, lobaplatin and oxaliplatin in calf thymus DNA in solution and in cultured human cells. *Carcinogenesis* **17,** 2763–2769.
15. Schmidt, W. and Chaney, S. G. (1993) Role of carrier ligand in platinum resistance of human carcinoma cell lines. *Cancer Res.* **53,** 799–805.
16. Scheeff, E. D. and Howell, S. B. (1998) Computer modeling of the primary cisplatin and oxaliplatin DNA adducts and relevance to mismatch repair recognition. *Proc. Am. Assoc. Cancer Res.* **39,** A1082.
17. Page, J. D., Husain, I., Sancar, A., and Chaney S. G. (1990) Effect of the diaminocyclohexane carrier ligand on platinum adduct formation, repair, and lethality. *Biochemistry* **29,** 1016–1024.
18. Nebel, S., Fink, D., Aebi, S., Nehme, A., Christen, R. D., and Howell, S.B. (1997) Role of the DNA mismatch repair proteins in the recognition of platinum DNA adducts. *Proc. Am. Assoc. Cancer Res.* **38,** A2402.
19. Vaisman, A., Varchenko, M., Umar, A., Kunkel, T. A., Risinger, J. I., Barrett, J. C., et al. (1998) The role of hMLH1, hMSH3, and hMSH6 defects in cisplatin and oxaliplatin resistance: correlation with replicative bypass of platinum-DNA adducts. *Cancer Res.* **58,** 3579–3585.
20. Fink, D., Nebel, S., Aebi, S., Zheng, H., Cenni, B., Nehme, A., et al. (1996) The role of mismatch repair in platinum drug resistance. *Cancer Res* **56,** 4881–4886.
21. Fink, D., Zheng, H., Nebel, S., Norris, P. S., Aebi, S., Lin, T. P., et al. (1997) In vitro and in vivo resistance to cisplatin in cells that have lost DNA mismatch repair. *Cancer Res.* **57,** 1841–1845.
22. Zwelling, L. A. and Kohn, K. W. (1982) In *Pharmacologic Principles of Cancer Treatment* (Chabner, B. ed.), W.B. Saunders, Philadelphia, pp. 309–339.
23. van der Vijgh, W. J. (1991) Clinical pharmacokinetics of carboplatin. *Clin. Pharmacokinet.* **21,** 242–261.
24. Duffull S. B. and Robinson, B. A. (1997) Clinical pharmacokinetics and dose optimisation of carboplatin. *Clin. Pharmacokinet.* **33,** 161–183.
25. Extra J. M., Marty, M., Brienza, S., and Misset J. L. (1998) Pharmacokinetics and safety profile of oxaliplatin. *Semin. Oncol.* **25(Suppl 5),** 13–22.
26. Gamelin, E., Bouil, A. L., Boisdron-Celle, M., Turcant, A., Delva, R., Cailleux A., et al. (1997) Cumulative pharmacokinetic study of oxaliplatin, administered every three weeks, combined with 5-fluorouracil in colorectal cancer patients. *Clin. Cancer Res.* **3,** 891–899.
27. Lokiec, F., Wasserman, E., Santoni, J., Mahjoubi, M., Misset, J. L., and Cvitkovic E. (1997) Pharmacokinetics (Pk) of the irinotecan (CPT-11)/oxaliplatin (LOHP) combination: preliminary data of an ongoing Phase I trial. *Proc. Am. Assoc. Cancer. Res.* **38,** 76.
28. Papamichael, D., Joel, S. P., Seymour, M. T., Richards, F., Bowerbank, M., and Slevin, M.L. (1998) Pharmacokinetic (PK) interaction between 5-fluorouracil (5-FU) and oxaliplatin (L-OHP). *Proc. Am. Soc. Clin. Oncol.* **17,** 202a.
29. Schilder, R. J., LaCreta, F. P., Perez, R. P., Johnson, S. W., Brennan, J. M., Rogatko, A. et al. (1994) Phase I and pharmacokinetic study of ormaplatin (tetraplatin, NSC 363812) administered on a day 1 and day 8 schedule. *Cancer Res.* **54,** 709–717.
30. Ribaud, P., Gouveia, J., Bonnay, M., and Mathe, G. (1981) Clinical pharmacology and pharmacokinetics of cis-platinum and analogs. *Cancer Treat. Rep.* **65(Suppl 3),** 97–105.
31. Mathe, G., Kidani, Y., Triana, K., Brienza, S., Ribaud, P., Goldschmidt, E., Ecstein, E., Despax, R., Musset, M., and Misset J. L. (1986) A phase I trial of *trans*-l-diaminocyclohexane oxalato-platinum (l-OHP). *Biomed. Pharmacother.* **40,** 372–376.
32. Extra, J. M., Espie, M., Calvo, F., Ferme, C., Mignot, L., and Marty, M. (1990) Phase I study of oxaliplatin in patients with advanced cancer. *Cancer Chemother. Pharmacol.* **25,** 299–303.
33. Brienza, S., Vignoud, J., Itzhaki, M., and Krikorian A. (1995) Oxaliplatin (L-OHP): Global safety in 682 patients. *Proc. Am. Soc. Clin. Oncol.* **14,** 209.
34. O'Rourke, T. J., Weiss, G. R., New, P., Burris, H., A. III, Rodriguez, G., Eckhardt, J., et al.

(1994) Phase I clinical trial of ormaplatin (tetraplatin, NSC 363812). *Anti-Cancer Drugs* **5,** 520–526.
35. Christian, M. C., Kohn, E., Sarosy, G., Link, C., Davis, P., Adamo, D., et al. (1992) Phase I pharmacologic study of ormaplatin (OP)/tetraplatin. *Proc. Am. Soc. Clin. Oncol.* **11,** 117.
36. Tutsch, K. D., Azoomanian, R. Z., Alberti, D., Fereraliend, C., Ralvins, H., I., and Spriggs, D. R. (1992) Phase I trial and pharmacokinetic study of ormaplatin. *Proc. Am. Assoc. Cancer Res* **33,** 56.
37. Levi, F. A., Hrushesky, W. J., Halberg, F., Langevin, T. R., Haus, E., and Kennedy B. J. (1982) Lethal nephrotoxicity and hematologic toxicity of cis-diamminedichloroplatinum ameliorated by optimal circadian timing and hydration. *Eur. J. Cancer Clin. Oncol.* **18,** 471–477.
38. Hrushesky W. J. (1985) Circadian timing of cancer chemotherapy. *Science* **228,** 73–75.
39. Caussanel, J. P., Levi, F., Brienza, S., Misset, J. L., Itzhaki, M., Adam, R., et al. (1990) Phase I trial of continuous venous infusion of oxaliplatin at circadian rhythm-modulated rate compared with constant rate. *J. Natl. Cancer Inst.* **82,** 1046–1050.
40. Diaz-Rubio, E., Sastre, J., Zaniboni, A., Labianca, R., Cortes-Funes, H., de Braud, F., et al. (1998) Oxalipatin as single agent in previously untreated colorectal carcinoma patients: a phase II multicentric study. *Ann. Oncol.* **9,** 105–108.
41. Becouarn, Y., Ychou, M., Ducreux, M., Borel, C., Berthault-Cvitkovic, F., Seitz, J. F., et al. (1998) Phase II trial of oxaliplatin as first-line chemotherapy in metastatic colorectal cancer patients. *J. Clin. Oncol.* **16,** 2739–2744.
42. Machover, D., Diaz-Rubio, E., de Gramont, A., Schilf, A., Gastiaburu, J. J., Brienza, S., et al. (1996) Two consecutive phase II studies of oxaliplatin (L-OHP) for treatment of patients with advanced colorectal carcinoma who were resistant to previous treatment with fluoropyrimidines. *Ann. Oncol.* **7,** 95–98.
43. Levi, F., Perpoint, B., Garufi, C., et al. (1993) Oxaliplatin activity against metastatic colorectal cancer. A five-day study of continuous venous infusion at circadian rhythm modulated rate. *Eur. J. Cancer* **9,** 1280–1284.
44. Levi, F., Misset, J. L., Brienza, S., Adam, R., Metzger, G., Itzhaki, M., et al. (1992) A chronopharmacologic phase II clinical trial with 5-fluorouracil, folinic acid, and oxaliplatin using an ambulatory multichannel programmable pump. High antitumor effectiveness against metastatic colorectal cancer. *Cancer* **69,** 893–900.
45. Levi, F., Dogliotti, L., Perpoint, B., Zidani, R., Giacchetti, S., Chollet, P., et al. (1997) A multicenter phase II trial of intensified chronotherapy with oxaliplatin (L-OHP), 5-fluorouracil (5-FU) and folinic acid (FA) in patients (pts) with previously untreated metastatic colorectal cancer. *Proc. Am. Soc. Clin. Oncol.* **16,** 266a.
46. Bertheault-Cvitkovic, F., Jami, A., Itzhaki, M., Brummer, P. D., Brienza, S., Adam, R., et al. (1996) Biweekly intensified ambulatory chronomodulated chemotherapy with oxaliplatin, fluorouracil, and leucovorin in patients with metastatic colorectal cancer. *J. Clin. Oncol.* **14,** 2950–2958.
47. Giachetti, S., Zidani, R., Perpoint, B., et al. (1997) Phase III trial of 5-fluorouracil (5-FU), folinic acid (FA) with or without oxaliplatin (OXA) in previously untreated patients (pts) with metastatic colorectal cancer. *Proc. Am. Soc. Clin. Oncol.* **16,** 229a.
48. Giacchetti, S., Brienza, S., Focan, C., Metouri, A., Perpoint, B., Faggiuolo, R., et al. (1998) Contribution of second line oxaliplatin (OXA)-chronomodulated 5-fluorouracil-folinic acid (CM-FU-FA) and surgery to survival in metastatic colorectal cancer patients (MCC PTS). *Proc. Am. Soc. Clin. Oncol.* **17,** 273a.
49. Levi, F. A., Zidani, R., Vannetzel, J. M., Perpoint, B., Focan, C., Faggiuolo, R., et al. (1994) Chronomodulated versus fixed-infusion-rate delivery of ambulatory chemotherapy with oxaliplatin, fluorouracil, and folinic acid (leucovorin) in patients with colorectal cancer metastases: a randomized multi-institutional trial. *J. Natl. Cancer Inst.* **86,** 1608–1617.
50. Levi, F., Zidani, R., and Misset, J. L. (1997) Randomised multicentre trial of chronotherapy

with oxaliplatin, fluorouracil, and folinic acid in metastatic colorectal cancer. *Lancet* **350,** 681–686.

51. de Gramont, A., Vignoud, J., Tournigand, C., Louvet, C., Andre, T., Varette, C., et al. (1997) Oxaliplatin with high-dose leucovorin and 5-fluorouracil 48-hour continuous infusion in pretreated metastatic colorectal cancer. *Eur. J. Cancer* **33,** 214–219.
52. de Gramont, A., Figer, A., Seymour, M., Homerin, M., LeBail, N., Cassidy, J., et al. (1998) A randomized trial of leucovorin (LV) and 5-fluorouracil (5FU) with or without oxaliplatin in advanced colorectal cancer. *Proc. Am. Soc. Clin. Oncol.* **17,** 257a.
53. Gerard, B., Bleiberg, H., Van Daele, D., Gil, T., Hendlisz, A., DiLeo, A., et al. (1998) Oxaliplatin combined to 5-fluorouracil and folinic acid: an effective therapy in patients with advanced colorectal cancer. *Anti-Cancer Drugs* **9,** 301–305.
54. Buechele, T., Schoeber, C., Kroening, H., Eckart, M., Lingenfelser, M., Respondek, G., et al. (1998) Weekly high-dose (HD) 5-fluorouracil (5-FU) and folinic acid (FA) with addition of oxaliplatin (LOHP) after documented progression under high-dose infusional 5-FU/FA in patients (PTS) with advanced colorectal cancer (CRC): a preliminary report. *Proc. Am. Soc. Clin. Oncol.* **17,** 287a.
55. Zeghari-Squalli, N., Misset, J. L., Cvitkovic, E., and Goldwasser, F., (1997) Mechanism of the in vitro synergism between SN38 and oxaliplatin. *Proc. Am. Assoc. Cancer Res.* **38,** 3.
56. Cvitkovic, E., Wasserman, E., Riofrio, M., Goldwasser, F., Mignard, D., Mahjoubi, M., et al. (1998) CPT-11/oxaliplatin (L-OHP): thymidylate synthase (TS) independent combination with efficacy in 5-FU refractory colorectal cancer (CRC) patients (PTS). *Proc. Am. Soc. Clin. Oncol.* **17,** 278a.
57. Fizazi, K., Soria, J. C., Bonnay, M., Ruffie, P., Ducreux, M., LeChevalier, T., et al. (1998) Phase I/II dose-finding and pharmacokinetic (PK) study of 'Tomudex' (T) in combination with oxaliplatin (O) in advanced solid tumors. *Proc. Am. Soc. Clin. Oncol.* **17,** 201a.
58. Chollet, P., Bensmaine, M. A., Brienza, S., Deloche, C., Cure, H., Caillet, H., et al. (1996) Single agent activity of oxaliplatin in heavily pretreated advanced epithelial ovarian cancer. *Ann. Oncol.* **7,** 1065–1070.
59. Dieras, V., Bougnoux, P., Petit, T., Chollet, P., Borel, C., Husseni, F., et al. (1998) Oxaliplatin (L-OHP) phase II study in platinum (PT) pretreated advanced ovarian cancer (AOC): preliminary results. *Proc. Am. Soc. Clin. Oncol.* **17,** 364a.
60. Misset, J. L., Chollet, P., Vennin, P., Laplaige, P., Lucas, V., Frobert, J., L., et al. (1998) Multicentric phase II-III trial of oxaliplatin (LOHP) versus cisplatin (P) both in association with cyclophosphamide (C) in the treatment of advanced ovarian cancer (AOC): toxicity efficacy results. *Proc. Am. Soc. Clin. Oncol.* **17,** 354a.
61. Kalla, S., Faivre, S., Bensmaine, M. A., Bourdon, O., Hauteville, D., Extra, J. M., et al. (1998) Paclitaxel (PXL)-oxaliplatin (L-OHP): a feasible active combination in heavily pretreated advanced ovarian carcinoma (ADOVCA) patients (PTS). *Proc. Am. Soc. Clin. Oncol.* **17,** 357a.
62. Soulie, P., Bensmaine, A., Garrino, C., Chollet, P., Brian, E., Fereres, M., et al. (1997) Oxaliplatin/cisplatin (L-OHP/CDDP) combination in heavily pretreated ovarian cancer. *Eur. J. Cancer* **33,** 1400–1406.
63. Garrino, C., Cvitkovic, E., Soulie, P., Llory, J. F., Musset, M., Fereres, M., et al. (1994) Preliminary report on the tolerance of transplatin (LOHP) cisplatin (CP) association alone (Bi) or in combination with ifosfamide and epirubicin (Bic) in platinum (PT) pretreated patients. *Proc. Am. Soc. Clin. Oncol.* **13,** 143.
64. Taamma, A., Cvitkovic, E., Soulie, P., et al. (1996) Feasibility trial of the taxol, oxaliplatin (L-OHP), and cisplatin (CDDP) combination in good prognosis recurrent ovarian cancer. *Ann. Oncol.* **7,** 75.
65. Bugat, R., Bekradda, M., Misset, J. L., Soulie, P., Chatelut, E., Canal, P., et al. (1998) Pharmacodynamics and pharmacokinetics (PK) of the carboplatin (CBDCA) oxaliplatin (L-OHP) combination in patients (PTS) with advanced malignancies: preliminary results of ongoing phase I trial. *Proc. Am. Soc. Clin. Oncol.* **17,** 236a.

66. Monnet, I., Brienza, S., Voisin, S., Gastiaburu, J., Armand, J. P., Cvitkovic, E., et al. (1993) Phase II study of oxaliplatin (L-OHP) in patients with advanced non small cell lung cancer (NSCLC): preliminary results. *Eur. J. Cancer* **29A (Suppl 6),** S163.
67. De Cremoux, H., Bekradda, M., Monnet, I., Soulie, P., Saltiel, S., Misset, J. L., et al. (1998) Preliminary report on oxaliplatin (L-OHP)/navelbine (NVB) phase I/II multicentric trial in patients (PTS) with advanced non small cell lung cancer (NSCLC), an active combination. *Proc. Am. Soc. Clin. Oncol.* **17,** 481a.
68. Garufi, C., Nistico, C., Brienza, S., Pace, R., Aschelter, A. M., Rotarski, M., et al. (1997) Oxaliplatin (L-OHP) activity in anthracycline (ANT)-resistant metastatic breast cancer (MBC) patients. *Proc. Am. Soc. Clin. Oncol.* **16,** 170a.
69. Gastiaburu, J., Brienza, S., Rotarski, M., Musset, M., DiPalma, M., Lemonnier M. P., et al. (1993) Oxaliplatin (L-OHP): a new platinum analog: active in refractory/relapsed intermediate and low grade non-Hodgkin lymphoma (NHL), a phase I-II study. *Eur. J. Cancer* **29A(Suppl 6),** S176.
70. Maugard-Louboutin, C., Fumoleau, P., Ibrahim, N., Bourdin, S., Resche, F., Lajat, Y., et al. (1993) Preliminary phase II trial of oxaliplatin (L-OHP) in malignant astrocytomas. *Eur. J. Cancer* **29A(Suppl 6),** S191.

11 Clinical Toxicology of Platinum-Based Cancer Chemotherapeutic Agents

Mark J. McKeage

CONTENTS

1. INTRODUCTION

The clinical toxicology of the platinum drugs is a subject area concerned with the adverse effects caused by platinum-based cancer chemotherapeutic agents in patients at doses conventionally used in cancer therapy. The topic includes the description of the organ systems involved in these adverse reactions and their frequency, severity, time-course, reversibility, and relationship to dose and administration schedule in patients. Of potential importance is information concerned with their biochemical mechanisms and relationships to pharmacokinetics because this knowledge can possibly lead to the development of mechanism-based or rational strategies for predicting or preventing clinical drug toxicity.

To this end, considerable progress has been made in improving the tolerance of platinum-based cancer chemotherapeutic agents since their introduction into human oncology 25 years ago. The development of methods of reducing their renal and gastrointestinal side effects has been key to the widespread clinical

From: *Platinum-Based Drugs in Cancer Therapy*
Edited by: L. R. Kelland and N. Farrell © Humana Press Inc., Totowa, NJ

application of platinum drugs in cancer therapy. Neurosensory toxicity and delayed nausea and vomiting remain problematic and are challenges for the future. In this chapter the clinical toxicology of the platinum-based cancer chemotherapeutic agents of current clinical interest (cisplatin, carboplatin, oxaliplatin, and oral JM216) will be reviewed with the focus on their adverse effect profiles when given as single agents.

2. CISPLATIN

2.1. Renal Effects

Nephrotoxicity was observed in the very first clinical trials of cisplatin carried out in the early 1970s, and clinical investigators commented at that time that the drug was too toxic to the kidney for general clinical use *(1)*. However, with the use of intravenous hydration and mannitol, the maximum tolerated dose of cisplatin was increased by threefold, and doses of 100 mg/m^2 were able to be given with acceptable levels of renal toxicity. Some patients with testicular cancer who had failed to respond to cisplatin given without hydration were noted to be sensitive to higher doses of cisplatin when given with hydration *(1)*.

Renal disturbances associated with cisplatin are manifest in patients by acute and/or chronic renal insufficiency and renal magnesium wasting. A rise in blood urea nitrogen and serum creatinine levels associated with decreased creatinine clearance are the usual initial manifestations of cisplatin nephrotoxicity *(2)*. Patients develop hypomagnesemia due to urinary loss of magnesium and disturbance of magnesium reabsorption mechanisms within the renal tubule *(2)*. The severity of nephrotoxicity depends on the dose of cisplatin, but there is no significant schedule dependence *(3)*. Renal damage is cumulative in that it becomes more severe with repeated cycles of treatment *(4)*.

Clinical trials have shown that the simultaneous administration of intravenous hydration, mannitol, and chloride-containing vehicles, as well as the avoidance of other nephrotoxic drugs, significantly reduces the incidence and severity of nephrotoxicity associated with cisplatin chemotherapy. A review by Comis *(3)* showed that the incidence of nephrotoxicity in patients treated with 50–75 mg/m^2 of cisplatin was 22.5% when hydration, mannitol, or diuretics were not used, but only 3.8% of patients experienced renal toxicity when nephroprotective measures were employed. At 100 mg/m^2 or more, 79% of patients experienced nephrotoxicity when hydration, mannitol, or diuretics are not used, compared with 24% to patients receiving nephroprotective measures. These maneuvers may protect against cisplatin nephrotoxicity by reducing the concentration of cisplatin in the renal tubule fluid, thereby lowering the exposure of renal tubule cells to the drug, or by preventing the hydrolysis of cisplatin and the formation of nephrotoxic biotransformation products *(4)*.

Current recommendations are that cisplatin be given in a chloride-containing vehicle, with intravenous fluid at 150–200 ml/h during and for 4–6 h after the drug, and with mannitol *(5)*.

Bissett and colleagues *(6)* studied the long-term renal sequelae of cisplatin treatment in 74 patients cured of testicular cancer at an average of 52 months after treatment. Creatinine clearance measurements calculated from the serum and 24-h urine creatinine values indicated that there was a significant deterioration in glomerular function associated with chemotherapy. The mean creatinine clearance before treatment was 130 mL/min (range, 41–233 mL/min); after treatment, the creatinine clearance was 101.5 mL/min (range, 49–338 mL/min; $p = 0.001$). Serum magnesium levels were normal in these patients assessed 52 months after therapy. Twenty-four percent of patients had raised blood pressure, but blood pressure abnormalities did not correlate with kidney function. Together, these data indicate that cisplatin is associated with a persistent fall in glomerular function that is not associated with abnormal blood pressure. Cisplatin-induced disturbances in renal tubular function are reversible.

Daugaard and Abildgaard *(4)* have reviewed the current understanding of the mechanisms involved in cisplatin-induced nephrotoxicity. Both vascular and tubular factors contribute to the pathogenesis of cisplatin renal toxicity. The damage is initiated by a renal tubule abnormality detectable early by decreased proximal reabsorption of sodium and water, followed 2–3 days later by reductions in renal blood flow and glomerular filtration rate. The main sites of histologic damage are in the distal part of the proximal tubule and in the distal tubule. The biochemical target of cisplatin in the kidney remains unclear. In short, the abnormal renal function in patients treated with cisplatin can be attributed to impairment of proximal and distal tubular reabsorption and increased vascular resistance.

A new nephroprotective agent, amifostine (Ethyol) was recently approved for use in patients to reduce the cumulative renal toxicity associated with repeated administration of cisplatin. A randomized trial reported by Kemp and colleagues *(7)* involved 242 patients with ovarian cancer treated with cisplatin (100 mg/m^2) and cyclophosphamide with or without amifostine (910 mg/m^2). At the sixth and final cycle of treatment, fewer patients treated with amifostine (13%) had 40% or greater reductions in creatinine clearance than the control arm (30%). The side effects associated with amifostine included vomiting, low blood pressure, somnolence, and sneezing. This study suggests that amifostine may have a role in the prevention of cumulative nephrotoxicity in patients treated with protracted high-dose (100 mg/m^2) cisplatin chemotherapy.

2.2. Gastrointestinal Effects

Nausea and vomiting are common and distressing side effects associated with cisplatin that not infrequently lead patients to be unable to comply with their cancer therapy regimen as prescribed. Cisplatin-induced nausea and vomiting is classified into two distinct types that differ in their responsiveness to antiemetic drugs and probably in their underlying emetic mechanism. Acute nausea and vomiting is defined as that occurring within the first 24 h of cisplatin administration and typically is intense but highly responsive to serotonin antagonist antiemetics drugs. Delayed nausea and vomiting associated with cisplatin is that occurring 24 h or more after giving cisplatin; it is usually less intense and less easily controlled with currently available antiemetic therapies that control acute nausea and vomiting.

A placebo-controlled antiemetic study conducted by Gralla and colleagues *(8)* provides a useful benchmark of the incidence and severity of acute nausea and vomiting associated with cisplatin when no antiemetic drugs are given. In this study the number of episodes of emesis, volume of emesis, and duration of nausea and vomiting were recorded during the first 24 h of giving cisplatin at a dose of 120 mg/m^2. In the placebo arm, the number of emetic episodes occurring in the first 24 h ranged from 5 to 25 (median, 10.5 episodes), the volume of emesis ranged from 250 to 1870 mL (median, 404 mL), the duration of nausea ranged from 0 to 19.2 h (median, 3.7 hs), and the duration of vomiting ranged from 2 to 17 h (median, 3.6 hs). This indicates that nausea and vomiting are very severe and occur in almost all patients given cisplatin without antiemetics at a dose of 120 mg/m^2. Typically, symptoms begin within 1–3 h of treatment and reach their worst 6–8 h after treatment.

Cubeddu et al. *(9)* carried out a randomized trial of the relationship between altered serotonin metabolism and acute emesis induced by cisplatin in patients receiving a selective antagonist of the serotonin type 3 receptor called ondansetron or placebo. The urinary excretion of 5-hydroxyindoleacetic acid (5-HIAA), a major metabolite of serotonin, was increased between 2 and 6 h after giving cisplatin. The increase in urinary 5-HIAA paralleled the onset of intense nausea and vomiting at 2–6 h after cisplatin in the patients not receiving ondansetron. Ondansetron significantly reduced the severity of nausea and vomiting and delayed its onset but did not effect the release of 5-HIAA into the urine. The findings of this study are consistent with the idea that serotonin release, probably from enterochromaffin cells in the gut wall, mediates the acute nausea and vomiting associated with cisplatin by interacting with serotonin type 3 receptors, possibly on afferent nerve fibers in the gut wall or within the central nervous system. The findings explain the effectiveness of ondansetron and other serotonin type 3 antagonists in the control of acute nausea and vomiting associated with cisplatin and provide insights into the role of serotonin in cisplatin-induced gastrointestinal toxicity.

Randomized clinical trials have established that ondansetron combined with dexamethasone is the most effective and least toxic antiemetic regimen currently available for the prevention of acute nausea and vomiting associated with cisplatin (reviewed in ref. *10*). Ondansetron and dexamethasone have largely replaced older antiemetic regimens based on high-dose metoclopramide because of the failure of the latter to control emetic symptoms in 30–40% of patients and the adverse effects associated with metoclopramide, e.g., sedation, diarrhea, dystonic reactions, akathisia, trismus, and oculogyric crisis. Crossover studies have shown that ondansetron-based antiemetic regimens are preferred by patients over metoclopramide-based protocols for the control of nausea and vomiting associated with cisplatin.

Tavorath and Hesketh *(11)* recently reviewed the literature on the current understanding and management of delayed nausea and vomiting occurring 24 h or more after cisplatin. These symptoms have been estimated to effect between 43 and 89% of patients and to peak between 48 and 72 h after cisplatin chemotherapy. A limited number of randomized trials have been carried out on antiemetic regimens for the control of delayed nausea and vomiting. At this time, the combination of oral dexamethasone (8 mg twice daily for 2 d and then 4 mg twice daily for 2 d) with oral metoclopramide (0.5 mg/kg 4 times daily for 4 d) is the best regimen currently available. Ondansetron has not proved superior to metoclopramide-based regiments in controlled studies for the control of gastrointestinal symptoms occurring 24 h or more after cisplatin administration.

2.2. Neurologic Effects

Neurotoxicity is now considered to be one of the most important side effects associated with cisplatin since the reduction of its renal and gastrointestinal side effects. Cisplatin-induced neurotoxicity most commonly occurs in the form of a peripheral neuropathy or ototoxicity, causing symptoms of numbness, tingling, and paresthesiae in the extremities, tinnitus, difficulty in walking, or deafness. Less common manifestations of cisplatin-induced neurotoxicity include Lhermitte's sign, retrobulbar neuritis, encephalitic symptoms, autonomic neuropathy, cerebral herniation, seizures, cortical blindness, opthalmologic effects, and vertigo *(12,13)*. This section focuses on the toxicity of cisplatin to peripheral sensory nerves. Ototoxicity is discussed in Section 2.4.

Gerritisen van der Hoop and colleagues *(14)* studied the frequency of peripheral neurotoxicity in patients treated with cisplatin by reviewing the literature and carrying out an analysis of toxicity data from their randomized trials of cisplatin in patients with ovarian cancer. Their review of the available literature on cisplatin-induced peripheral neurotoxicity indicated that this side effect occurred in 47.5% of patients given cisplatin. In the analysis of the toxicity data from 292 patients with ovarian cancer that were treated with cisplatin in randomized controlled studies, the overall incidence of peripheral neurotoxicity of any severity grade was also 47%. These two studies indicate that peripheral neurotoxicity develops in about half of the patients treated with cisplatin at conventional doses.

Thompson and colleagues *(15)* carried out a prospective study of the neurologic signs and symptoms occurring in patients receiving cisplatin. The first signs of peripheral neurotoxicity were decreased vibration sense in the toes and loss of the ankle jerks after a mean cumulative dose of 400 mg/m^2. With further treatment, paresthesias occurred in the feet, which were painful in some patients, and the deficits in vibration sense and deep tendon reflexes became more profound and progressed proximally.

Ultimately, peripheral neurotoxicity is the major factor that limits the dose and number of repeated treatments of cisplatin that can be given. A study of high-dose cisplatin in patients with ovarian cancer carried out by Ozols and Young *(16)* found that peripheral neurotoxicity occurred in all patients after two doses of high-dose cisplatin. Further cycles of treatment were associated with the onset of gait disturbances, difficulty with manual dexterity, and difficulty with ambulation due to profound deficits in proprioception.

Hovestadt et al. *(17)* attempted to define the time-course of cisplatin-induced peripheral neurotoxicity after the cessation of treatment by documenting the neurologic signs and symptoms and the vibration perception thresholds in 18 patients with ovarian carcinoma for 2 years after completing a course of cisplatin-based chemotherapy. The results of this study showed that there was significant worsening of the signs and symptoms of cisplatin-induced neurotoxicity and vibration perception threshold in the first 4 months after stopping cisplatin treatment. After 4 months there was some improvement in these parameters, but recovery was generally incomplete. Bissett and colleagues *(6)* documented persisting sensory neuropathy in 23 of 74 patients, 52 months after cisplatin-based chemotherapy for testicular cancer. Therefore peripheral neurotoxicity induced by cisplatin is characterized by deterioration in the first 4 months after stopping treatment; subsequent improvement but recovery is generally incomplete.

The biochemical mechanisms involved in cisplatin-induced peripheral neurotoxicity are poorly understood. Gregg and colleagues *(18)* studied the possible role of platinum deposition in neurologic tissues by correlating the concentration of platinum in various tissues with the clinical symptoms and histologic damage in patients treated with cisplatin. The concentrations of platinum in tissues from the peripheral nervous system (dorsal root ganglia, peripheral nerves) were higher than those in tissues from the central nervous system (brain, spinal cord). High platinum concentrations in dorsal root ganglia and peripheral nerves were associated with clinical symptoms and histologic evidence of peripheral neurotoxicity. These findings support the idea that platinum accumulation in dorsal root ganglia and peripheral nerves leads to damage to the cell bodies and axons of sensory neurons that reside in these tissues located outside the blood-brain barrier.

Alberts and Noel *(19)* recently reviewed the various attempts that have been made to prevent cisplatin-induced peripheral neurotoxicity in patients. Several different agents have been studied for this purpose including nucleophilic sulfur thiols, adrenocorticotropic hormone (ACTH) homologs with neurotrophic activity, and calcium channel antagonists. To demonstrate their neuroprotective effects, and to determine their possible effects on antitumor activity and survival, prospective randomized controlled trials are required that are preferably blinded and placebo controlled.

Kemp and colleagues *(7)* undertook a randomized controlled trial of amifostine, a thiol-cytoprotective agent, to evaluate its protective effects against cisplatin- and cyclophosphamide-induced toxicities including peripheral neurotoxicity. Two hundred and forty-two patients with ovarian cancer receiving cisplatin (100 mg/m^2) and cyclophosphamide were randomized to receive amifostine (910 mg/m^2) or no amifostine. After the last cycle of chemotherapy, the incidences (% of patients) of neurologic toxicity in the amifostine and no-amifostine arms respectively were as follows: grade 0, 45% vs 33%; grade 1, 24% vs 26%; grade 2, 24% vs 29%; and grade 3, 7.3% vs 12.5%. Although the difference between the two arms in the incidence of peripheral neurologic toxicity reached statistical significance, the clinical relevance of the effect is probably small.

Gandara et al. *(20)* carried out a randomized placebo-controlled study of another thiol-chemoprotective agent, diethyldithiolcarbamate, in 221 patients receiving cisplatin (100 mg/m^2) in combination with cyclophosphamide or etoposide. The incidence of peripheral neurotoxicity was similar in the two groups. Moreover, withdrawal for chemotherapy toxicity and nephrotoxicity was more frequent in the group receiving diethyldithiolcarbamate.

An Italian group *(21)* have carried out a randomized double-blind placebo-controlled study of the neuroprotective effects of glutathione, an endogenous thiol containing tripeptide (glutamyl-cysteinyl-glycine) in 50 patients with gastric cancer receiving a dose-intensive regimen of cisplatin (40 mg/m^2/week) with fluorouracil, epirubicin, and leucovorin. Clinical and electrophysiologic evaluation of neurotoxicity at 9 and 15 weeks showed significantly less toxicity in the glutathione arm. It is uncertain whether the neurotoxicity was prevented or simply delayed in onset since the toxicity evaluation was not continued into the posttreatment interval when symptoms and signs commonly deteriorate.

Smyth et al. *(22)* have reported another randomized trial of glutathione in patients receiving cisplatin (100 mg/m^2) for the treatment of ovarian cancer. Neurotoxicity was evaluated in this trial during the course of treatment but not in the posttreatment interval. In a symptom checklist scored by patients there was a statistically significant difference in the response to a question about tingling and numbness in the hands and feet favoring the glutathione group. The incidence of neurotoxicity scored by the physician, however, was similar in the glutathione and placebo groups (no. of patients): grade 0, 41 vs 45; grade 1, 34 vs 27; grade 2, 2 vs 2; and grade 3, 0 vs 0. To date, clinical trials of glutathione given in conjunction with cisplatin have not been reproducible in demonstrating a neuroprotective effect.

Nimodipine is a dihydropyridine calcium channel antagonist that has shown neuroprotective activity in a model system of cisplatin peripheral neurotoxicity. A randomized double-blind placebo-controlled study of nimodipine in patients with ovarian cancer receiving cisplatin was discontinued by Cassidy and colleagues *(23)* before its completion because of the toxicity of the neuroprotective agent. Many patients receiving nimodipine were unable to comply with the treatment because of nausea and vomiting symptoms. Neurotoxicity scores 27 weeks after commencing chemotherapy in 40 patients who completed the trial showed a highly significant difference in the severity of neurotoxicity favoring the placebo group. This suggests that nimodipine may enhance rather than protect the neurotoxicity associated with cisplatin. The experience of these investigators is a sobering example of some of the difficulties involved with clinical trials of neuroprotective agents given in conjunction with cancer chemotherapy.

ORG 2766 is an analog of ACTH with neurotrophic activity that has been extensively investigated for the prevention of cisplatin-induced peripheral neurotoxicity. Initial clinical trials of ORG 2766 were encouraging, but subsequent studies have failed to reproduce evidence of neuroprotection in patients receiving cisplatin. For example, in a study reported by Roberts et al. *(24)* neurotoxicity was monitored by vibration perception threshold (VPT) in women with ovarian cancer receiving cisplatin (75–100 g/m^2). VPT continued to deteriorate after the cisplatin therapy had been completed, and there was no significant difference in VPT measurements between the ORG 2766 and placebo groups.

2.4. Ototoxicity

Ototoxicity symptoms associated with cisplatin include tinnitus (ringing in the ears) and hearing difficulties *(25)*. Typically, tinnitus is high-pitched, intermittent, and not particularly bothersome to most patients. The usual hearing complaints include difficulty hearing in noisy environments, difficulty hearing the telephone ringing, or difficulty following a telephone conversation.

Changes in hearing thresholds on audiometric testing are very common in patients receiving cisplatin *(26)*. The abnormalities are usually bilateral and occur at high frequencies but may involve the middle frequencies involved in speech communication in some patients. Audiometric changes are more frequent than ototoxic symptoms and are not necessarily predictive of an imminent change in hearing. Opinions vary as to the value of audiometric monitoring of cisplatin therapy.

Bokemeyer and colleagues *(27)* recently studied the hearing symptoms and audiograms of 86 patients treated with cisplatin for testicular cancer after a minimum follow-up period of 15 months. Seventeen (20%) patients had persisting symptoms of tinnitus (10 patients), hearing loss (3 patients), or both (3 patients) that were slightly or mildly annoying in 14 patients and very disturbing in only 3 patients. An additional nine patients experienced hearing symptoms that reversed completely during or after chemotherapy. Significant abnormalities on audiogram were observed in 57 patients (60%), whereas hearing symptoms were not always associated with significant changes on the audiogram. The most important factor predicting persistent ototoxicity symptoms was a cumulative cisplatin dose of 600 mg/m^2 or more. These findings were in keeping with a literature review carried by Bokemeyer and colleagues *(27)* showing that the literature values for the incidence of cisplatin-associated tinnitus, deafness, and pathologic audiograms in patients with testicular cancer range from 2 to 65%, 3 to 25%, and 28 to 77%, respectively.

The mechanism involved in the ototoxic effects of cisplatin are poorly understood. Histopathologic studies show the loss of inner and outer hair cells of the basal turns of the cochlear, degeneration of the stria vascularis, and loss of spinal ganglion cells *(28)*. Saito and colleagues *(29)* recently published evidence for cisplatin metabolites mediating the ototoxic effect of this drug. Exposure of isolated cochlear hair cells to cisplatin that had been incubated with S9 fractions of guinea pig liver resulted in toxicity, but hair cell viability remained under conditions in which enzymatic activity was suppressed.

3. CARBOPLATIN

Carboplatin has a chemical structure similar to that of a cisplatin, except that it has a cyclobutane dicarboxylate leaving group in place of the two chloride leaving groups of cisplatin. Carboplatin's mode of action involves the generation of platinum-DNA adducts that are similar in their nature to those formed by cisplatin. The major differences between carboplatin and cisplatin are their stability in biologic fluids and the rate of their reactions with biologic macromolecules.

The best data currently available on the clinical spectrum of adverse effects associated with carboplatin is a database compiled by the Antitumor Clinical Research Department of the Bristol-Myers Company *(30)*. The database contains toxicity information from 710 patients who received single-agent carboplatin as part of Phase II and III clinical trials, with data analyzed according to World Health Organization (WHO) toxicity scales. An analysis of the frequency (% of patients) of adverse effects associated with carboplatin showed that myelosuppression in the form of leukopoenia (55%), thrombocytopenia (32%), and anemia (59%) were common but that infection (4%), bleeding (6%), or the need for transfusion of blood products (21%) occurred infrequently. The majority of patients experienced gastrointestinal symptoms, most frequently in the form of nausea and vomiting (53%) or nausea alone (25%). In contrast to cisplatin, the incidence of abnormalities of serum creatinine (7%), peripheral neurotoxicity (6%), or clinical ototoxicity (1.1%) associated with carboplatin were low.

3.1. Pharmacokinetics

Duffull and Robinson *(31)* and van der Vijgh *(32)* have compiled reviews of the literature concerned with the clinical pharmacokinetics of carboplatin. During the first 10–12 h after carboplatin administration, the plasma concentration-time profiles of intact carboplatin and ultrafiltrate platinum overlap, suggesting that most of the freely exchangeable drug in plasma is in the form of carboplatin and that little or no metabolites are present in the systemic circulation. The clearance of carboplatin is highly variable between patients, but it correlates with the creatinine clearance and other measures of glomerular filtration rate. Carboplatin is excreted in the urine, and cumulative urinary excretion accounts for between 43 and 78% of the dose. Renal clearance is comparable to glomerular filtration rate, indicating that the drug is cleared by renal filtration with only limited tubular reabsorption or secretion. The greater chemical stability and slower plasma protein and tissue binding of carboplatin compared with cisplatin mean that its distribution and elimination half-lives are longer than those of cisplatin. However, at the maximum tolerated doses of cisplatin (100 mg/m^2) and carboplatin (400 mg/m^2), the amount of platinum retained in the body bound to tissues and plasma proteins is similar for both compounds. The volume of distribution of carboplatin approximates the volume of extracellular fluid.

3.2. Hematologic Effects

Myelosuppression was the dose-limiting toxicity in the Phase I clinical trials of carboplatin *(33,34)*. At the maximum tolerated dose, the effect on platelets (thrombocytopenia) was more marked than the effect on the white blood cells (leukopoenia). Typically, the platelet count fell to its lowest level 3 weeks after treatment and then recovered by 4 weeks after treatment.

The severity of thrombocytopenia is highly variable between patients treated with carboplatin at the maximum tolerated dose. Several factors have been identified that were associated with severe thrombocytopenia in Phase I *(33,34)* or subsequent clinical investigations *(35)*. Patients that are elderly (>70 years) and/or have a low creatinine clearance (<60 mL/min), low pretreatment platelet count, poor performance status, or history of prior chemotherapy are at greater risk of severe thrombocytopenia than patients without these factors. A reduction of the carboplatin dose may avoid unacceptable levels of thrombocytopenia in patients having one or more risk factors for severe toxicity.

3.3. Relationship Between Hematotoxicity and Carboplatin AUC

Jodrell and colleagues *(36)* studied the relationship between carboplatin-induced hematotoxicity and carboplatin exposure [area under the curve (AUC)] using data from 989 patients with ovarian cancer entered in clinical studies of single-agent carboplatin who had glomerular filtration rate (GFR) measurements by ^{51}Cr EDTA or creatinine clearances. The carboplatin AUC in each patient was calculated using a reorganized form of the Calvert formula, carboplatin AUC = dose/(GFR + 25). Patients were ranked according to their AUC into a series of cells, and the proportions of patients with grade 1, 2, 3, or 4 thrombocytopenia and leukopoenia were calculated for each cell. Fits to sigmoidal E_{max} models were obtained when the probability of hematotoxicity was related to the carboplatin AUC. In patients who had no prior chemotherapy, the probability of grade 3 or 4 thrombocytopenia at AUC cells 4–5, 6–7, and 8–9 were 4, 20, and 48% respectively. As the carboplatin AUC approached 10, the probability of grade 3 or 4 thrombocytopenia was 100%. In the same group of patients, the probabilities of grade 3 or 4 leukopoenia at the AUC cells of 4–6, 6–7, and 8–9 were 1, 7, and 30%, respectively.

Huizing et al. *(35)* have also studied the relationship between the severity of carboplatin-induced thrombocytopenia and carboplatin exposure using sigmoidal E_{max} equations. In their studies, thrombocytopenia was expressed as the percent decrease in platelet count rather than the probability of obtaining a certain severity grade of toxicity. According to the parameters of their model, the AUC_{50} (AUC predicted to yield a 50% decrease in platelet count) was 4 mg/min/mL, and the Hill constant was 1.9.

Newell et al. *(37)* also found a significant sigmoidal relationship between thrombocytopenia (expressed as a percentage of the pretreatment count) and carboplatin AUC in 22 children aged 3 months to 15 years. The AUC_{50} in this pediatric population was 6 mg/min/mL, which is higher than in adults *(37)*. This finding suggests that the sensitivity of the bone marrow to the effects of carboplatin may be less in children than in adults.

3.4. Prediction of Carboplatin-Induced Thrombocytopenia

Egorin and colleagues *(38)* generated a pair of equations for calculating the dose of carboplatin for individual patients based on patient factors that they or others identified to influence the severity of thrombocytopenia, e.g., creatinine clearance, pretreatment platelet count, status of prior chemotherapy, and body surface area. Two separate equations were derived, one for previously untreated patients:

$$\text{dosage (mg/m}^2) = 0.091\left(\frac{CrCl}{BSA}\right)(\%\text{ reduction in platelet count}) + 86$$

and another for patients who had received prior chemotherapy:

$$\text{dosage (mg/m}^2) = 0.091\left(\frac{CrCl}{BSA}\right)[(\%\text{ reduction in platelet count}) \text{ -}17] + 86$$

where CrCl is creatinine clearance in mL/min and BSA is body surface in m^2. A figure must be entered in these equations for a desired and acceptable level of platelet toxicity in the individual concerned. The equations were prospectively validated by evaluating their precision in 38 courses of carboplatin and 23 patients. The actual decrease in platelet count was compared with that predicted from the calculation of the dose of carboplatin. There was a high correlation between predicted and observed reductions in platelet count ($r \geq 0.94$), and the data formed a line very close to the line of identity.

The relationship between drug concentration and drug effect is often best described by a sigmoidal curve that is defined by the Hill equation where E_{max} is the maximal possible effect, EC_{50} is the concentration of drug producing 50% of the maximal effect, C is concentration, and H is the Hill constant;

$$\% \text{ effect} = \frac{E_{max} \cdot C^H}{[EC_{50}{}^H + C^H]}$$

Huizing and colleagues *(35)* described such a relationship between the thrombocytopenia induced by carboplatin and the carboplatin AUC where the EC_{50} (or AUC_{50}) was 4 mg/min/mL and the Hill constant was 1.9. Assuming that the maximal possible effect (E_{max}) of carboplatin on the platelet count was a 100% reduction in platelet count, the parameters can be introduced into the Hill equation as follows:

$$\% \text{ reduction in platelet count} = \frac{100 \cdot AUC^{1.9}}{[4^{1.9} + AUC^{1.9}]}$$

or

$$\% \text{ reduction in platelet count} = \frac{100 \cdot AUC^{1.9}}{[13 + AUC^{1.9}]}$$

From this equation, it is possible to predict the percentage by which the platelet count will fall in an individual patient if the carboplatin AUC in that individual is known.

It is possible to predict the carboplatin AUC achieved in an individual patient using the Calvert *(39)* or Chatelut *(40)* formulas, and in doing so, introduce these values into the Hill equation for carboplatin-induced thrombocytopenia. Using a reorganized Calvert formula, the carboplatin AUC can be simply calculated from the carboplatin dose (mg) and the patient's renal function where GRF is glomerular filtration rate:

$$\text{carboplatin AUC} = \frac{dose}{(GFR + 25)}$$

Alternatively, carboplatin clearance (mL/min) for an individual patient may be calculated using the Chatelut formula, where wt is body weight in kilogram, age is years, sex = 0 if male or 1 if female, and serum creatinine concentration is expressed in μM:

$$\text{clearance} = (0.134 \times wt) + \frac{[218 \times wt\,(1 - 0.00457 \times age) \times (1 - 0.314 \times sex)]}{\text{serum creatinine concentration}}$$

Carboplatin AUC can then be calculated by introducing carboplatin clearance and dose values into the following equation:

$$AUC = \frac{dose}{clearance}$$

3.5. Gastrointestinal Effects

Nausea and vomiting are common side effects associated with carboplatin. In the toxicity database compiled by the Antitumor Clinical Research Department of the Bristol-Myers Company, 53% of patients experienced nausea and vomiting, and an additional 25% of patients experienced nausea without vomiting *(30)*. In Phase I studies of carboplatin *(33,34)*, nausea and vomiting was a dose related adverse effect and tended to come on 6–12 h after carboplatin administration and resolve by 24 h.

du Bois and colleagues *(41)* have studied the metabolism of serotonin in patients receiving carboplatin since serotonin release has been implicated in acute nausea and vomiting associated with cisplatin. The urinary excretion of the serotonin metabolite 5-HIAA increased after treatment with carboplatin by an average of 35%. Urinary 5-UIAA levels peaked at 12 h after treatment. Combining carboplatin with alkylating agents increased both the urinary excretion of 5-HIAA and severity of emesis. These findings suggest the involvement of serotonin in the nausea and vomiting associated with carboplatin and provide a rationale for giving serotonin antagonists with carboplatin.

An Italian group *(42)* has reported a prospective randomized double-blind trial comparing a serotonin antagonist (granisetron) given alone with dexamethasone alone or granisetron combined with dexamethasone in 408 patients receiving moderately emetogenic chemotherapy including 56 patients treated with carboplatin at doses ≥ 300 mg/m^2. Granisetron and dexamethasone were more effective than either antiemetic agent given alone in the complete or major protection of nausea and vomiting on d 1–3. Constipation and hot flushes were more common in patients receiving the combination of antiemetics. Although most patients in this study were given chemotherapy not including carboplatin, it is some of the best evidence currently available to support the treatment policy of giving a serotonin antagonist in combination with dexamethasone to prevent the nausea and vomiting associated with carboplatin.

4. OXALIPLATIN

Oxaliplatin is the R,R-isomer of a diaminocyclohexane platinum(II) complex containing an oxalato leaving group. Similar to other platinum complexes, oxaliplatin's mode of action involves the generation of aquated platinum species within cells and the formation of DNA adducts *(43)*. Oxaliplatin has shown significant antitumor activity in patients with advanced stage colorectal cancer when given alone or in combination with 5-fluororacil *(44)* and is approved for clinical use in France for this indication.

Misset *(45)* and Extra et al. *(46)* have recently reviewed the safety profile of oxaliplatin in more than 2000 patients who were given the drug in clinical trials. Oxaliplatin does not appear to cause significant ototoxicity or nephrotoxicity or to require nephroprotective measures *(45)*. Hematological toxicity is generally mild when oxaliplatin is given as a single agent but was dose related in Phase I dose-finding clinical trials *(46)*. Of 124 patients given oxaliplatin as a single agent, grade 3 or 4 anemia, thrombocytopenia, or neutropenia occurred in 3, 2, and 1% of patients, respectively *(45)*. The major toxicities associated with oxaliplatin, however, are nausea and vomiting, as well as peripheral sensory neurotoxicity.

4.1. Gastrointestinal Effects

In the initial Phase I clinical trials of oxaliplatin *(46)*, almost all patients experienced nausea and vomiting, and these symptoms were of grade 3 or 4 severity in over 50% of patients. Diarrhea also occurred but was less frequent (24% of courses) and less severe than emesis. Gastrointestinal toxicity was not dose related at doses ranging from 45 to 200 mg/m^2 and is not influenced by the duration of the drug infusion. Antiemetics were not given routinely during this study until the dose level of 90 mg/m^2, and many patients had been previously exposed to emetogenic chemotherapy; these factors may have increased the frequency and severity of nausea and vomiting.

Subsequent experience with oxaliplatin *(45)* given in conjunction with antiemetics including serotonin antagonists has shown less gastrointestinal toxicity. In 262 patients treated with oxaliplatin alone, the overall incidence of nausea and vomiting was 64.9%, and only 10.7% of patients experienced grade 3 or 4 toxicity. Diarrhea occurred in 30.4% of patients and was of grade 3 or 4 severity in only 4% of patients. The incidence and severity of nausea, vomiting, and diarrhea increases when oxaliplatin is combined with 5-fluororacil. This experience indicates that gastrointestinal symptoms are of mild to moderate severity and manageable with modern antiemetic regimes in most patients treated with oxaliplatin as a single agent.

4.2. Peripheral Neurotoxicity

Peripheral neurotoxicity is a very common side effect associated with oxaliplatin. Eighty-five to 95% of patients treated with the drug experience neurosensory symptoms to some degree *(45)*.

The most common symptoms *(43,45,46)* are paresthesias (spontaneous abnormal tingling sensations often described by patients as pins and needles) and dysesthesias (abnormal and unpleasant sensations felt when the skin is touched) that are induced or exacerbated by the cold, such as when patients touch cold surfaces or drink cold fluids. Typically, these symptoms occur in the fingers, hands, toes, and lips, but many also involve the legs, forearms, mouth, and throat. Severe oxaliplatin neurotoxicity may be associated with sensory ataxia causing walking and handwriting difficulties, or transient laryngospasm and a feeling of difficulty breathing or swallowing.

Neurosensory symptoms typically come on during the drug infusion and persist for a variable time but have normally resolved within 7 d of the first dose of oxaliplatin *(43,46)*. A progressive increase in the duration and intensity of symptoms occurs with further administration of oxaliplatin. At the end of the course of treatment, there is a tendency for the neurotoxicity symptoms to resolve *(45)*. After 6 months, the symptoms have completely disappeared in 18% of patients and partially disappeared in 35% of patients. Twelve months after treatment, the symptoms have completely disappeared in 41% of patients, partially disappeared in 41% of patients, and not changed in 18% of patients.

In Phase I studies, oxaliplatin-induced neurotoxicity was shown to be dose related *(46)*. At doses of 90 mg/m^2 or less, neurotoxicity was not observed. On the first cycle of treatment of higher doses, however, 50, 64, 71, and 100% of patients experienced neurotoxicity symptoms at 135, 150, 175, and 200 mg/m^2, respectively. The severity of neurotoxicity is dependant on the cumulative dose of oxaliplatin given. Severe neurotoxicity, manifest as functional motor disturbances or sensory ataxia, occurred in 10, 50, and 75% of patients receiving cumulative doses of 780, 1170, and 1560 mg/m^2, respectively *(43)*.

Levi and colleagues *(44)* found that the commonly used WHO and National Cancer Institute-Common Toxicity Criteria (NCI-CTC) grading systems for neurosensory toxicity were inadequate for scoring the severity of oxaliplatin neurotoxicity. They developed an oxaliplatin-specific scale whereby grade 0 is no symptoms; grade 1 is when paresthesias and/or dysesthesias (induced by the cold) are present with complete regression within 1 week; grade 2 is when paresthesiae and/or dysesthesiae are present with complete regression within 21 days; grade 3 is when paresthesias and dysesthesias have incompletely regressed at day 21; and grade 4 is when paresthesias and/or dysesthesias are associated with functional consequences *(45)*. In this scoring system, the severity of toxicity is assigned solely on the basis of the duration of symptoms and whether symptoms are associated with functional difficulties. Intensity of the symptoms or the presence of neurologic deficits, such as glove and stocking sensory loss or reduced tendon reflexes, are not taken into account.

The mechanism of the neurotoxicity associated with oxaliplatin and other platinum diaminocyclohexane complexes is poorly understood. Screnci and colleagues *(47)* hypothesized that the lipophilic diaminocyclohexane ligand, which has two chiral centers and three possible isomeric forms, could be important for their accumulation and toxicity in peripheral nerves. They prepared the pure R,R- and S,S-enantiomers of oxaliplatin and some other platinum diaminocyclohexane (DACH) complexes and studied their neurotoxicity in a rat model. Both R,R- and S,S-enantiomers of oxaliplatin caused slowing of sensory nerve conduction velocity during repeated dose treatment in this model, but the R,R-enantiomer (the constituent of the clinical preparation of oxaliplatin) caused neurotoxicity at an earlier time and at lower cumulative doses than its S,S-enantiomer. There was no enantiomeric selectivity in the concentrations of platinum in samples of sciatic nerve, dorsal root ganglia, spinal cord, or brain taken at the end of the experiment despite differences between the enantiomers in their neurotoxicity. The investigators concluded that Pt (DACH) complexes such as oxaliplatin exhibit enantiomeric selectivity of their peripheral neurotoxicity possibly due to stereoselective interactions on or within large proprioceptive neurons since their accumulation in nerve tissue is similar.

4.3. Chronomodulation of Oxaliplatin Toxicity

Researchers from France have been investigating the idea of modulating the clinical toxicities of oxaliplatin by giving the drug as a continuous infusion at variable dosing rates based on circadian rhythms rather than at a constant rate. Causanell and colleagues *(48)* carried out a Phase I clinical study of oxaliplatin in which patients were treated with a 5-d continuous infusion and randomly assigned to either a constant infusion rate or a dosing rate altered in a sinusoidal fashion with peak delivery at 1600 h coinciding with circadian rhythms. The incidence of neutropenia, neurotoxicity, nausea, and vomiting was lower with chronomodulation of the oxaliplatin infusion rate. Higher doses were able to be given, and more patients were able to complete the planned treatment with the chronomodulated infusion.

These findings have been confirmed in a randomized controlled study reported by Levi et al. *(44)* of oxaliplatin (20–25 $mg/m^2/pd$) given over 5 consecutive d in combination with 5-fluorouracil and folinic acid to patients with metastatic colorectal cancer. In all, 186 patients were randomly assigned to either constant infusion rates of oxaliplatin, 5-fluororacil, and folinic acid or control. The incidence of severe neurotoxicity associated with functional impairment was 16% in patients treated by chronotherapy vs 31% in the control arm ($p < 0.01$). The incidence of vomiting was the same in both groups. Treatment had to be withdrawn, mainly for neurotoxicity, more frequently in the constant infusion group. Tumor responses occurred in 51% of patients in the chronotherapy group vs 29% of the control group ($p = 0.003$).

4.4. Pharmacokinetics

The pharmacokinetics of oxaliplatin have been studied using inductively coupled plasma mass spectrometry *(43,49)*. In blood, oxaliplatin is sequestered into free, protein-bound, and erythrocyte-bound platinum. The pharmacokinetics of platinum in plasma ultrafiltrate reveal a large volume of distribution

(582 L) and high clearance (10.1 L/h). Biotransformation products appear in plasma ultrafiltrate including (DACH)$PtCl_2$, (DACH)$PtClH_2O$, (DACH)Pt(methionine), and (DACH)Pt(glutathione). About half of the dose is excreted in the urine.

Gamelin et al. *(49)* studied the pharmacokinetics of oxaliplatin given at a dose of 130 mg/m^2 over 2 h for eight courses. Platinum did not accumulate in plasma or plasma ultrafiltrate but showed progressive accumulation in red blood cells with repeated courses. It may be that the lack of accumulation of oxaliplatin in plasma explains the reversibility of its neurotoxicity and the lack of cumulative nephrotoxicity. Correlations between platinum concentrations and neurotoxicity showed no clear relationship. However, patients experiencing anemia had higher red blood cell levels than those who did not have anemia.

5. JM216

JM216 is a new platinum analog that is given by mouth rather than intravenously. It differs from cisplatin, carboplatin, and oxaliplatin by being a platinum(IV) complex rather than platinum(II) complex. This feature may make the molecule more stable, which could be important as it moves through the contents of the gastrointestinal tract. JM216 is also more lipophilic than the other platinum drugs currently of clinical interest, a feature that may aid its absorption through the membranes of the gastrointestinal wall.

Currently, a limited amount of information is available on the effects of oral JM216 in patients. The best indication of its clinical toxicity profile comes from recent reports of Phase II trials *(50,51)*. Hematological toxicity is common, in the form of thrombocytopenia and neutropenia, and the major nonhematologic toxicities of oral JM216 are nausea, vomiting, diarrhea, and constipation. It appears that toxicity to the hearing, kidney, or peripheral nerves occur infrequently in patients treated with oral JM216.

Recently, some preliminary results of a clinical trial were reported in abstract form providing details on the comparative adverse effect profiles of oral JM216 and intravenous cisplatin *(51)*. In this study, 31 patients with advanced non-small cell carcinoma of the lung were randomly assigned treatment with either oral JM216 (120 mg/m^2/d on d 1–5) or cisplatin (100 mg/m^2 iv on d 1). Grade III and IV toxicities occurred with the following frequencies (% of courses) in patients treated with JM216 and cisplatin, respectively: thrombocytopenia, 25 or 0%; leukopoenia, 18 and 2%; neutropenia, 17 and 0%; nausea, 28 and 60%; vomiting, 13 and 44%; nephrotoxicity, 2 and 15%; and neurotoxicity, 0 and 2%. These data suggest that grade III or IV hematologic toxicities occur more frequently in patients treated with oral JM216 than in those receiving intravenous cisplatin but that nonhematologic toxicities involving the gastrointestinal, renal, and neurosensory systems are less common than with cisplatin.

5.1. Hematologic Effects

During Phase I trials of oral JM216 given once daily for 5 consecutive d at doses ranging from 30 to 140 $mg/m^2/d$, the severity and incidence of thrombocytopenia and neutropenia was dose related, and these toxicities were the major dose-limiting factors present at the maximum tolerated dose *(52)*. Hematologic toxicity was more severe in patients who had been previously treated with chemotherapy compared with chemotherapy-naive patients. Platelet and neutrophil nadirs occurred between 17 and 21 d after treatment and had recovered to normal in most patients by 28 d. Neutropenia associated with sepsis or thrombocytopenia associated with hemorrhage occurred infrequently.

5.2. Gastrointestinal Effects

In Phase I trials antiemetics were given in conjunction with oral JM216 in an attempt to reduce nausea and vomiting symptoms *(52)*. The antiemetic regimen was oral dexamethasone 4 mg given 3 times daily with oral metoclopramide 20 mg given 4 times daily or ondansetron 8 mg once daily for 5 d. Despite these emetics, nausea and vomiting occurred on 50–65% of courses. The symptoms were not related to the dose of JM216 given, and most often they were of grade 1 severity. Nausea usually came on after 24 h of starting the 5-d course of oral JM216 and usually lasted 5 d. Vomiting typically came on 75 h after starting the treatment and lasted 1 d. Diarrhea was dose related and lasted usually 2 d on average.

Subsequent Phase II experience with JM216 has provided a clearer picture of the frequency of gastrointestinal symptoms in patients receiving JM216 *(50)*. Antiemetic treatment was not specified for this trial, and several different antiemetic treatment regimens were used. In 17 patients, the frequencies (% of patients) of ≥ grade 2 nausea, vomiting, diarrhea, and constipation were 41, 47, 24, and 18%, respectively. This suggests that gastrointestinal symptoms associated with oral JM216 are mild or absent in most patients when the drug is given in conjunction with oral antiemetic therapy.

5.3. Pharmacokinetics

The pharmacokinetics of platinum after oral administration of JM216 were studied as part of its Phase I clinical trial *(52)*. The pharmacokinetic parameters of platinum in plasma ultrafiltrate at the recommended dose for Phase II studies (100 $mg/m^2/d$ x 5) were as follows: C_{max} d 1, 61 ± 37 mg/L; d 5, 81 ± 39 mg/L: T_{max}, d 1, 1.7 ± 1.2 h and 5, 1.9 ± 0.7 h; $AUC_{o\text{-}t}$ d 1 0.44 ± 0.2 mg/h/L and d 5, 0.76 ± 0.3 mg/h/L; $t_{1/2}$; d 1, 7.7 ± 3.3 h and d 5, 12 ± 4.7 h). There was accumulation of platinum in plasma and plasma ultrafiltrate with repeated daily dosing. There was a linear relationship between JM216 dose and the plasma ultrafiltrate AUC; the T_{max}, $t^1/_2$, and urinary recovery (4.7–6.2%

of the dose) showed no dose-related changes. These findings indicate that the pharmacokinetic behavior of oral JM216 is dose independent at doses of 30–140 mg/m^2.

There was considerable variability between subjects in the plasma ultrafiltrate platinum AUC and in the severity of thrombocytopenia at the dose of JM216 recommended for Phase II studies *(52)*. However, these pharmacokinetic and pharmacodynamic parameters were significantly related in a relationship described by a sigmoidal E_{max} equation with the following parameters: E_{max}, 5.6% (platelet nadir expressed as the % of pretreatment platelet count; AUC_{50}, 0.82 mg/h/L; Hill slope, 1.1; and R^2, 0.831. This finding suggests that the between-subject variability of the hematotoxicity of oral JM216 may be due to its pharmacokinetic variability.

A further complexity in the pharmacokinetic behavior of JM216 in patients has been demonstrated by Raynaud and co-workers *(53)* in studies of the metabolic profile in plasma ultrafiltrate after the oral administration of JM216. These investigators have identified a total of six platinum-containing platinum species in the plasma ultrafiltrate of patients, including four that had been previously identified during in vitro incubations in plasma and two that had not been seen in vitro. No parent JM216 was seen in plasma ultrafiltrate taken from patients given the drug. Further studies of the biotransformation of JM216 have been hampered by their low concentrations in vivo and methodologic difficulties in their analysis. Their individual pharmacokinetic properties and role in mediating the effects of JM216 in patients remain to be fully characterized.

6. COMPARATIVE ADVERSE EFFECT PROFILES

6.1. Gastrointestinal Effects

Nausea and vomiting are common adverse effects associated with all the platinum derivatives currently of clinical interest. These symptoms occur more frequently with cisplatin than with carboplatin *(30)* or oral JM216 *(51)* and have been associated with oxaliplatin as well. Antiemetic treatment with 5-hydroxytryptamine type 3 receptor antagonists in combination with dexamethasone reduces emetic symptoms occurring within the first 24 h of chemotherapy to manageable levels in most patients. Serotonin release appears to be the major emetic mechanism operating within the first 24 h of platinum-based chemotherapy. Diarrhea and constipation also occur in patients treated with cisplatin, carboplatin, oxaliplatin, and oral JM216 but may be due at least in part to the side effects of antiemetic drugs given with the chemotherapy.

6.2. Hematologic Effects

Myelosuppression is the dose-limiting adverse effect associated with carboplatin and the newer orally administered analog JM216. The myelosuppression associated with carboplatin is highly variable but is predicted by the carboplatin AUC, renal function, prior treatment, performance status, and pretreatment white blood cell and platelet counts *(5)*. Similarly, myelosuppression associated with JM216 is highly variable but is related to the free plasma AUC *(52)*. Otherwise, carboplatin (and possibly JM216) have favorable nonhematologic toxicity profiles and are well accepted by patients.

6.3. Neurosensory Effects

Peripheral sensory neurotoxicity is currently the major dose-limiting side effect of cisplatin but is poorly understood. Neurotoxicity symptoms and signs come on after cumulative doses of 300 mg/m^2 or more and worsen during the first 1–4 months after treatment. Long-term survivors of testes and ovarian cancer frequently have permanent signs or symptoms of cisplatin-induced peripheral nerve damage.

Oxaliplatin is also associated with dose-limiting cumulative sensory neuropathy, but the toxicity differs from that of cisplatin in its time-course, exacerbating factors, reversibility, and schedule dependency. Oxaliplatin neurotoxicity is characterized by paresthesias and dysesthesias of the extremities, lips, mouth, and throat coming on during the infusion and reversing within minutes to d after the end of the infusion. The symptoms may be brought on or worsened by exposure to the cold. The incidence and severity of neurotoxicity associated by oxaliplatin is reduced by chronomodulated administration schedules.

Cisplatin frequently causes ototoxic symptoms and audiometric abnormalities, but tinnitus and symptomatic hearing loss are often reversible at cumulative doses less than 600 mg/m^2 *(27)*. Other platinum analogs very uncommonly cause clinically significant ototoxicity at conventional doses.

6.4. Renal Effects

Nephrotoxicity seriously limited the early clinical experience with cisplatin; however, the use of intravenous hydration, mannitol, and chloride-containing drug vehicles has reduced kidney damage to acceptable levels. Long-term survivors of cisplatin treatment typically have mild-to-moderate deficits in glomerular filtration and normal renal tubular function. The other platinum analogs of current clinical interest neither induce significant nephrotoxicity nor require neuroprotective measures.

7. CONCLUSIONS

Since the introduction of the antitumor platinum complexes into human oncology in the early 1970s, considerable progress has been made in understanding their clinical toxicology and in the development of preventive and predictive techniques for improving their safety and tolerance by patients. Advances in three areas, in particular, have been key to reducing their host toxicities to manageable levels:

1. Intense acute nausea and vomiting associated with serotonin release within the first 24 h of giving cisplatin or other platinum derivatives is essentially abolished in most patients by antiemetic therapy with selective serotonin type 3 receptor antagonists in combination with dexamethasone.
2. Thrombocytopenia associated with carboplatin is readily predictable from an individual's renal function, carboplatin clearance, prior treatment history, performance status, and pretreatment platelet count. Individualized dosing of carboplatin based on these patient factors (especially renal function and carboplatin clearance) achieves more consistent levels of hematotoxicity compared with giving doses calculated according to the patient's body surface area.
3. The use of intravenous hydration, mannitol, and chloride-containing drug vehicles with cisplatin to reduce the exposure of renal tubule cells to this drug or its toxic biotransformation products has significantly reduced the clinical nephrotoxicity associated with this platinum agent to acceptable levels.

8. FUTURE CHALLENGES

Significant challenges remain, concerned with the clinical toxicology of platinum derivatives, particularly in the control of neurosensory toxicities and delayed nausea and vomiting.

8.1. Neurosensory Toxicity

Neurosensory symptoms resulting from peripheral sensory neurotoxicity or ototoxicity are common in patients treated with cisplatin and oxaliplatin. For some patients, symptoms such as numbness or pins and needles in the hands or feet or ringing in the ears represent a mild annoyance, whereas for others the symptoms may be painful or associated with proprioceptive or hearing disabilities. Neurosensory toxicity, particularly in the form of peripheral sensory neuropathy, is the major factor limiting the amount of cisplatin and oxaliplatin (both single and cumulative doses) that can be given.

The molecular and biochemical mechanisms underlying the peripheral neurotoxicity of cisplatin and oxaliplatin are poorly understood. It is not appreciated why cisplatin and oxaliplatin neurotoxicity should differ in time-course, reversibility, exacerbating factors, and schedule dependence or why other platinum analogs do not damage peripheral neurons. It is not understood why a subset of large proprioceptive postmitotic sensory neurons are selectively damaged by these agents. Until such mechanistic information becomes available, the development of neuroprotective strategies will remain largely empirical.

To date, randomized clinical trials have failed to demonstrate the reproducible evidence of prevention of cisplatin neurotoxicity by thiols, neurotrophic factors, or calcium channel antagonists. The trials have highlighted a number of potential difficulties with carrying out studies of putative neuroprotective agents during cancer chemotherapy, such as (1) how to measure neurotoxicity; (2) when to measure neurotoxicity; (3) adverse effects of the neuroprotective agent, and; (4) the possibility of pharmacokinetic and pharmacodynamic interactions between the neuroprotective and chemotherapeutic agents.

8.2. Delayed Nausea

Nausea and vomiting occurring 24 h or more after chemotherapy is frequent in patients treated with cisplatin, and possibly in patients treated with other platinum analogs. The currently recommended antiemetic regimen for delayed emesis [oral metoclopramide (0.5 mg/kg 4 times daily for 4 d) and dexamethasone (8 mg twice daily for 2 d followed by 4 mg twice daily for the next 2 d)] controls symptoms in only 50% of patients and is associated at times with metoclopramide adverse effects, i.e., sedation, diarrhea, and extrapyramidal reactions. Serotonin antagonists have limited efficacy in the control of emesis after 24 h, suggesting that emetic mechanisms other than serotonin release occur at this time. Identifying those mechanisms and better antiemetic regimens for delayed nausea and vomiting is now a priority.

ACKNOWLEDGMENTS

I would like to thank Kavita Hussein for her very skillful secretarial assistance.

REFERENCES

1. Krakoff, I. H. (1979): Nephrotoxicity of cis-dichlorodiammineplatinum(II). *Cancer Treat. Rep.* **63,** 1523–1525.
2. Weiss, R. B. and Poster, D. S. (1982) The renal toxicity of cancer chemotherapeutic agents. *Cancer Treat. Rev.* **9,** 37–56.
3. Comis, R. L. (1980): Cisplatin nephrotoxicity: the effect of dose, schedule, and hydration scheme, in *Cisplatin: Current Status And New Developments* (Prestayko, A. W. et al. eds.), Academic, Orlando, FL, pp. 485–494.
4. Daugaard, G. and Abildgaard, U. (1989) Cisplatin nephrotoxicity. *Cancer Chemother. Pharmacol.* **25,** 1–9.
5. Blachley, J. D. and Hill, J. B. (1981) Renal and electrolyte disturbances associated with cisplatin. *Ann. Intern. Med.* **95,** 628–632.
6. Bissett, D., Kunkeler, L., Zwanenberg, L., Paul, J., Gray, C., Swan, I. R. C., et al. (1990) Long-term sequelae of treatment for testicular germ cell tumors. *Br. J. Cancer* **62,** 655–659.
7. Kemp, G., Rose, P., Lurain, J., Berman, M., Manetta, A., Roullet, B., et al. (1996) Amifostine pretreatment for protection against cyclophosphamide-induced and cisplatin-induced toxicities: results of a randomized control trial in patients with advanced ovarian cancer. *J. Clin. Oncol.* **14,** 2101–2112.
8. Gralla, R. J., Itri, L. M., Pisko, S. E., Squillante, A. E., Kelsen, D. P., Braun, D. W., et al. (1981) Antiemetic efficacy of high-dose metoclopramine: randomized trials with placebo and prochlorperazine in patients with chemotherapy-induced nausea and vomiting. *N. Engl. J. Med.* **9,** 905–909.

9. Cubeddu, L. X., Hoffman, I. S., Fuenmayor, N. T., and Finn, A. L. (1990) Efficacy of ondansetron (GR 38032F) and the role of serotonin in cisplatin-induced nausea and vomiting. *N. Engl. J. Med.* **322,** 810–816.
10. Del Favero, A., Roila, F., and Tonato, M. (1993) Reducing chemotherapy-induced nausea and vomiting: current perspective and future possibilities. *Drug Safety* **9,** 410–428.
11. Tavorath, R. and Hesketh, P. J. (1996) Drug treatment of chemotherapy-induced delayed emesis. *Drugs* **52,** 639–648.
12. Hamers, F. P. T., Gispen, W. H., and Neijt, J. P. (1991) Neurotoxicity side effects of cisplatin. *Eur. J. Cancer* 27:372–376.
13. Cersosimo, R. J. (1989) Cisplatin neurotoxicity. *Cancer Treat. Rev.* **16,** 195–211.
14. Gerritsen van der Hoop, R., Van Der Burg, M. E. L., Ten Bokkel Huinink, W. W., Van Houwelingen, J. C., and Neijt, J. P. (1990) Incidence of neuropathy in 395 patients with ovarian cancer treated with or without cisplatin. *Cancer* **66,** 1697–1702.
15. Thompson, S. W., Davies, L. E., Kornfeld, M., Hilgers, R. D., and Standefer, J. C. (1984) Cisplatin neurotoxicity: clinical, electrophysiolic, morphologic and toxicologic studies. *Cancer* **54,** 1269–1275.
16. Ozols, R. F. and Young, R. C. (1985) High-dose cisplatin therapy in ovarian cancer. *Semin. Oncol.* **12,** 21–30.
17. Hovestadt, A., Van Der Berg, M. E., Verbiest, H. B., Van Putten, W. L., and Vecht, C. J. (1992) The course of neuropathy after cessation of cisplatin treatment combined with org2766 or placebo. *J. Neurol.* **239,** 143–146.
18. Gregg, R. W., Molepa, J. M., Monpetit, V. J. A., Mikael, N. Z., Redmond, D., Gadia, M., et al. (1992) Cisplatin neurotoxicity: the relationship between dosage, time and platinum concentration in neurological tissues, and morphologic evidence of toxicity. *J. Clin. Oncol.* **10,** 795–803.
19. Alberts, D. S. and Noel, J. K. (1995) Cisplatin-associated neurotoxicity: can it be prevented? *Anti-Cancer Drugs* **6,** 369–383.
20. Gandara, D. R., Natishas, W. A., Adelson, M. D., Lichtman, S. M., Podczaski, E. S., Yanovich, S., et al. (1995) Randomized placedo-controlled multicentre evaluation of diethyldithiolcarbamate for chemoprotection against cisplatin-induced toxicities. *J. Clin. Oncol.* **13,** 490–496.
21. Cascinu, S., Cordella, L., Ferro, E. D., Fronzoni, M., and Catakino, G. (1995) Neuroprotective effect of reduced glutathione on cisplatin-based chemotherapy in advanced gastric cancer: a randomized placebo-controlled trial. *J. Clin. Oncol.* **13,** 26–32.
22. Smyth, J. F., Bowman, A., Perren, T., Wilkinson, P., Prescott, R. J., Quinn, K. J., et al. (1997) Glutathione reduces the toxicity and improves quality of life of women diagnosed with ovarian cancer treated with cisplatin: results of a double-blind randomized trial. *Ann. Oncol.* **8,** 569–573.
23. Cassidy, D., Paul, J., Soukop, M., Habeshaw, T., Reed, N. S., Parkin, D., et al. (1998) Clinical trials of nimodipine as a potential neuroprotector in ovarian cancer patients treated with cisplatin. *Cancer Chemother. Pharmacol.* **41,** 161–166.
24. Roberts, J. A., Jenison, E. L., Kim, K. M., Clarkepearson, D., and Langlebean, A. (1997) A Randomized, multicentre, double-blind, placebo-controlled dose-finding study of ORG 2766 in the prevention or delay of cisplatin-induced neuropathies in women with ovarian cancer. *Gynecol. Oncol.* **67,** 172–177.
25. Melmamed, L. B., Selim, M. A., and Schuchman, D. (1985) Cisplatin ototoxicity in gynaecology cancer patients. *Cancer* **55,** 41–43.
26. Laurell, G. and Jungnelius, U. (1990) High-dose cisplatin treatment: hearing loss and plasma concentrations. *Laryngoscope* **100,** 724–734.
27. Bokemeyer, C., Berger, C. C., Hartmann, J. T., Kollmannsberger, C., Schmoll, H., Kuczyk, M. A., et al. (1998) Analysis of risk factors for cisplatin-induced ototoxicity in patients with testicular cancer. *Br. J. Cancer* **77,** 1355–1362.

28. Hinojosa, R., Riggs, L. C., Strauss, M., and Matz, G. J. (1995) Temporal bone histopathology of cisplatin ototoxicity. *Am. J. Otol.* **16,** 731–740.
29. Saito, T., Yamada, T., Manabe, Y., Yamamoto, T., and Saito, H. (1996) Cisplatin metabolites and their toxicity on isolated cochlear outer hair cells in vitro. *Acta Otolaryngol.* **116,** 561–565.
30. Canetta, R., Rozencweig, M., and Carter, S. K. (1985) Carboplatin: the clinical spectrum to date. *Cancer Treat. Rev.* **12(Suppl. A),** 125–136.
31. Duffull, S. B. and Robinson, B. A. (1997) Clinical pharmacokinetics and dose optimisation of carboplatin. *Clin. Pharmacokinet.* **33,** 161–183.
32. Van Der Vijgh, W. J. F. (1991) Clinical pharmacokinetics of carboplatin. *Clin Pharmacokinet* **21,** 242–261.
33. Calvert, A. H., Harland, S. J., Newell, D. R., Siddik, Z. H., Jones, A.C., McElwain, T.J., et al. (1982) Early clinical trials with cis-diammine-1,1-cyclobutane dicarboxylate platinum II. *Cancer Chemother. Pharmacol.* **9,** 140–147.
34. Van Echo, D. A., Egorin, M. J., Whitacre, M. Y., Olman, E. A., and Aisner, J. (1984) Phase I and pharmacological trial of carboplatin daily for 5 d. *Cancer Treat. Rep.* **68,** 1103–1114.
35. Huizing, M. T., Van Warmerdam, L. J. C., Rosing, H., Schaefers, M. C. W., Lai, A., Helmerhorst, T. J. M., et al. (1997) Phase I and pharmacologic study of the combination paclitaxel and carboplatin as first-line chemotherapy in stage III and IV ovarian cancer. *J. Clin. Oncol.* **15,** 1953–1964.
36. Jodrell, D. I., Egorin, M. J., Canetta, R. M., Langenberg, P., Goldbloom, E. P., Burroughs, J. N., et al. (1992) Relationships between carboplatin exposure and tumor response and toxicity in patients with ovarian cancer. *J. Clin. Oncol.* **10,** 520–528.
37. Newell, D. R., Pearson, A. D. J., Balmanno, K., Price, L., Wyllie, R. A., Keir, M., et al. (1993) Carboplatin pharmacokinetics in children: the development of a pediatric dosing formula. *J. Clin. Oncol.* **11,** 2314–2323.
38. Egorin, M. J., Van Echo, D. A., Olman, E. A., Whitacre, M. Y., Forrest, A., and Aisner, J. (1985) Prospective validation of a pharmacologically based dosing scheme for the cis-diamminedichloroplatinum(II) analog diamminecyclobutanedicarboxylatoplatinum. *Cancer Res.* **45,** 6502–6506.
39. Calvert, A. H., Newell, D. R., Gumbrell, L. A., O'Reilly, S., Burnell, M., Boxall, F. E., et al. (1989) Carboplatin dosage: prospective evaluation of a simple formula based on renal function. *J. Clin. Oncol.* **7,** 1748–1756.
40. Chatelut, E., Canal, P., Brunner, V., Chevreau, C., Pujol, A., Boneu, A., et al. (1995) Prediction of carboplatin clearance from standard morphological and biological characteristics. *J. Natl. Cancer Inst.* **87,** 573–580.
41. Du Bios, A., Vach, W., Siebert, C., Holy, R., Ledergerber, M., Wechsel, U., et al. (1997) The relationship between parameters of serotonin metabolism and emetogenic potential of platinum-based chemotherapy regimens. *Support Care Cancer* **5,** 212–218.
42. The Italian Group For Antiemetic Research (1995) Dexamethasone, granisetron or both for the prevention of nausea and vomiting during chemotherapy for cancer. *N. Engl. J. Med.* **332,** 1–5.
43. Extra, J. M., Marty, M., Brienza, S., and Misset, J. (1998) Pharmacokinetics and safety profile of oxaliplatin. *Semin. Oncol.* **25,** 13–22.
44. Levi, F., Zidani, R., and Misset, J. (1997) randomized multicentre trial of chronotherapy with oxaliplatin, fluorouracil and folinic acid in metastatic colorectal cancer. *Lancet* **350,** 681–686.
45. Misset, J. (1998) Oxaliplatin in practice. *Br. J. Cancer* **77,** 4–7.
46. Extra, J. M., Espie, M., Calvo, F., Ferme, C., Mignot, L., and Marty, M. (1990) Phase I study of oxaliplatin in patients with advanced cancer. *Cancer Chemother. Pharmacol.* **25,** 299–303.
47. Screnci, D., Er, H. M., Hambley, T. W., Galettis, P., Brouwer, P. and McKeage, M. J. (1997)

Stereo-selective peripheral sensory neurotoxicity of diaminocyclohexane platinum enantiomers related to ormaplatin and oxaliplatin. *Br. J. Cancer* , **76,** 502–510.

48. Caussanel, J., Levi, F., Brienza, S., Misset, J., Itzhaki, M., Adam, R., et al. (1990) Phase I trial of 5-d continuous venous infusion of oxaliplatin at circadian rhythm-modulated rate compared with constant rate. *J. Natl. Cancer Inst.* **82,** 1046–1050.
49. Gamelin, E., Le Boul, A., Boisdron-Celle, M., Turcant, A., Delva, A., Cailleux, A., et al. (1997) Cumulative pharmacokinetic study of oxaliplatin administered every three weeks combined with 5-fluorouracil in colorectal cancer patients. *Clin. Cancer Res.* **3,** 891–899.
50. Judson, I. R., Cerny, T., Epelbaum, R., Dunlop, D., Smyth, J., Schaefer, B., et al. (1997) Phase II trial of the oral platinum complex JM216 in non-small-cell lung cancer: an EORTC early clinical studies group investigation. *Ann. Oncol.* **8,** 604–606.
51. Fokkema, E., Lunenberg, J., Van Putten, J. W. G., Van Rijswijk, R. E. N., Weil, C., and Groen, H. J. M. (1998) Randomized phase II study of oral JM216 versus intravenous cisplatin in non-small cell lung cancer (NSCLC): preliminary results. *Proc. Am. Soc. Clin. Oncol.* **17,** 483 (abstract)
52. McKeage, M. J., Raynaud, F., Ward, J., Berry, C., O'Dell, D., Kelland, L. R., et al.(1997) Phase I and pharmacokinetic study of an oral platinum complex given daily for 5 d in patients with cancer. *J. Clin. Oncol.* **15,** 2691–2700.
53. Raynaud, F. I., Mistry, P., Donaghue, A., Poon, G., Kelland, L. R., Barnard, C. F. J., et al. (1996) Biotransformation of the platinum drug JM216 following oral administration to cancer patients. *Cancer Chemother. Pharmacol.* **38,** 155–162.

12 Toxicology and Regulatory Aspects of Platinum Drugs

Diana L. Clark, Paul A. Andrews, D. D. Smith, Joseph J. DeGeorge, Robert L. Justice, and Julie G. Beitz

CONTENTS

1. INTRODUCTION

The goals of preclinical toxicology studies for oncology drugs are (1) to identify a starting dose that is both safe and that minimizes the number of patients treated with ineffective doses, (2) to identify important potential clinical toxicities, and (3) to assist in the design of human dosing regimens and escalation schemes *(1)*. Toward these goals, studies are performed in animals to estimate the human maximally tolerated dose (MTD) and characterize drug-induced toxicities. Studies in both rodents and non-rodents to support Phase I trials have been expected by the U.S. Food and Drug Adminstration (FDA) since 1982 *(2,3)*. In contrast, since 1981 clinical trials conducted under the auspices of the Cancer Research Campaign and the European Organization for the Research and Treatment of Cancer have relied on preclinical testing in rodents only for oncology drugs *(4)*. The European Agency for the Evaluation of Medicinal Products has recently formalized this rodent-only approach as only acceptable for entry of cytotoxic oncology drugs with known mechansims of action into Phase I trials. For drugs with novel mechanisms of action, studies in rodents and non-rodents are currently expected *(5)*.

From: *Platinum-Based Drugs in Cancer Therapy*
Edited by: L. R. Kelland and N. Farrell © Humana Press Inc., Totowa, NJ

The success of the rodent-only approach for preclinical testing of anticancer drugs, including alkylating, tubulin-binding, DNA-binding, and antiendocrine agents, has been examined *(6,7)*. For these drugs, unacceptable toxicities were never encountered at the Phase I starting dose. Although the acceptance of rodent-only toxicology studies may have decreased the expense and time of the nonclinical development of an anticancer agent, for some drugs this approach may have led to extended development times in the Phase I setting *(6)*. Regarding the use of both rodents and non-rodents in preclinical testing of anticancer agents, as practiced in the United States, Grieshaber and Marsoni *(2)* have documented the success of this approach for seven drugs developed by the U.S. National Cancer Institute. More extensive analyses examining this approach have not been reported.

To examine the regulatory practices of the FDA, including the use of both rodents and non-rodents for preclinical testing of cancer drugs, we evaluated how well rodents (mice and rats) and non-rodents (dogs) estimated the starting dose, predicted human toxic doses, and predicted the spectrum of toxicities experienced by patients exposed to the platinum anticancer agents. Data for this analysis were garnered either from studies submitted to the FDA supporting investigational new drugs or from the biomedical literature *(8–19)*. Due to confidentiality restrictions, we are prevented from identifying the specific platinum analogs in this document. Only preclinical and clinical studies employing single-dose drug administration schedules are presented here. Eleven of the 12 drugs were administered intravenously, and the remaining drug was orally administered.

In this chapter, we report the following findings: (1) calculation of the starting dose based on 1/10 the rodent LD_{10} may be too conservative for platinum anticancer drugs, (2) either rodents or dogs may be used to predict safely the starting doses of platinum drugs in humans, and (3) rodents and dogs were equally accurate for predicting dose-limiting toxicities in humans.

2. DETERMINATION OF STARTING DOSES FROM PRECLINICAL TOXIC DOSES

The starting dose for first-in-human studies of anticancer agents in the United States is 1/10 the rodent LD_{10}, provided this dose is tolerated in a non-rodent, usually a dog *(1)*. If this dose is not tolerated in the non-rodent, then the starting dose is defined as one-sixth the non-rodent toxic dose high (TDH), which we define as the highest nonseverely toxic dose (HNSTD). Severe toxicities include convulsions, coma, bloody diarrhea, and death. This algorithm for determining the starting dose was examined in the context of both safety and trial efficiency. If a starting dose is too high, the first humans exposed to the agent would experience unacceptable toxicities. On the other hand, if a starting dose is too low, then an unacceptable number of escalation steps would be required before reaching the human MTD for the drug.

2.1. Sources of LD_{10}s, TDHs, and MTDs

In oncology drug development, the human MTD for a drug is believed to be estimated by that dose that causes lethality or severe toxicity in 10% of rodents (LD_{10}) or by the highest nonlethal dose in dogs (TDH). Therefore, the term MTD_{animal} refers to either a rodent LD_{10} or a dog TDH in this chapter. Not all 12 platinum anticancer agents examined had an LD_{10} determination from mice and rats and a TDH determination for dogs: 11 drugs had LD_{10} determinations in mice, 9 drugs had LD_{10}s defined in rats, and 9 drugs had TDH determinations in dogs. One drug was excluded from quantitative comparisons since Phase I trials were terminated before an accurate MTD was reached.

LD_{10}s in rodents were determined by probit analysis or, if insufficient data were available for a probit calculation, the LD_{10} was determined as that dose that actually caused 10% lethality in the animals. If an LD_{10} was not available by either of these approaches, then the LD_{10} was taken as the highest nonlethal dose.

All preclinical doses were normalized to body surface area (mg/m^2). Although there is evidence that dose normalization to body surface area may not be the most accurate for this drug class *(20)*, body surface area normalization is the convention for oncology drugs. LD_{10} values reported in mg/kg in mice and rats were multiplied by 3 and 6, respectively, and the dog TDH values were multiplied by 20 to convert from mg/kg to mg/m^2 *(21)*. The MTD values used in the analysis were defined and reported by the investigators and therefore may be above or equal to the recommended Phase II dose. When the preclinical or clinical studies provided equivocal results, final values were chosen while investigators were blinded to the corresponding animal or human value.

2.2. Starting Dose Safety

Applying the starting dose algorithm to the 12 platinum analogs would have provided a safe starting dose for every drug. One-tenth the rodent LD_{10} or one-sixth the dog TDH was significantly below the MTD for every drug. In no case would the MTD have been reached with this hypothetical starting dose.

2.3. Phase I Trial Efficiency

In addition to the safety of the starting dose, the efficiency of dose escalation trials must also be considered. An excess of dose escalations to reach the MTD causes many patients to be exposed to nontherapeutic doses, prolongs the trial, and is unnecessarily costly. For determining the efficiency of the Phase I trials, the average number of dose levels required to reach the MTD from the starting dose was calculated assuming a modified Fibonacci escalation scheme. The starting dose for this calculation was determined according to the process discussed above and may not reflect the actual starting dose. Likewise, the actual escalation scheme and the subsequent number of dose levels needed to reach the MTD, may have differed from this hypothetical model.

Table 1
Effect of Starting Dose on Theoretical Phase I Trial Efficiency[a]

	Fraction of LD_{10} or TDH[b]		
Animal	*1/10 or 1/6[c]*	*1/3*	*Difference*
Mouse	8.7 ± 1.8 (6–11)	4.7 ± 1.5 (3–7)	4.0
Rat	7.6 ± 1.9 (4–10)	3.7 ± 1.3 (2–6)	3.9
Most sensitive rodent	9.0 ± 1.5 (7–11)	4.8 ± 1.5 (3–7)	4.2
Dog	5.6 ± 1.7 (3–7)	3.3 ± 0.9 (2–4)	2.3

[a]Number of modified Fibonacci dose levels required to reach the MTD if the starting dose were determined from one-third the LD_{10} or TDH versus one-tenth the LD_{10} or one-sixth the TDH.
[b]Mean ± SE (range)
[c]One-tenth the rodent LD_{10} or one-sixth the non-rodent TDH.

Determining the starting dose from rodents would have required an average of 7.6–9.0 dose levels to reach the MTD; a starting dose determined from one-sixth of the TDH would have required an average of 5.6 dose levels to reach the MTD (Table 1). The data available suggest that an alternative model would have been acceptable for these 12 platinum anticancer agents. Selecting one-third of the LD_{10} for the most sensitive rodent species or one-third of the TDH for dogs (rather than 1/10 or 1/6, respectively) for the starting dose would have permitted both safe and efficient Phase I trials under a modified Fibonacci dose escalation scheme. Using one-third of the LD_{10} of the most sensitive rodent species for the starting dose would have allowed the MTD to be reached in an average of 4.2 fewer dose levels than if the starting dose was chosen using the conventional method of 1/10 the rodent LD_{10}. The higher starting dose would have still allowed a reasonable degree of safety since a minimum of two additional dose levels would have been evaluated prior to reaching the MTD. Similarly, using one-third of the dog TDH as the starting dose would have resulted in an average of 2.3 fewer dose levels to reach the MTD, compared with a starting dose of one-sixth the TDH.

Several approaches have been proposed to optimize the efficiency of Phase I testing of oncology drugs. Simon et al. *(22)* recently published an analysis that supported the use of a dose-doubling escalation scheme and single-patient cohorts to define the MTD more rapidly with fewer patients. The modified continual reassessment *(23)* and pharmacokinetically guided *(24,25)* dose escalation methods have also been proposed to "to escalate quickly" to the MTD. Alternatively, the time and patients needed to define the MTD could be minimized by simply beginning trials at higher doses *(26,27)*. The data for these platinum drugs show that starting doses could have been up to three times higher without compromising patient safety. It remains to be determined whether higher starting doses could be safely used for other oncology drug classes.

3. PREDICTIVE VALUE OF PRECLINICAL SPECIES

In addition to evaluating the starting doses determined by preclinical toxic doses, it is also useful to examine the accuracy of rodents or non-rodents in estimating the human MTD. This is a fundamental assumption in starting dose determinations, but we wish to examine explicitly the toxic dose levels reported in preclinical and clinical settings. In addition, we wish to examine whether preclinical studies also accurately forecast side effects or toxicities that are encountered when the drug is administered to humans.

3.1. Quantitative Evaluation of Toxic Dose Levels in Preclinical Species

To evaluate how well LD_{10}s and TDHs reported in experimental animals approximated human MTDs, we developed a measure of the predictive value and then applied this measure to platinum drugs for which both human MTD and estimated human MTD based on animal doses are known. Linear regressions, descriptive statistics, and hypothesis testing were calculated using SAS (SAS Institute, Cary, NC).

3.1.1. Relative Differences Between Preclinical LD_{10} or TDH and Clinical MTD

The relative differences of MTDs, which compare preclinical LD_{10}s or TDHs (MTD_{animal}) with actual MTDs (MTD_{human}), were determined for each drug and for each species. The formula for the relative differences is shown below:

$$\text{relative difference of MTD} = (MTD_{animal} - MTD_{human})/MTD_{human} \times 100$$

The sign of the relative difference indicates whether the preclinical results were greater than or less than the human MTD. A positive value indicates that the animal LD_{10} or TDH overpredicted the human MTD and, conversely, a negative value indicates that the animal data underpredicted the human MTD. A relative difference of zero implies that MTD_{animal} was equal to MTD_{human}.

In general, the animal MTDs underpredicted human MTDs for these platinum drugs (Fig. 1). All the relative differences were negative except for a single drug in the mouse, a single drug in the rat, and two drugs in the dog. One drug overpredicted the MTD (i.e., had a positive relative difference) in both the mouse and the dog, but the relative difference was negative for this drug in the rat. The drug that had the single positive relative difference in the rat had a negative relative difference in mice; relative difference data for this drug were not available in the dog.

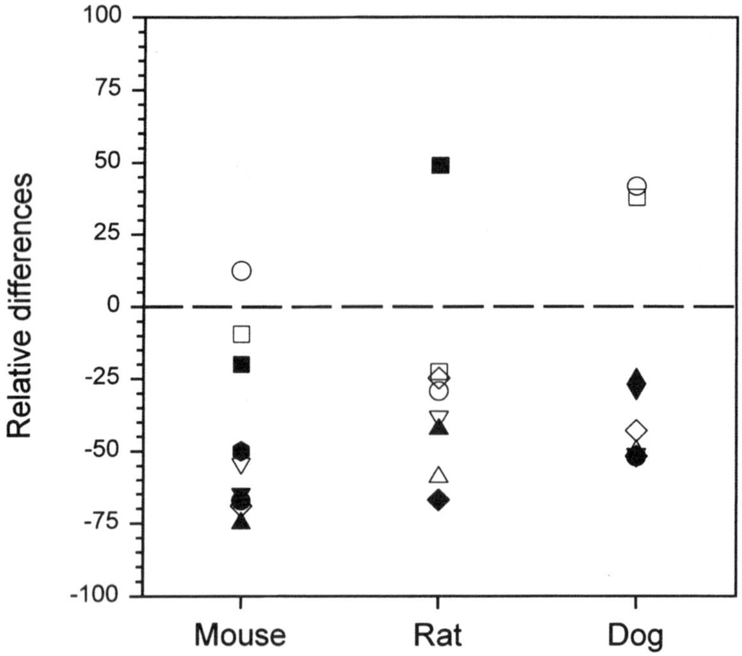

Fig. 1. Relative difference of human MTD from the MTD predicted by animals. The relative difference is defined as $(MTD_{animal} - MTD_{human}) / MTD_{human} \times 100$. All doses were expressed in mg/m^2 for platinum anticancer drugs administered on a single dose schedule. Each symbol corresponds to the same drug in all three species.

The mean relative differences ± SE for the mouse, rat, and dog were − 46.5 ± 9.5, − 29.2 ± 12.5, and − 32.4 ± 11.3, respectively. Based on these means of relative differences, MTD_{dog} and MTD_{rat} are each closer to zero and hence better predictors of MTD_{human} than MTD_{mouse}. However, there were no statistically significant differences between species with respect to the means of relative differences (ANOVA, $p = 0.36$). This implies that, when considering the mean relative differences, one species was not superior to the others in estimating the human MTD, rather all species generally underpredicted the human MTD for this drug class.

3.1.2. MTD Prediction Based on Preclinical LD_{10} or TDH

The relative difference measure examines the direct relationship between preclinical and clinical MTDs. However, it fails to describe the relationship of toxic dose levels between preclinical species and humans. For example, it does not address whether a meaningful correlation between mouse LD_{10}s and human MTDs exists other than relative comparisons between drugs. To address this, we performed a linear regression between the predicted human MTD de-

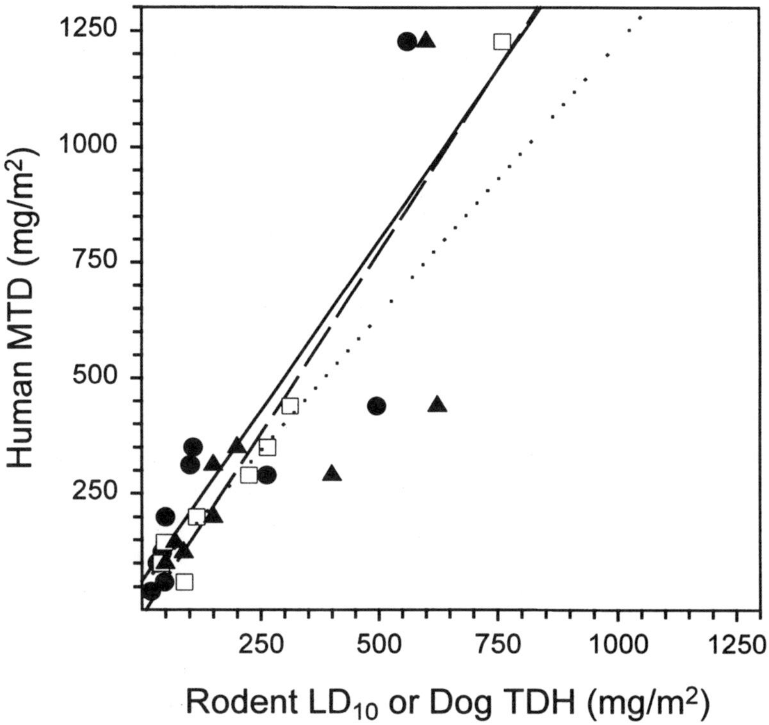

Fig. 2. Collective comparisons of animal estimates of the MTD with the actual MTD. All doses were expressed in mg/m^2. Linear regression lines were calculated and are included in the graph. Mouse (—, ●), Rat (— — —, □), Dog (•••••, ▲), most sensitive rodent (—••).

rived from each of the preclinical species (rodent LD_{10} or dog TDH) and the known human MTD. If there was a direct correspondence between the preclinical and clinical MTD, we would expect a slope of 1.0 and a *y*-intercept of 0.0 for the linear regression line. We tested whether there was a significant difference between the regression line and the line of unity (i.e., the line defined by $MTD_{human} = MTD_{animal}$ or $y = x$) using *F*-tests for the slope and intercept parameters using generalized linear modeling methodology. If an LD_{10} has a marked departure from the line of unity with respect to human MTD, this may imply that the LD_{10} does not necessarily have a one-to-one correspondence with human MTD, and therefore the ability of this preclinical species to predict human MTD may be questionable.

Plots of human MTD versus the rodent LD_{10} and dog TDH appear in Fig. 2, as well as the corresponding regression lines for each species. The most-sensitive rodent group was constructed by selecting the lowest LD_{10} in either mice or rats. Table 2 shows the slopes and intercepts of the regression lines, as well as their r^2 values. The *p*-values in Table 2 correspond to the hypothesis test of

Table 2
Linear Regression Results Between Preclinical Species and Humans (see Fig. 1)

Animal	*y-Intercept*	*Slope*	r^2	*p value of departure from y = x*
Mouse	60.7 ± 82.9	1.47 ± 0.32	0.722	0.165
Rat	−12.8 ± 31.8	1.57 ± 0.10	0.977	0.001
Most sensitive rodent	30.7 ± 44.7	1.90 ± 0.21	0.901	0.026
Dog	57.0 ± 126.2	1.26 ± 0.39	0.640	0.240

whether each regression line is statistically different from the line of unity. Any *p*-value less than 0.05 implies that the given regression line produces an improved fit over $y = x$. The results are described in the following subsections.

3.1.2.1. Rodents and Humans. The slopes of the regression line for all three rodent groups (mice, rats, and most-sensitive rodents) are approximately 1.5 or greater (Table 2). The regression line for rat LD_{10} and human MTD is a particularly good fit ($r^2 = 0.98$); however, the estimated regression line is statistically different from the line of unity ($y = x$; $p = 0.001$). Although LD_{10} values determined from rats composed the minority of points in the most-sensitive rodent data set, the linear regression line comparing most-sensitive rodent LD_{10}s with human MTDs is also statistically significantly different from $y = x$ ($p = 0.026$). This suggests that human MTDs are not necessarily directly scalable from LD_{10}s from rats or the most-sensitive species. In contrast to the rat and most-sensitive rodent groups, the regression line for the mouse does not differ statistically significantly from the line of unity. However, the regression fit for the mouse is worse than the rat and most-sensitive rodent group, as evidenced by the r^2 value.

3.1.2.2. Non-Rodents and Humans. Out of the four groups of preclinical toxic doses examined, dog TDHs generated the regression line that had the largest *p*-value ($p = 0.240$). This implies that it best approximated the human MTD. However, the r^2 value indicates that the regression line for dog TDH vs human MTD was also the most variable. Comparing all preclinical predictions for the human MTD, it appears from the limited data that the more robust the regression line is, the more likely it will diverge from $y = x$ in this analysis. Clearly, additional data are required to explore this more fully.

3.2. Qualitative Evaluation of Preclinical Species

In addition to predicting the human MTD and the appropriate starting dose for Phase I trials, preclinical studies may also forecast side effects or toxicities that will be encountered when the drug is administered to humans. Preclinical and clinical studies differ in their design and execution. First, there are no dose-limiting toxicities (DLTs) *per se* identified in animals, as it is often difficult to distinguish which of numerous toxic findings are the most deleterious to the animals. It follows that it is impossible to determine whether a dose-limiting toxicity in humans was predicted to be dose limiting from studies in animals. Instead, what is able to be determined is whether the toxicity was evident or not in preclinical studies. Nonetheless, as dose-limiting toxicities are of the most concern to the clinician, it is helpful to separate dose-limiting from non-dose-limiting toxicities in assessing the predictability of preclinical studies.

Second, studies of multiple cycles of drug administration are most often not performed in experimental animals. If a toxicity is cumulative and only evident after more than one cycle of drug exposure, then it will not be detected in single-dose studies in animals conducted for U.S. regulatory purposes. However, for the current analysis, whether the toxicity was evident in the first or a subsequent cycle of drug administration in humans was not taken into consideration.

For these platinum drugs, not every drug had preclinical studies that investigated end-organ toxicity in all three experimental species. Mouse end-organ toxicity data were available for 7 of the 12 drugs; rat end-organ toxicity findings were available for 10 drugs; and dog end-organ toxicity findings were reported for 11 drugs. Preclinical end-organ toxicity data in three experimental species were available for three drugs. Furthermore, the predictability of preclinical studies in animals can only be investigated when the toxicity has been reported in humans and a corresponding study performed in the preclinical species. Thus, the number of comparisons for which we are able to determine predictability is variable according to the particular toxicity. This is reflected in the variability of the denominator of the reported values in Tables 3 and 4. Conversely, false predictions of toxicities from preclinical studies can only be determined if the drug did not cause the toxicity in humans and a corresponding study was performed in the preclinical species. Unfortunately, the number of platinum drugs that have studies satisfying both of these criteria is rather small. Therefore, this analysis is intended to be descriptive rather than conclusive.

Included in our analysis are toxicities that were evident from clinical, laboratory, and histopathologic findings. The absence of a preclinical finding may have resulted from the design of the study rather than its true absence (e.g., serum chemistry was not measured, which might have detected renal toxicity). Additionally, this is a retrospective analysis. Non-reporting of a toxicity is not a guarantee that the toxicity was not observed. This is especially true for toxicities reported in humans. Very often, only grade 3 or 4 toxicities in clinical trials are published and discussed. More minor toxicities are not consistently reported, especially in a patient population with a terminal illness.

Toxicities observed in Phase I trials of platinum anticancer drugs were predominantly hematologic, gastrointestinal, renal, or neurologic in origin. DLTs for the platinum anticancer drug class were limited to myelosuppression (nine

Table 3
Number of Drugs in Which the Dose-Limiting Toxicities Encountered in Phase I Trials of Platinum Anticancer Drugs Were Predicted from Preclinical Studies[a]

	Correctly predicted by			
Dose-limiting toxicity	*Mice*	*Rats*	*Rodents*	*Dogs*
Hematologic	6/6	5/5	11/11	7/8
Renal	0/0	1/1	1/1	1/1
Neurologic	1/1	1/2	2/3	1/2
Total	7/7	7/8	14/15	9/11

[a]The denominator equals the number of drugs in which the toxicity was reported in clinical studies and corresponding preclinical studies were performed.

drugs), neurologic toxicities (two drugs), and damage to the kidney (one drug). Whereas gastrointestinal distress was often a serious toxicity in humans for this drug class, the use of antiemetics and hydration of the patients enabled investigators to prevent gastrointestinal toxicities from becoming dose limiting.

3.2.1. Toxicities Predicted by Preclinical Species

Importantly, the DLT (either myelosuppression, nephrotoxicity, or neurotoxicity) in this class of drugs was predicted preclinically in most of the corresponding preclinical studies. Human DLTs were observed in 100% (7/7) of the relevant mouse studies, 87% (7/8) of the relevant rat studies (14/15 of the rodent studies combined), and 82% (9/11) of the relevant dog studies (Table 3). We compared the total number of DLTs correctly predicted by rodent studies vs the total number of DLTs correctly predicted by dog studies using Fisher's exact test. The p-value for this test was 0.556, and this implies that there is no difference between rodent and dog studies with respect to predicting DLTs correctly.

Every platinum anticancer drug caused myelosuppression when administered to patients; however, the myelosuppression was not always dose limiting. Every drug caused leukopenia in humans, 11/12 drugs caused thrombocytopenia, and 4/12 drugs also caused anemia. Among those animals that exhibited hematologic toxicity, a similar distribution of myelosuppression was reported. Overall, rodents (mouse and rat combined) predicted hematologic toxicity (whether dose limiting or not) in 13/15 (87%) of the corresponding human studies, and dogs predicted myelosuppression in 9/11 (82%) analogous studies in humans (Table 4).

It is difficult to compare nephrotoxicity between animals and humans for this class of drugs since patients often received prophylactic measures to prevent nephrotoxicity (e.g., hydration and/or forced diuresis), whereas experimental animals did not. Nephrotoxicity in humans, usually evidenced by

Table 4
Number of Drugs in Which the Toxicities (Dose-Limiting or Non-Dose-Limiting) Encountered in Phase I Trials of Platinum Anticancer Drugs Were Correctly Predicted by Preclinical Studies[a]

Toxicity (non-DLT and DLT	*Mouse*	*Rat*	*Rodent*	*Dog*
Hematologic	6/7	7/8	13/15	9/11
Renal	0/0	2/2	2/2	3/3
Neurologic	1/1	3/4	4/5	1/5
Gastrointestinal	3/7	5/8	8/15	9/11

[a]The denominator equals the number of drugs in which the toxicity was reported in clinical studies and corresponding preclinical studies were performed.

increased blood urea nitrogen or decreased creatinine clearance, was reported for three drugs. Two of the human nephrotoxic drugs had toxicity studies performed in rats, and renal damage was observed with both of them. All drugs causing human nephrotoxicity were also nephrotoxic to dogs. There were no studies in mice that assessed kidney damage for the three human nephrotoxic drugs.

Although difficult to detect and interpret in the oncology drug development setting, neurotoxicity with platinum drugs was often predicted by the animal studies. Neurotoxicity was detected in Phase I trials of five drugs as evidenced by parasthesia, myalgia, or coma. Investigations in rats were performed with four of these five neurotoxic drugs. For three of these drugs, rats exhibited neurotoxicity (e.g., ptosis, ataxia, tremor, or coma). Toxicology studies in both mice and rats were performed with only one of the neurotoxic drugs. Ptosis, trembling, or seizures were observed in the mice, but not in the rats for this drug. The dog appeared to be less susceptible to measurable neurotoxicity: only one of the five drugs caused neurotoxicity (e.g., tremor, ataxia).

Every platinum anticancer drug also caused gastrointestinal toxicities (nausea and vomiting) in patients. As mentioned previously, this was not a DLT, due to coadministration of antiemetics. Rodents (8/15; 53%) manifested gastrointestinal distress as diarrhea, and dogs exhibited either vomiting or diarrhea in 9/11 (82%) of the studies.

3.2.2. Incorrect Toxicity Predictions

Another way to assess the predictive value of preclinical studies is to determine the rate of false predictions, that is, when a toxicity is apparent in the preclinical setting but not evident in humans exposed to the same drug. Four drugs caused elevated liver enzymes in dogs (Table 5). One of these drugs also caused hepatotoxicity in rats. However, no liver toxicity has been reported in the

Table 5
Number of Drugs in Which the Toxicity Was Reported Preclinically, but Not Reported Clinically[a]

	No. of drugs in which the toxicity was reported in humans	*No. of drugs in which the toxicity was reported in preclinical species but not in humans[a]*			
		Mouse	*Rat*	*Rodent*	*Dog*
Hematologic	12/12	0/0	0/0	0/0	0/0
Gastrointestinal	12/12	0/0	0/0	0/0	0/0
Renal	3/12	1/7	4/6	5/13	5/8
Hepatic	0/12	0/7	1/8	1/15	4/11
Neurologic	5/12	0/6	0/4	0/10	0/6
Pulmonary	0/12	1/7	2/8	3/15	1/11
Dermal	1/12	1/7	2/7	3/14	1/10
Cardiac	0/12	0/7	0/8	0/15	1/11

[a]The denominators equal the number of preclinical studies performed only for those drugs in which the toxicity was *not* observed in humans

Phase I setting with these platinum analogs, despite being reported in both a rodent and a non-rodent. Rats and dogs also suffered renal toxicity from four and five, drugs respectively; two of the four drugs caused kidney damage in both rats and dogs. One drug caused renal damage in all three experimental species (mice, rats, and dogs). Nephrotoxicity was not reported in Phase I trials for any of these drugs. However, patients were most often pretreated to prevent nephrotoxicity, so it is difficult to interpret these observations.

Although pulmonary toxicity was never reported in humans during a Phase I trial, pulmonary edema and hemorrhage were reported in mice and dogs for one drug, and dyspnea was reported in the rat for two additional drugs. Only one preclinical study suggested cardiotoxicity from platinating agents: dogs exhibited bradycardia with one drug, although no cardiotoxicity has been reported in patients. The presence of a toxicity in both a rodent and a non-rodent did not necessarily increase the likelihood that the toxicity would be experienced by patients in a Phase I trial.

3.3. Summary

There was no statistically significant difference among the preclinical species in the relative difference for the preclinical estimate of the MTD and the actual MTD. This implies that one species was not superior to the others in estimating the human MTD, rather all species generally underpredicted the MTD. This is consistent with the findings from the starting dose evaluation. Moreover, the starting dose is determined from the LD_{10} or TDH values, and we determined that 1/10 of the LD_{10} or 1/6 of the TDH allowed a safe starting dose, yet one that would have required several dose escalations to reach the MTD for some platinum anticancer drugs.

Comparing the collective ability of preclinical species to predict the human MTD, the regression line generated with dog TDH values more closely approximated the line of unity than the lines generated with mice, rats, or most-sensitive rodent LD_{10} values. This implies that there is a direct correspondence between dog TDH and clinical MTD values. However, the regression coefficient for this line was notably smaller than the regression coefficient for rodents. In fact, it appears from the limited data that the more robust the regression line is that compares preclinical LD_{10} or TDH values with human MTDs, the more likely it will diverge from $y = x$. More data are required to test this hypothesis.

When comparing toxic doses between species, another factor to consider is whether the exposures [areas under the curve (AUCs)] at the preclinical and clinical MTDs were equivalent for these drugs. Perhaps, if AUCs at toxic doses rather than the toxic doses themselves were compared between species (as in Fig. 1), a different pattern of accuracy might have been observed, as Collins et al. *(28)* has reported for three platinum anticancer agents. Such an analysis was precluded for the entire dataset, however, since plasma levels of ultrafilterable platinum were not available in more than one species for most of these drugs.

There was no obvious difference between species in the accuracy of the prediction of human toxicities in response to platinum anticancer drugs. Hematologic and gastrointestinal toxicities were observed preclinically and clinically for most drugs; however, there were few opportunities to evaluate the ability of preclinical species to predict neurologic and renal toxicities in humans. Additionally, there was no obvious difference between the rate of false predictions when comparing one species with another.

4. CONCORDANCE BETWEEN PRECLINICAL SPECIES

Although the extrapolation of doses in preclinical species to human doses is an important consideration, it is also useful to measure the consistency of preclinical species. Specifically, we wish to examine whether there is consistency in the information provided by mice and rats and whether there is a difference in the information provided by rodents and non-rodents. In this section, we discuss this question in both a quantitative and qualitative sense.

4.1. Quantitative Evaluation Between Preclinical Species

The regulatory practice of requesting toxicologic assessments in a second species is based on the supposition that the second species, whether a rodent or a non-rodent, may provide findings alternative to those of the first species.

We refer the reader to Section 3.1., in which we introduced measures to examine the predictive value of preclinical species. We apply the same methodology in this section, but in this setting, we relate preclinical species to each other instead of relating each preclinical species to humans. Performing an ANOVA to compare the mean of the relative differences for these groups, however, is not particularly instructive since there is no meaningful interpretation of the hypothesis that the means are equal among our set of pairwise groupings. It is more instructive to consider the relative differences separately for each set of species.

4.1.1. Relative Differences Between Preclinical LD_{10} and TDH

We used relative difference to measure the agreement between rodent LD_{10}s or between rodent LD_{10}s and dog TDHs. The four comparisons that we examined were mouse vs rat, mouse vs dog, rat vs dog, and most-sensitive rodent vs dog. When comparing mice vs rats, we calculated:

$$\text{relative difference} = (LD_{10,\,mouse} - LD_{10,\,rat})/LD_{10,\,rat} \times 100.$$

When comparing any rodent group vs. dogs the relative difference was given by $(LD_{10,\,rodent} - TDH)/TDH \times 100$. Figure 3 shows the relative differences among these four species combinations. For mice vs rats, six of the eight drugs have mouse LD_{10}s ranging from 41 to 80% of the rat LD_{10}. The mean relative difference ± SE in this case was -20.3 ± 14.2. When we consider the three rodent vs dog comparisons using relative differences, we see that only two drugs in rat had larger LD_{10}s than the TDH in the dog. In all other cases, the TDH value was higher than the corresponding rodent LD_{10}. This implies that dogs were generally less sensitive than rodents in this set of platinum anticancer drugs.

4.1.2. LD_{10} or TDH Prediction Based on Single Rodent LD_{10}

Plots of rat vs mouse LD_{10} and dog TDH vs mouse, rat, or most-sensitive rodent LD_{10} appear in Fig. 4, as well as the corresponding regression lines. We again consider regression as a method of quantifying the relationships between preclinical species. In this setting, our regression models use LD_{10} from the smaller species to predict the LD_{10} or TDH of the larger species. Table 6 shows the slopes and intercepts of the regression lines, as well as their r^2 values. The p-value column in Table 6 corresponds to the hypothesis test of whether each regression line is statistically different from the line of unity. The interpretation of these hypothesis tests and their corresponding p-values is the same as in Section 3.1.2.

4.1.2.1. Comparability Between Rodents. Eight of the 12 platinum anticancer drugs had LD_{10} determinations in both mice and rats. The linear regression line comparing the LD_{10}s was not significantly different than the line of unity ($p = 0.083$), and therefore we may conclude that there is a general one-to-one agreement in LD_{10} doses between rodents. This would imply that performing a toxicologic assessment in a second rodent may not yield any additional useful information for regulatory purposes.

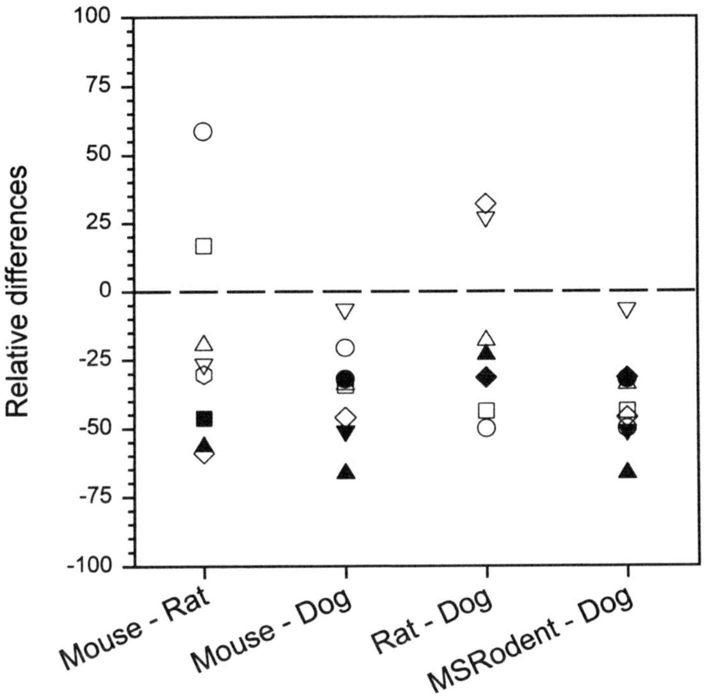

Fig. 3. Relative difference of preclinical "MTDs". After normalization of the doses to mg/m^2, the LD_{10}s between mice and rats and the rodent (mouse, rat, and most-sensitive rodent) LD_{10}s with the dog TDH were compared for the same drug. Each symbol corresponds to the same drug in all species.

4.1.2.2. Comparability Between Rodents and Non-Rodents. The results of the dog TDH vs three rodent LD_{10} regressions appear in Table 6. The regression of dog vs mouse resulted in the slope closest to 1.0, but the *p*-value to test divergence from $y = x$ was significant at $p = 0.002$. This is largely because the intercept of this regression was statistically different from zero. This implies that there is an agreement between the findings in mice and dogs, but this agreement does not follow the model TDH = $LD_{10,\ mouse}$.

In contrast, there was no statistically significant departure from $y = x$ with the dog TDH vs rat LD_{10} regression ($p = 0.23$). The regression slope was less than 1.0 for this comparison, which implies that dogs are more sensitive than rats to platinum anticancer agents. However, only two drugs had positive relative differences when comparing rat LD_{10}s and dog TDHs (Fig. 3), and so the influence of these two drugs forced the regression slope to be less than 1.0. It should also be noted that the dose of one of these two drugs was greater than 600 mg/m^2 for both species, which is substantially larger than the five drugs with negative relative differences.

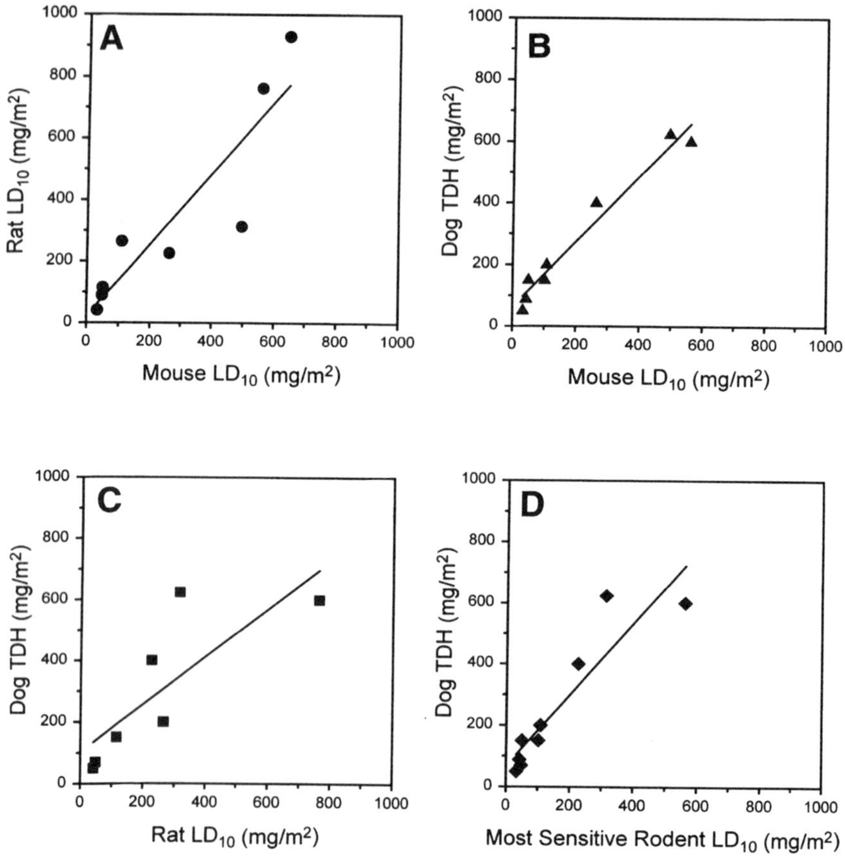

Fig. 4. Linear regression of preclinical "MTDs" comparing mouse and rat **(A),** mouse and dog **(B),** rat and dog **(C),** and most-sensitive rodent and dog **(D)** after doses were normalized to mg/m^2.

In the case of most-sensitive rodent vs dog, the slope of the regression line reflected the tendency of dogs to be less sensitive than rodents (Fig. 3). The p-value for divergence from $y = x$ approached statistical significance ($p = 0.061$). This is consistent with the large difference between most-sensitive rodent and dog slopes when using each species to predict human MTD (Table 2).

4.2. Concordance of Toxicities Between Preclinical Species

Determining the agreement of toxicity manifestations between preclinical species is difficult due to the small number of directly comparable preclinical studies performed with these drugs. Eleven of the 12 drugs had toxicity assessments performed in either mice or rats. In only four drugs were end-organ toxicities examined in both mice and rats. Despite the small number of com-

Table 6
Linear Regression Results Between Preclinical Species (see Fig. 4)

Animals	*y-Intercept*	*Slope*	r^2	*p value for departure from y = x*
Rats vs mice	24.0 ± 82.0	1.15 ± 0.22	0.815	0.083
Dogs vs mice	57.7 ± 22.1	1.05 ± 0.07	0.974	0.002
Dogs vs rats	78.7 ± 97.4	0.79 ± 0.27	0.678	0.234
Dogs vs most-sensitive rodent	60.8 ± 47.6	1.15 ± 0.20	0.843	0.061

parisons possible, the greatest concordance between studies in mice and rats was with hematologic toxicities (Table 7). Only one drug was consistent in producing nephrotoxicity or gastrointestinal toxicity in both rodents. Ten drugs were examined in dogs plus a rodent (mouse or rat). Combining the findings in mice and rats and comparing the toxicities reported in rodents with toxicities reported in non-rodents, the greatest concordance was also with hematologic toxicities.

4.3. Summary

When we compared rodent LD_{10} with non-rodent TDH values, we found that the rodent LD_{10} value was almost always lower than the TDH value for the same drug. However, mouse or rat LD_{10} values were not statistically different from dog TDH values when collectively examined via linear regression. Qualitatively, there are insufficient data to determine the likelihood of observing a toxicity due to platinum anticancer drugs in one species if the toxicity was observed in another preclinical species. Generally, with the small number of cases that we are able to compare, the agreement between preclinical species was not great for nonhematologic toxicities.

5. CONCLUSIONS AND REGULATORY CONSEQUENCES

To determine the value of rodent and non-rodent toxicology studies in oncology drug development, we retrospectively examined submissions to the FDA and reports in the biomedical literature. By comparing quantitative and qualitative findings between experimental species and humans, we evaluated the current regulatory practices at the FDA. Specifically, we examined more closely the algorithm for choosing a starting dose and toxicologic evaluations in both a rodent and a non-rodent prior to initiating trials in humans. We chose the platinum anticancer agents as the initial drug class to examine. In summary, we conclude that safe and efficient starting doses could have been obtained by

Table 7
Number of Drugs in Which Toxicities Were Observed in Both Mice and Rats or in Both Rodents and Dogs[a]

Toxicity	*Mouse and rat*	*Rodent and dog*
Hematologic	3/4	7/10
Renal	1/4	4/8
Neurologic	0/1	1/4
Gastrointestinal	1/3	5/9

[a]The denominator equals the number of drugs in which a toxicity was observed in one species of the pair and a toxicity assessment was performed in the alternate species.

using larger fractions, such as one-third rather than 1/10, of the rodent LD_{10} or dog TDH for these platinum anticancer drugs. Additionally, similar information was available from preclinical toxicologic studies conducted in rodents and non-rodents. From the data we examined, there was no obviously superior preclinical species for estimating the clinical MTD or predicting toxicities in humans exposed to these platinum anticancer drugs. Between preclinical species, rodent LD_{10} values were generally lower than dog TDH values. There were limited data to evaluate the agreement between species with regard to toxicities, but generally, the concordance between preclinical species for non-hematologic toxicities was not particularly striking.

Based on these findings, it is not apparent that toxicologic studies in dogs provide additional information to that obtained from toxicologic characterizations in rodents. We therefore encourage potential sponsors of new platinum analogs to discuss with the Division of Oncology Drug Products within the FDA rodent-only toxicology testing prior to submitting an IND to the Agency. Considerations for proceeding with rodent-only toxicology would include (1) the structural similarity of the novel platinum agent with those agents that were examined in this analysis, (2) the spectrum of toxicities that were observed in those preclinical studies that were performed, and (3) any other relevant preclinical findings.

ACKNOWLEDGMENTS

We wish to acknowledge that data for these analyses were supplied by ASTA Medica (Hackensack, NJ), Bristol-Myers Squibb (Wallingford, CT), Lederle Laboratories (Philadelphia, PA), National Cancer Institute (Bethesda, MD), Parke-Davis Pharmaceutical Research Division (Ann Arbor, MI), Dr. Roman Perez-Soler (Houston, TX), and Sanofi Pharmaceuticals (Malvern, PA). We thank these sponsors for their gracious permission to publish their data in this format. We also thank Gary Gensinger for designing the database used to store the collected information. **Note:** This article is not an official Food and Drug Administration (FDA) guidance or policy statement. No official support or endorsement by the FDA is intended or should be inferred.

REFERENCES

1. DeGeorge, J. J., Ahn, C. -H., Andrews, P. A., Brower, M. E., Giorgio, D. W., Goheer, M. A., et al. (1998) Regulatory considerations for preclinical development of anticancer drugs. *Cancer Chemother. Pharmacol.* **41,** 173–185.
2. Grieshaber, C. K. and Marsoni, S. (1986) Relation of preclinical toxicology to findings in early clinical trials. *Cancer Treat. Rep.* **70,** 65–72.
3. Lowe, M. C. and Davis, R. D. (1984) The current toxicology protocol of the National Cancer Institute, in *Fundamentals of Cancer Chemotherapy* (Helmann, K. and Carter, S. K. eds.), McGraw-Hill, New York, pp. 228–235.
4. Burtles, S. S., Newell, D. R., Henrar, R., and Connors, T. A. (1995) Revisions of general guidelines for the preclinical toxicology of new cytotoxic anticancer agents in Europe. *Eur. J. Cancer* **31A,** 408–410.
5. European Agency for the Evaluation of Medicinal Products (1998) Note for guidance on the pre-clinical evaulation of anticancer medicinal products. *CPMP/SWP/997/96*, London.
6. Connors, T. A. and Pinedo, H. M. (1997) Drug development in Europe, in *Anticancer Drug Development Guide: Preclinical Screening, Clinical Trials and Approval* (Teicher, B. A., ed.), Humana, Totowa, NJ, pp. 271–288.
7. Burtles, S. S., Jodrell, D. I., and Newell, D. R. (1998) Evaluation of "rodent-only" preclinical toxicology for Phase I trials of new cancer treatments—the Cancer Research Campaign (CRC) experience. *Proc. Am. Assoc. Cancer Res.* **39,** 363.
8. Koeller, J. M., Trump, D. L., Tutsch, K. D., Earhart, R. H., Davis, T. E., and Tormey, D. C. (1986) Phase I clinical trial and pharmacokinetics of carboplatin (NSC 241240) by single monthly 30-minute infusion. *Cancer* **57,** 222–225.
9. Theriault, R. L., Cohen, I. A., Esparza, L., Kowal, C., and Raber, M. N. (1993) Phase I clinical evaluation of [SP-4–3(R)]-[1,1-cyclo-butanedicarboxylato(2-)](2-methyl-1,4-butanediamine-N,N) platinum in patients with metastic solid tumors. *Cancer Chemother. Pharmacol.* **31,** 333–337.
10. DeConti, R. C., Toftness, B. R., Lange, R. C., and Creasey, W. A. (1973) Clinical and pharmacological studies with cis-diamminedichloroplatinum(II). *Cancer Res.* **33,** 1310–1315.
11. Ceulemans, F., Trouet, A., Duprez, P., Vindevogel, A., Alaerts, P., Hammershaimb, L., et al. (1989) Phase I study of a new water soluble platinum containing antitumor agent CL 287,110 (CL) in advanced cancer patients (pts.). *Proc. Am. Assoc. Cancer Res.* **30,** 283.
12. Creaven, P. J., Madajewicz, S., Pendyala, L., Mittelman, A., Pontes, E., Spaulding, M., et al. (1983) Phase I clinical trial of cis-dichloro-trans-dihydroxy-bis-isopropylamine platinum (IV) (CHIP). *Cancer Treat. Rep.* **67,** 795–800.
13. McKeage, M. J., Mistry, P., Ward, J., Boxall, F. E., Loh, S., O'Neill, C., et al. (1995) A phase I and pharmacology study of an oral platinum complex, JM216: dose-dependent pharmacokinetics with single-dose administration. *Cancer Chemother. Pharmacol.* **36,** 451–458.
14. Perez-Soler, R., Lopez-Berestein, G., Lautersztain, J., Al-Baker, S., Francis, K., Macias-Kiger, D., et al. (1990) Phase I clinical and pharmacological study of liposome-entrapped cis-bis-neodecanoato-*trans*-R,R-1,2-diaminocyclohexane platinum (II). *Cancer Res.* **50,** 4254–4259.
15. Fiebig, H. H., Moss, K., Henss, H., Ludolph, D., Meyberg, F., Aulenbacher, P., et al. (1994) Phase I clinical trial of lobaplatin (D-19466) after intravenous bolus injection. *Onkologie* **17,** 142–148.
16. Extra, J. M., Espie, M., Calvo, F., Ferme, C., Mignot, L., and Marty, M. (1990) Phase I study

of oxaliplatin in patients with advanced cancer. *Cancer Chemother. Pharmacol.* **25,** 299–303.
17. Tanis, B. C., Vermorken, J. B., Ten Bokkel Huinink, W. W., Klein, I., Gall, H. E., van Oosterom, A. T., et al. (1991) Phase I study of spiroplatin. *Eur. J. Cancer* **27,** 268–273.
18. O'Rourke, T. J., Weiss, G. R., New, P., Burris, H. A., Rodriguez, G., Eckhardt, J., et al. (1994) Phase I clinical trial of ormaplatin (tetraplatin, NSC 363812). *Anti-Cancer Drugs* **5,** 520–526.
19. Dodion, P. F., de Valeriola, D., Crespeigne, N., Kantrowitz, J. D., Piccart, M., Wery, F., et al. (1991) Phase I clinical and pharmacokinetic study of zeniplatin, a new platinum complex. *Ann. Oncol.* **2,** 589–596.
20. Clark, D. L., Andrews, P. A., DeGeorge, J. J., Justice, R. L., and Beitz, J. G. (1998) Extrapolating starting doses using $mg/kg^{0.77}$ instead of mg/m^2 would have allowed more efficient Phase I trials for platinum anticancer drugs. *Proc. Am. Assoc. Cancer Res.* **39,** 363.
21. Freireich, E. J., Gehan, E. A., Rall, D. P., Schmidt, L. H., and Skipper, H. E. (1966) Quantitative comparison of toxicity of anticancer agents in mouse, rat, hamster, dog, monkey and man. *Cancer Chemother. Rep.* **50,** 219–244.
22. Simon, R., Freidlin, B., Rubinstein, L., Arbuck, S. G., Collins, J., and Christian, M. C. (1997) Accelerated titration designs for Phase I clinical trials in oncology. *J. Natl Cancer Inst.* **89,** 1138–1147.
23. Faries, D. (1994) Practical modifications of the continual reassessment method for phase I cancer clinical trials. *J. Biopharm. Stat.* **4,** 147–164.
24. Collins, J., Zaharko, D. S., Dedrick, R. L., and Chabner, B. A. (1986) Potential roles for preclinical pharmacology in phase I clinical trials. *Cancer Treat. Rep.* **70,** 73–80.
25. EORTC Pharmacokinetics and Metabolism Group (1987) Pharmacokinetically guided dose escalation in phase I clinical trials. Commentary and proposed guidelines. *Eur. J. Cancer Clin. Oncol.* **23,** 1083–1087.
26. Mani, S. and Ratain, M. (1997) New phase I trial methodology. *Semin. Oncol.* **24,** 253–261.
27. Verweij, J. (1996) Starting dose levels for phase I studies. *Ann. Oncol.* **7,** 13–18.
28. Collins, J., Grieshaber, C. K., and Chabner, B. A. (1990) Pharmacologically guided phase I clincial trials based upon preclinical drug development. *J. Natl Cancer Inst.* **82,** 1321–1326.

IV NEW PLATINUM DRUGS OF THE FUTURE

13 New Platinum Drugs

The Pathway to Oral Therapy

Lloyd R. Kelland

Contents

1. INTRODUCTION

Around 120 years elapsed between the original chemical identification of Peyrone's chloride [*cis*-diamminedichloroplatinum(II), now known as cisplatin] and the realization of its potent anticancer properties in the late 1960s and introduction into clinical oncology in the early 1970s. Since then, there has been an explosion of activity aimed at optimizing the antitumor potential of this class of inorganic coordination complex. Many hundreds of cisplatin analogs have been described, concentrating on two broad themes: (1) attempts to reduce the severe side effects of the parent drug (namely, nephrotoxicity, nausea and vomiting, and neurotoxicity); and (2) attempts to find agents active against cisplatin-resistant tumors.

Shortly after the early clinical trials with cisplatin, a collaborative research program was established between the Drug Development Section of the Institute of Cancer Research (ICR; Sutton, UK) and the Johnson Matthey Company (JM). The initial aim of this collaboration was to discover a less toxic but equally efficacious platinum analog. The resulting lead compound was *cis*-diammine, 1,1-cyclobutane dicarboxylato platinum (II), carboplatin, Paraplatin®, marketed by Bristol Myers Squibb *(1)*. Carboplatin entered clinical trial at the Royal Marsden Hospital, London, in 1981 and has been shown,

From: *Platinum-Based Drugs in Cancer Therapy*
Edited by: L. R. Kelland and N. Farrell © Humana Press Inc., Totowa, NJ

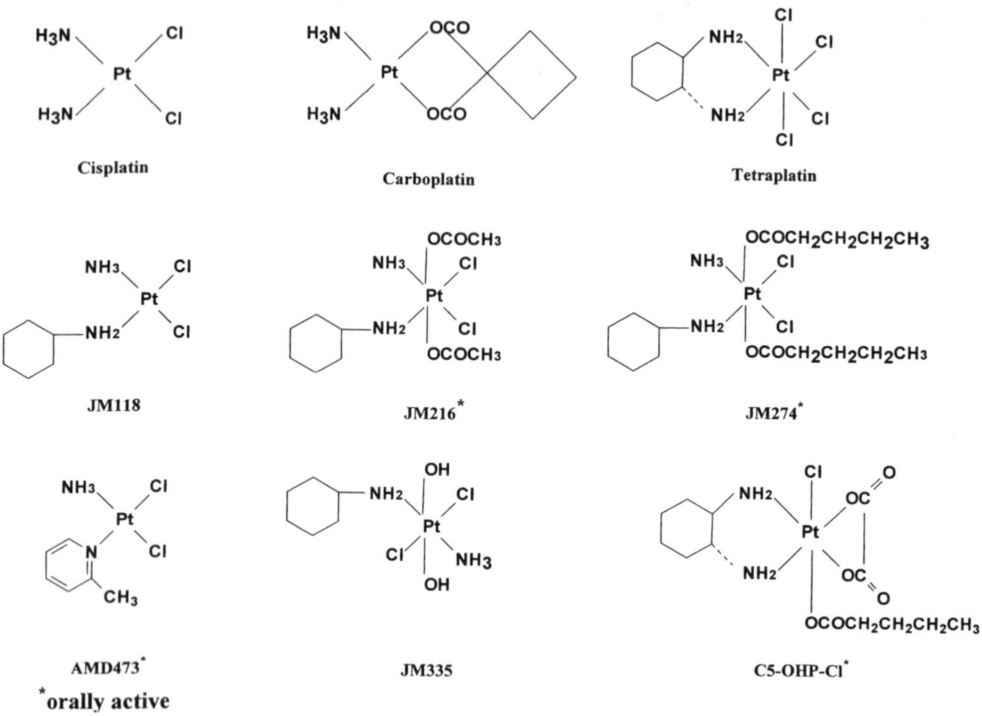

Fig. 1. Chemical structures of cisplatin, carboplatin, and tetraplatin; JM compounds 118, 216, 274, 473 and 335; and orally active compounds JM-216, -274, AMD473, and C5-OHP-Cl.

at least in most tumor types, to fulfil the above-mentioned desired criteria (myelosuppression is the dose-limiting toxicity). Carboplatin remains the only cisplatin analog to be widely registered. Indeed, in the United States, it has now essentially replaced cisplatin as front-line therapy for many tumor types. In 1991, the Drug Development Section of the ICR, JM, and the Royal Marsden Hospital were jointly awarded the Queen's Award for Technological Achievement for the development of carboplatin.

This chapter describes platinum drug development from the ICR/JM collaboration perspective, post carboplatin. Initially, the major focus of research concerned the discovery of orally administerable platinum complexes. Arising from the collaboration, the first orally active platinum compound to enter clinical trial, JM216 [*bis*-acetato ammine dichloro(cyclohexylamine) platinum(IV)], entered the clinic in 1992. Post JM216, the focus has been on agents that circumvent cisplatin resistance. The first "lead" compound was JM335 [*trans*-ammine (cyclohexylamine) dichlorodihydroxo platinum(IV)], and the second was JM473 [AMD473, ZD0473, *cis*-amminedichloro(2-methylpyridine) platinum(II)],

which entered a phase I clinical trial in 1997. The preclinical chemical, biologic, pharmacologic, and, where applicable, clinical properties of these three "JM" compounds are described (see Fig. 1 for structures).

2. 1983–1992: CARBOPLATIN TO JM216, THE FIRST ORAL PLATINUM

The success of the less toxic cisplatin analog, carboplatin, provided early testimony to the importance of addressing patient quality of life in the chemotherapy of cancer. This is particularly the case with palliative therapy and in permitting combinations with other cytotoxics. Both cisplatin and carboplatin are administered by intravenous infusion; some patients have a "fear of the needle." Therefore, the idea of developing an orally available platinum drug with "carboplatin-like" side effects emerged shortly after the introduction of carboplatin itself into Phase I. Preclinical studies began by determining the antitumor properties of "standard" platinum drugs of the time, cisplatin, carboplatin, and CHIP [*cis*-dichloro-*trans*-dihydroxy-*bis*-(isopropylamine) platinum(IV)] in mice bearing the subcutaneous (sc) murine ADJ/PC6 plasmacytoma *(2)*. This tumor had been widely used in defining the structure-activity rules for platinum analogs *(3)*, including in the discoveries of carboplatin and CHIP, and was widely believed to predict well for clinical activity *(4)*.

Although antitumor activity by the oral route can be demonstrated for cisplatin and carboplatin in mice bearing ADJ/PC6 *(2)* (Table 1), the low level of absorption makes this impractical in patients. This is illustrated (Table 1) by the reduction in therapeutic index [TI; the ratio of the median lethal dose, (LD_{50}), and the dose causing a 90% reduction in tumor mass (ED_{90})] when these drugs are administered orally compared with intraperitoneally (ip). Cisplatin and carboplatin are both less toxic *and* less active when given orally with their therapeutic indices being lower. Carboplatin possesses a greater aqueous solubility than cisplatin, which, although desirable for an intravenously administered drug of lower potency, the resulting low organic/aqueous partition coefficients are far from ideal for oral absorption. Indeed, oral bioavailability studies in mice indicated values of only 11–15% for carboplatin, with the major part (60–80%) of the dose excreted in the feces *(2)*. Nevertheless, a pilot clinical trial of oral carboplatin in two patients (with drug made up in lemonade syrup) was conducted in the Netherlands and reported in 1989 *(5)*. Confirming the mouse studies, poor absorption with a bioavailability of only 4–5% (and severe gastrointestinal toxicity) was observed.

Thus, it became clear that, to achieve clinically useful oral bioavailability with a platinum complex, novel chemistry was required. During the remainder of the 1980s, the collaborative studies between ICR and JM concentrated on preclinical studies (again largely using the ADJ/PC6 tumor) with a variety of asymmetric platinum (II) and (IV) complexes, the so-called mixed amines. Primarily, these

Table 1
Oral vs Intraperitoneal Antitumor Activity: ADJ/PC6 Murine Plasmacytoma

	Oral			*Intraperitoneal*		
Compound	*LD_{50} (mg/kg)*	*ED_{90} (mg/kg)*	*TI*	*LD_{50} (mg/kg)*	*ED_{90} (mg/kg)*	*TI*
Cisplatin	140	24	5.8	11.3	0.6	18.8
Carboplatin	235	99	2.4	180	14.5	12.4
Tetraplatin	480	45	10.6	22.5	0.8	28
JM118	140	11	13	14	1	14
JM216	330	5.8	56.9	30	5.7	5.3
JM274	1120	3.6	311	14	5	2.8
AMD473	560	6.2	90.3	43	3	14.3

were made to provide optimal physicochemical properties compared with corresponding *bis*-substituted complexes. It was also thought that platinum complexes with asymmetric carrier ligands might bind to alternative regions of DNA or in a different spatial orientation than cisplatin/carboplatin. Additional human tumor models, largely concentrating upon ovarian cancer, were also established during this period. These in vitro *(6)* and in vivo xenograft *(7)* models were to become increasingly important in the ICR Drug Development Programme (see below). Two events in the late 1980s then stimulated the rapid realisation of a lead oral platinum suitable for clinical trial: (1) the synthesis of the platinum (IV) ammine/amine dicarboxylates, and (2) the signing of a 5-year research agreement in December 1989 among ICR, JM, and Bristol Myers, the first objective of which was to take an oral platinum into phase I.

2.1 The Ammine/Amine Platinum (IV) Dicarboxylates

Oral versus ip dosing with platinum (II) mixed amine complexes (such as JM118 shown in Table 1) to mice bearing the ADJ/PC6 tumor produced similar results to those described for cisplatin and carboplatin, i.e., no gain in therapeutic index. Similar results were exhibited by platinum(IV) dihydroxo complexes, e.g., JM149 (the Pt IV dihydroxo homolog of JM118: TI ip of 44, TI oral of only 7). As the amine ligands of platinum complexes had been shown in early structure-activity relationship studies to be essential for antitumor activity *(3)*, it was considered that modification of this part of the structure would probably be detrimental to antitumor activity. Thus, to improve oral absorption, chemistry concentrated on platinum(IV) complexes and, specifically, modification of the axial ligands from dihydroxo (as in JM149) to more lipophilic, neutral complexes. Although the synthesis of the target molecules was not straightforward [since platinum(IV) molecules are relatively inert to substitution under most conditions] this was overcome by exploiting the strong nucleophilic character after binding to platinum of the oxygen atom of the hydroxo ligand (as in CHIP and JM149). This then allowed participation in reactions with appropriate electrophiles while the inertness of the bond with platinum prevented the structure from breaking down. Specifically, for most of the resulting dicarboxylate series, reaction of the platinum(IV) dihydroxo complex with an acid anhydride as the electrophile was used. Stirring at ambient temperature for several hours achieved essentially 100% conversion to dicarboxylate products containing simple alkyl and aryl axial ligands *(8)*. Carbamate and carbonate complexes were also obtained by reaction with isocyanates and pyrocarbonates, respectively, as electrophiles.

JM216 (containing acetato axial ligands and ammine/cyclohexylamine carrier ligands) was one of the first of around 30 platinum(IV) mixed amine dicarboxylates to be evaluated against the ADJ/PC6 tumor (Table 1). There was tangible excitement when this result was produced since, for the first time, a clear gain in TI was observed by oral versus ip dosing: TI of 57 with oral dosing but only 5 by the ip route. Interestingly, the antitumor effectiveness (ED_{90}) was maintained while there was a substantial reduction in toxicity. Before long, as additional complexes were tested, there was a surfeit of molecules exhibiting marked oral antitumor activity. Some, such as JM274 (see Fig. 1 for structure), exhibited a TI in this model of over 300 (Table 1).

The preclinical properties of the lead platinum(IV) mixed amine dicarboxylates were first described at the 6th International Symposium on Platinum and other Metal Coordination Complexes in Cancer Chemotherapy at San Diego in January, 1991 *(9,10)*. Octanol/water partition coefficients ranging from 0.1 for JM216, to 7 for JM229 (propionato homolog), and up to 41 for JM221 (butryato homolog) were reported *(9)*. JM221 exhibited a TI by the oral route in mice bearing the ADJ/PC6 of 54 *(9)*. Absorption in the mouse was shown to be substantially higher for the dicarboxylates: 71% dose absorbed over 48 h for JM216 and 76% for JM221, vs only 22% for carboplatin *(10)*.

To select one dicarboxylate compound for clinical trial from the 20 plus showing good oral antitumor activity against the ADJ/PC6, two additional series of experiments were then conducted in parallel. These were oral dosings to nude mice bearing human ovarian carcinoma xenografts of varying responsiveness to cisplatin and emesis-inducing properties in the ferret model (as mice do not possess an emetic response). All of the 10 most orally active compounds in the ADJ/PC6 experiments showed marked (60 days growth delay or greater) oral antitumor activity against the cisplatin-sensitive PXN/100 model *(11)*. Conversely, all compounds were less active against a tumor (SKOV-3) that also did not respond to cisplatin, although JM216, JM221, and JM244 [*bis*-benzoato ammine dichloro (n-propylamine) platinum(IV)] induced growth delays of greater than 10 days. With three xenografts of intermediate responsiveness to cisplatin (OVCAR-3, HX/110, and PXN/109T/C), good activity was observed with JM216, JM244, JM225 (*bis*-acetato ammine dichloro [cyclopentylamine) platinum(IV)], and JM269 (as for JM225 and JM216 but cycloheptylamine), whereas JM274 (see Fig. 1 for structure) was less active.

At the time, significant emphasis was placed on the results of the ferret emesis studies in the final selection process. It is possible that today, with the proven clinical benefit of the 5-hydroxytryptamine 3 5-HT_3 receptor antagonist antiemetics, more emphasis on absorption and antitumor activity might have prevailed. However, after JM221 and JM244 were shown to be highly emetic in this model compared with the acetato series of JM216, JM225, and JM269 *(10)*, these two compounds were dropped. Notably, the three remaining acetato compounds were shown to be comparably emetogenic to carboplatin and less so than either JM244/JM221 or cisplatin.

The final choice among JM216, JM225, and JM269 rested with a combination of head-to-head antitumor studies of the three compounds (administered by oral gavage) vs equitoxic iv cisplatin and carboplatin using four human ovarian carcinoma xenografts *(11,12)*. These studies confirmed that the dicarboxylates produced broadly comparable antitumor activity to that of cisplatin and carboplatin. Other studies using additional tumor models (A2780 human ovarian xenograft and M5076 murine reticulosarcoma) were conducted within Bristol Myers *(13)*. JM216 appeared to be most active against the M5076 tumor.

Overall, the final choice of JM216 represented a compromise of good oral antitumor activity (at least comparable to iv carboplatin in most models), low emetic properties in the ferret, and favorable physicochemical properties (especially compared with the much less aqueous soluble JM269). JM216 possesses a solubility in water of around 0.3 mg/mL and in saline of 0.4 mg/mL. Also, in relation to possible reactions in the stomach prior to absorption, the compound showed good stability in acid (a half-life of several hours in 1 *M* hydrochloric acid).

2.2. JM216- Preclinical Properties

2.2.1. Rodent Toxicology

As the initial goal of the oral program was to develop a compound with carboplatin-like toxicology and comparable antitumor activity, rodent toxicology studies were an important part of the preclinical program. In mice receiving a single oral dose of 200 mg/kg, myelosuppression was the dose-limiting toxicity, with leukopenia the prominent effect. A nadir occurred at d 2–10 post treatment but with recovery by d 14. In addition, mild thrombocytopenia and anemia were observed. In contrast, on repeated dosing (55 mg/kg daily for 5 d), thrombocytopenia was more pronounced (nadir by d 14 but again with recovery, by d 30 *(14)*.

Two nonmyelosuppressive toxicities of particular concern with platinum compounds are nephrotoxicity (as observed with cisplatin) and neurotoxicity [which led to the abandonment of tetraplatin (Ormaplatin®—see Fig. 1 for structure—from Phase I)]. However, in contrast to cisplatin, JM216 at a maximum tolerated dose, like carboplatin, was shown to be devoid of nephrotoxicity in mice and rats *(15)*. Neurotoxicity was assessed in the rat using a sensory nerve conduction velocity model *(16)*. Tetraplatin (ip at a dose of 1 mg/kg, twice weekly for 6 weeks) and cisplatin (ip at a dose of 2 mg/kg, twice weekly for 6 weeks) caused a significant slowing of sensory nerve conduction (14 and 17% decreases, respectively). Conversely, JM216 (po at a dose of 25 mg/kg for 20 weeks) caused no reduction in sensory nerve conduction velocity.

Histologic abnormalities in mice following maximum tolerated doses of po JM216 occurred only in the intestinal tract. Villus atrophy, crypt tip necrosis, and reduced frequency of crypt mitosis was observed, although this was similar in severity to that observed with cisplatin or carboplatin. However, measures of mucosal damage (sucrase, threhalase, and maltase) revealed no damage *(14)*. Although tissue distribution studies revealed high platinum levels in the liver (and kidney), both alkaline phosphatase and alanine aminotransferase measurements were unaffected, suggestive of no liver damage.

2.2.2. Further Antitumor Studies

The most significant preclinical antitumor studies in relation to the clinical findings (see below) involved a study of administering oral JM216 by different dosing schedules *(17)*. Using the PXN/109T/C ovarian xenograft, the antitumor activity of JM216 was compared according to the following schedules; 100 or 200 mg/kg single dose every 21 d, 40 or 60 mg/kg daily for 5 d every 21 d, 40 or 60 mg/kg daily for 5 d, every 28 d, and 9.5 or 14.5 mg/kg daily. The main findings are shown in Fig. 2. In contrast to previously reported observations with carboplatin and cisplatin, the antitumor effect of JM216 was significantly improved by splitting the dosing into a daily schedule for 5 d. However, antitumor benefit was lost on daily chronic dosing. Maximum growth delays were 30 d in the single-dose arm and only 16 d in the chronic daily arm, but 91 days in the daily for 5 d every 21 d group and 65 d in the daily for 5 d every 28 d group.

A second preclinical in vivo antitumor study of subsequent clinical significance involved combining JM216 with oral etoposide *(18)*. Therapeutic synergy was apparent in the ascitic P388 leukemia model but not in the M5076 sc reticulosarcoma model. Of interest was that, in the combination arm, only about 25% of each drug's maximum tolerated dose could be safely given. This combination is now being evaluated in Phase I.

2.2.3. Mechanistic Studies

Growth inhibition studies using a variety of human cancer cell lines showed that JM216 was similar in potency to cisplatin itself and more potent than carboplatin; mean IC_{50} values in μM were 1.7 for JM216, 3.5 for cisplatin, and 26.3 for carboplatin *(12,19)*. In terms of pattern of response across cell lines,

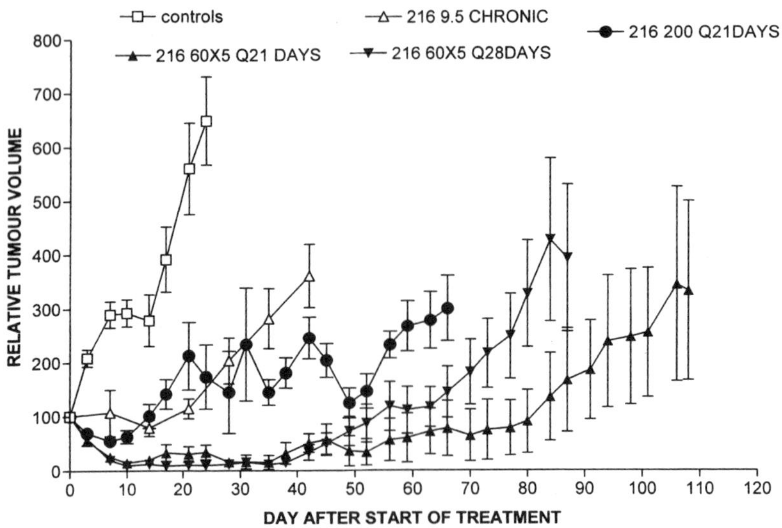

Fig. 2. Comparative oral antitumor activity of JM216 administered to mice bearing the PXN/109T/C human ovarian cancer xenograft. □, control, untreated; ●, 200 mg/kg every 21 days; ▲, 60 mg/kg daily for 5 days every 21 days; ▼, 60 mg/kg daily for 5 days every 28 days; and △, 9.5 mg/kg daily. (Data replotted from ref. *17*).

JM216 appeared to behave similarly to cisplatin and carboplatin. Although not a central issue in the selection process, JM216 did show complete circumvention of acquired cisplatin resistance in the 41McisR ovarian cancer cell line *(12)* and HX/155cisR cervical cancer cell line *(19)* (see below). The DNA binding properties of JM216 on naked DNA or within tumor cells appeared broadly similar to those of cisplatin, although there may be some differences in the nature of the DNA adducts *(20)*. However, as described below, interpretation of these findings is complicated because of the rapid and complex biotransformation of the parent drug.

Acquired resistance to JM216 was established in vitro in two human ovarian carcinoma cell lines *(21)*. Whereas some resistance mechanisms common to cisplatin were observed, the results suggested that, in comparison to cisplatin, acquired resistance to JM216 may be less likely to occur through reduced drug transport.

2.2.4. Biotransformation Studies

JM216 is one of only a few platinum(IV) complexes to enter clinical trial. Since reduction of platinum(IV) to -(II) is widely presumed to be required before reaction with target DNA, the reduction rate needs to be a compromise between maintaining the parent molecule for uptake and distribution and reducing to platinum(II) species sufficiently rapidly to achieve reaction with DNA.

Biotransformation studies have been performed under both in vitro conditions [incubation in 5 m*M* ascorbate *(9)*, plasma (22)] and in vivo [within cancer cell lines *(23)*, in rodents *(24)*, and in patients *(25)*]. Overall, a complex pattern of biotransformation has emerged. Sampling of patient's plasma following dosing with JM216 revealed six platinum-containing peaks and no parent drug (Fig. 3A) *(25)*. Four metabolites have been identified: JM118 [*cis*-ammine dichloro (cyclohexylamine) platinum (II)], the major metabolite seen in patients, JM383 [*bis*-(acetato) ammine (cyclohexylamine) dihydroxo platinum(IV)], and JM518, JM559 isomers of [*bis*-(acetato)amminechloro(cyclohexylamine)hydroxo platinum(IV)] *(22,25)*. In tumor cells, the proportion of each of the biotransformation products was dependent on intracellular levels of glutathione *(23)*, suggesting that conjugation with glutathione represents a major detoxification pathway for JM216.

2.2.5. JM216 Clinical Trials

JM216 entered clinical trial at the Royal Marsden Hospital in August 1992 as a single oral dose with the drug delivered in dry filled capsules every 21 d. Starting with 60 mg/m^2, the equivalent one-tenth of the mouse LD_{10}, the dose was escalated up to 700 mg/m^2 *(26)*. Due to limited absorption/dissolution of the drug, no dose-limiting toxicity was reached, however. Plasma platinum pharmacokinetics were linear up to only the 120 mg/m^2 dose level; thereafter the area under the curve (AUC) increased less than proportionally with dose. Some evidence of myelosuppression (leukopenia, thrombocytopenia) was reported. Emesis was mild and controllable, and there was no significant neuro-, oto-, or nephrotoxicity. From 37 patients treated, there was some evidence of antitumor efficacy in three patients with advanced ovarian cancer.

In an attempt to overcome the apparent saturable absorption observed with the bolus schedule, a second Phase I trial using a daily dosing schedule for 5 d began in March, 1993 *(27)*. As mentioned above, the use of this split-dose schedule was also supported by antitumor studies in xenografts. Starting at a dose of 20 mg/m^2/d, a maximum tolerated dose of 140 mg/m^2/d was reached, with thrombocytopenia and leukopenia the dose-limiting toxicities. This myelosuppression was noncumulative and reversible with the nadir from d 17 to 21 and recovery by d 28. There was good control of emesis through the use of prophylactic administration of oral dexamethasone with either metoclopramide or ondansetron. In contrast to the single-dose trial, the pharmacokinetic parameters AUC and C_{max} increased linearly with dose for both total and ultrafiltrable platinum, although considerable interpatient variability was seen. The recommended doses for Phase II studies were 100 mg/m^2/d in patients previously treated with platinum drugs and 120 mg/m^2/d in previously untreated patients.

A final Phase I trial conducted at the Royal Marsden involved twice daily dosing, 12 h apart *(28)*. Nineteen patients received doses between 150 and 350 mg/m^2 twice daily. However, a less than proportional increase in AUC was observed with increasing doses and, as a result, the maximum tolerated dose was not reached.

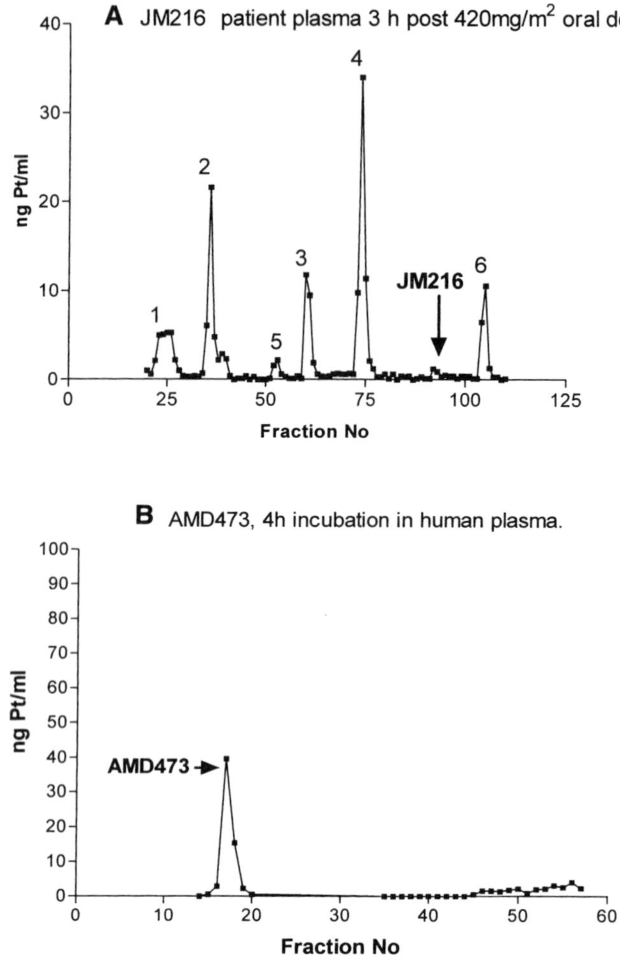

Fig. 3. Comparative biotransformation (shown as platinum peaks following separation by HPLC) of **(A)** JM216 in patient plasma 3 h after an oral dose of 420 mg/m^2 and **(B)** AMD473 4 h after incubation in human plasma.

Two patients with mesothelioma had stable disease and received six cycles. Toxicities were similar to those observed in the other Phase I trials. Overall, these Phase I trials confirmed that a daily schedule for 5 d was optimal for JM216.

Phase II trials with JM216 (BMS 182751), all using the daily schedule for 5 d, have been or are being conducted in non-small cell lung cancer (NSCLC) *(29)*, small cell lung cancer (SCLC) *(30)*, and hormone-refractory prostate cancer (HRPC) *(31)*. The EORTC early clinical trials group Phase II trial in NSCLC showed that JM216 afforded useful palliation in some patients but that overall, the drug did not possess significant antitumor activity against this generally chemoresistant disease. In contrast, responses were observed in patients presenting with previously untreated SCLC. The overall response rate was 5/16 (31%), with 5 partial responses and 5 with stable disease. Notably, responses have been reported in patients with HRPC; of nine patients with measurable disease, one had a partial response and six had stable disease. Seven patients (32%) had greater than 50% reductions in the prostate cancer marker, prostate-specific antigen (PSA) for more than 28 d. The drug was generally well tolerated, and a Phase III trial with and without prednisone is planned. Reports of trials in additional diseases, including ovarian cancer and in combination with radiation, are still awaited.

3. 1992–1997: JM216 TO JM335 TO JM473/AMD473/ZD0473

During 1991, as JM216 was being prepared for clinical trial (preclinical toxicology, formulation), the ICR/JM, Bristol Myers research agreement continued with the further aim of discovering a "third-generation" platinum drug possessing activity against cisplatin-refractory disease. Many reports describing mechanisms of resistance to cisplatin in cell lines repeatedly exposed to cisplatin began to emerge from the late 1980s onwards. In these cell lines, three major causes of resistance were observed: decreased drug transport, increased intracellular levels of thiols, especially glutathione or metallothioneins, and increased adduct removal from DNA and tolerance (for review, see ref. *32*). Acquired cisplatin resistance was also generated and studied in the ICR cisplatin-sensitive human ovarian carcinoma cell lines 41M and CH1 *(6)*. Fortuitously, acquired resistant lines emerged with differing major underlying mechanisms of resistance, 41McisR being resistant mainly due to reduced drug transport, *(33)* and CH1cisR being resistant through a post-DNA binding mechanism *(34)*. The A2780/A2780cisR lines were also added, A2780cisR being resistant through a combination of decreased transport, increased glutathione, and increased adduct removal from DNA *(32)*. Across eight "parent" human ovarian carcinoma cell lines, we observed an excellent correlation (*r* of 0.91) between cisplatin cytotoxicity (which ranged by over 100-fold) and glutathione levels *(35)*. Also, a statistically significant positive correlation was observed between in vitro sensitivity to cisplatin and corresponding in vivo xenograft responsiveness (r of 0.88, $n = 8$) *(36)*. Focusing on these cisplatin-resistant cell line models and various in vivo models (including xenograft counterparts to the cell lines), a preclinical evaluation cascade for the discovery of a broader spectrum third-generation platinum complex was established (Fig. 4) and put into practice.

Compounds were sought that circumvented acquired cisplatin resistance in vitro against a panel of eight human ovarian carcinoma cell lines (41M, 41McisR; A2780, A2780cisR; CH1, CH1cisR; and two intrinsically cisplatin-resistant lines, SKOV-3 and HX/62). Thereafter, an initial dose-finding in vivo study was performed in conventional mice bearing the ADJ/PC6 sc tumor prior to more extensive in vivo experimentation in nude mice bearing sc xenografts

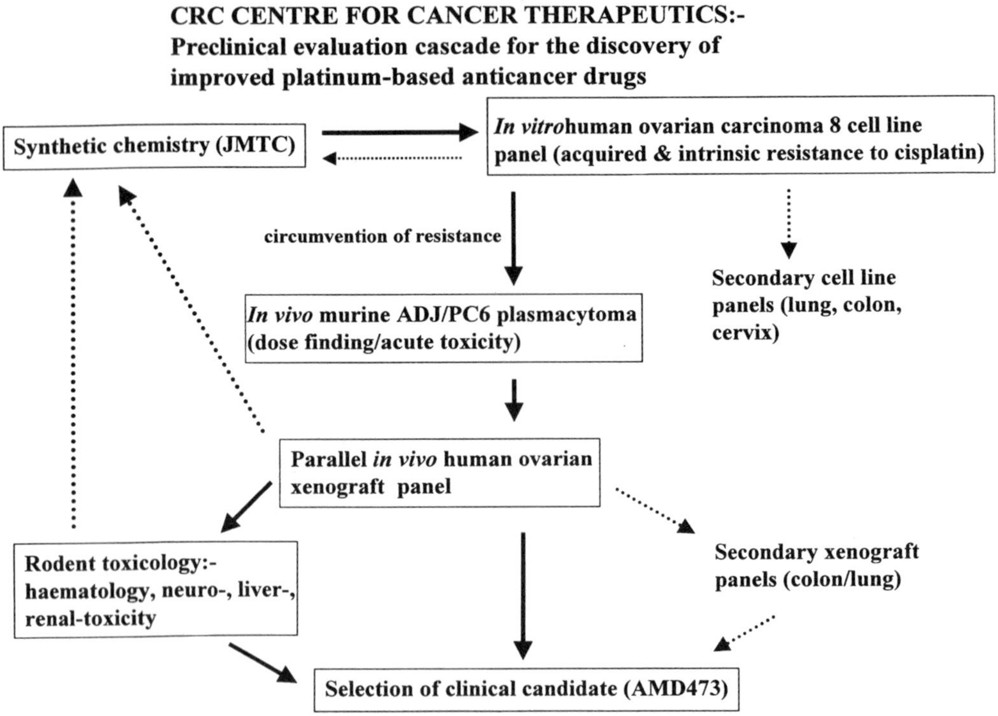

Fig. 4. CRC Centre for Cancer Therapeutics, Institute of Cancer Research Preclinical Evaluation Cascade for the discovery of "third-generation" platinum complexes.

of predetermined sensitivity to cisplatin. Importantly, an early assessment of toxicology in rodents was included with special regard to neurotoxicity, nephrotoxicity, and liver toxicity.

From 1991 to 1995, more than 500 compounds were studied against the eight-cell line ovarian panel using the sulphorhodamine B growth inhibition assay as used by the National Cancer Institute Drug Screening Program. The first "lead" compound to emerge was the *trans*-platinum(IV) complex, JM335 (see Fig. 1 for structure). A major paradigm for structure-activity relationships of platinum complexes is that *trans*-platinum complexes are inactive as antitumor agents (e.g., ref *3*). However, by the early 1990s, Farrell and co-workers (*37*) had first shown that certain *trans*-platinum compounds possessed interesting antitumor properties, at least in vitro.

3.1. Preclinical Properties of JM335

Initial in vitro experiments with JM335 revealed that the compound was comparably cytotoxic to cisplatin itself (mean IC_{50} of 3.1 μM for JM335) and over 50-fold more potent than transplatin. Moreover, against the three pairs of lines, partial to full circumvention of acquired cisplatin resistance was observed; resistance factors were 1.1 for the 41M pair, and 1.9 for the CH1 pair, but 7.1 for the A2780 pair *(38)*.

Mechanistic studies with JM335 revealed DNA binding properties distinct from those of cisplatin. Interestingly, for a platinum complex, JM335 induced DNA single-strand breaks in the CH1 cell line, although interstrand crosslinks were detectable in SKOV-3 cells *(20)*. DNA extracted from cells exposed to JM335 was not recognized by a monoclonal antibody raised against *cis*-platinated DNA. The kinetics of apoptosis was shown to be more rapid for JM335 with its *cis*-isomer in CH1 cells and, at high 10 x IC_{50} JM335 concentrations, death appeared to occur by a nonapoptotic mechanism *(39)*.

Structure-activity relationship studies identified a total of 14 *trans* complexes that showed in vivo antitumor activity against the ADJ/PC6 model. All were platinum(IV) complexes (13 possessing axial dihydroxo ligands) and, when tested, all their respective platinum(II) or platinum(IV) tetrachloro counterparts were inactive *(40)*. JM335 was the first *trans*-platinum complex to demonstrate marked antitumor activity against several human ovarian carcinoma xenografts, including an impressive 64-d growth delay against the PXN/100 model *(38)*. However, when compared with the activity of cisplatin itself, JM335 was disappointingly less active *(40)*, resulting in the compound not being selected for clinical trial. Since cross-resistance in the A2780cisR cell line (see above) was shown to be associated with high levels of GSH *(38)*, it was reasoned that the relative lack of in vivo activity of JM335 may be due to inactivation by thiols. This provided an impetus to designing platinum analogs with reduced affinity toward thiols (see below).

3.2. JM473/AMD473

The most significant lead to emerge from the cascade was JM473 (AMD473; see Fig. 1 for structure). The chemical rationale for the synthesis of AMD473 was based on having a platinum compound with reduced susceptibility to inactivation by elevated intracellular thiol concentrations. As mentioned above, the two intrinsically cisplatin-resistant cell lines HX/62 and SKOV-3 and the acquired cisplatin-resistant line A2780cisR had been shown to possess high levels of the intracellular thiol, glutathione, compared with the relatively sensitive lines *(35,38)*. In an attempt to decrease inactivation by thiols, increased steric bulk was introduced at the platinum center, thereby shifting the substitution reaction pathway more toward a dissociative rather than associative mechanism.

3.2.1. Circumvention of Acquired Cisplatin Resistance

Relative to all the platinum compounds evaluated against the eight-cell line panel AMD473 showed particularly promising in vitro properties *(41)*. A comparison of potencies against the three pairs of ovarian lines in the panel (as well as two additional pairs) for carboplatin, JM216, and AMD473 is shown in Fig. 5. In common with the clinical observations, a high degree of cross-resistance was observed between cisplatin and carboplatin in all five pairs. With the exception of the HX/155 cervical cancer pair of lines, AMD473 showed comparable (e.g., in the transport-deficient 41McisR) or superior circumvention of acquired cisplatin resistance than JM216. This was particularly evident in the A2780cisR line, in which glutathione is known to play a role in resistance.

In vitro growth inhibition studies revealed AMD473 to be intermediate in potency (mean IC_{50} of 8.1 μM) between that of cisplatin (mean IC_{50} of 2.6 μM) and carboplatin (mean IC_{50} of 20.3 μM) across the cell line panel. Notably, across the National Cancer Institute 60-cell line panel, the COMPARE analysis indicated that AMD473 possesses a distinct pattern of response from all other platinum agents and was "COMPARE negative" (no compound with a Pearson coefficient of greater than 0.7 *(41)*.

3.2.2. In Vivo Antitumor Properties

In the first in vivo study, good antitumor activity was observed following a single ip administration of AMD473 to mice bearing the ADJ/PC6 tumor *(42)* (Table 1). The ED_{90} dose was 3 mg/kg, whereas severe toxicity was not observed until a dose of 43 mg/kg was used (TI of 14.3). However, interest in AMD473 was stimulated following the observation of activity against the ovarian xenograft panel, including in some secondary models possessing acquired resistance to cisplatin *(42)*. Activity was also observed against CH1 ovarian xenografts that had regrown following initial treatment with cisplatin *(42)*.

In addition, AMD473 represents the first platinum(II) complex to demonstrate good oral antitumor activity. In mice bearing the ADJ/PC6 tumor, a TI of 90 was obtained (Table 1). Antitumor activity following oral dosing (greater activity than either iv administered cisplatin or carboplatin or orally administered JM216) was also observed against the acquired cisplatin-resistant CH1cisR xenograft *(42)*.

3.2.3. Rodent Toxicology and Pharmacology

The dose-limiting toxicity of AMD473 in mice (and rats) is myelosuppression (leukopenia and thrombocytopenia). Moreover, no renal toxicity, liver toxicity, or neurotoxicity has been observed *(42)*. Hence, the toxicity in rodents is more like carboplatin than cisplatin. Platinum pharmacokinetics following iv administration to mice showed a biexponential decay in plasma with a rapid distribution ($t_{1/2\alpha}$ of 24 min) followed by a slow elimination ($t_{1/2\beta}$ of 44 h). Following oral dosing, platinum absorption was rapid (T_{max} of 0.5 h), with a bioavailability of 40% *(42)*. Platinum accumulated mainly in the liver, kidney, and spleen. Biotransformation studies involving incubations in human plasma, exposure to tumor cells, and dosing to mice have been performed. In contrast to the rapid and complex biotransformation observed with JM216 (see above),

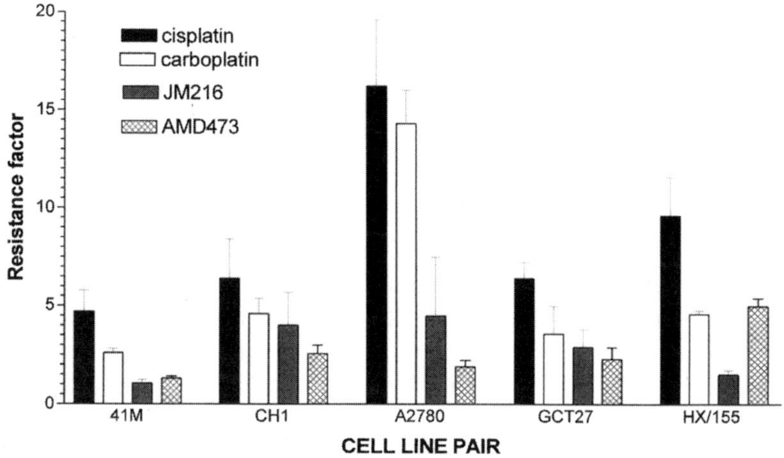

Fig. 5. Comparative cross-resistance profiles for the 41M/41McisR, CH1/CH1cisR, A2780/A2780cisR (ovarian), GCT27/GCT27cisR (testicular), and HX155/HX155cisR (cervical) pairs of human tumor cell lines for cisplatin itself, carboplatin, JM216, and AMD473. Resistance factor = IC_{50} resistant/parent lines determined from 96-h drug exposure SRB assay. Error bars = SEM, *n* = >3.

parent AMD473 was detectable up to 6 h post administration (ip or oral) to mice or 4 h following incubation in human plasma (Fig. 3b). The drug is mainly biotransformed to aquated activation products *(43)*. Again, in contrast to results obtained for JM216 *(23),* only AMD473 itself was detectable within human ovarian carcinoma cells; no glutathione adduct was formed *(43)*.

3.2.4. Mechanistic Studies

As predicted, AMD473 was shown to be less reactive than cisplatin toward the sulphur-containing molecules methionine and thiourea *(44)*. Moreover, in the presence of 5 m*M* glutathione, AMD473 binding to salmon sperm DNA was significantly less affected than cisplatin binding *(44)*. When glutathione levels were artificially raised in an ovarian cancer cell line, the degree of protection of cytotoxicity was less for AMD473 compared with cisplatin *(41)*. Platinum transport studies following exposure of the 41M and A2780 pair of lines to AMD473 showed, in contrast to results obtained with cisplatin, equal intracellular drug levels in the parent and acquired resistant lines *(41)*. Although, as with other platinum drugs, the compound's mechanism of action probably involves binding to DNA, the DNA binding properties of AMD473 differ from those of cisplatin. On naked DNA, several adducts unique to AMD473 were observed *(44)*. Within cells, DNA interstrand crosslinks were formed much more slowly in cells exposed to AMD473 compared with cisplatin (peak formation of 5 h for cisplatin versus 14–24 h for AMD473) *(41)*.

A polyclonal antibody raised to DNA adducts of AMD473 showed no crossreactivity with cisplatin-DNA adducts *(45)*. As with other DNA-damaging agents, induction of p53 was observed in p53 wild-type cell lines following exposure to IC_{50} concentrations of AMD473. The rate of induction, however, was markedly slower and lasted longer than with cisplatin *(41)*.

3.2.5. Synthesis

AMD-473 is prepared by a modified Dhara synthesis *(46)* by a method similar to that described for the preparation of the platinum(II) precursor of JM216 *(8,9)*. Potassium amminetrichloroplatinate(II) is reacted with 2-picoline in the presence of iodide at ambient temperature, resulting in precipitation of the desired isomer [PtCl(I)(NH_3)(2-picoline)]. In the second step, the iodide ligand is removed by reaction with silver ions in water at ambient temperature, and treatment of the resulting aqua platinum complexes with chloride yields [$PtCl_2$(NH_3)(2-picoline)]. There is retention of stereochemistry at platinum, thus yielding the pure *cis* isomer, which may be recrystallized from dilute hydrochloric acid.

3.2.6. Clinical Trials

During the course of the above preclinical studies, a new Canadian venture capital-backed company, AnorMED, spun out of the biomedical division of Johnson Matthey. With all rights to JM473 and analogs being returned to JM at the end of the agreement with Bristol Myers Squibb in 1994, the now renamed AMD473 was chosen for late-stage preclinical development. In 1996, based largely on the preclinical evidence of in vivo activity against acquired cisplatin resistance and a favorable toxicology profile, AMD473 was selected for a Phase I clinical trial under the auspices of the UK Cancer Research Campaign.

The initial, single-dose intravenous administration, Phase I study began at the Royal Marsden NHS Trust Hospital in November, 1997. Subsequently, in April, 1998, the drug was licensed to Zeneca for continuing clinical development and renamed ZD0473.

4. OTHER ORALLY ACTIVE PLATINUMS

In the past 2 years, platinum derivatives of the platinum(II) 1,2diaminocyclohexane (DACH) complex, oxaliplatin, (Eloxatin®) have been reported. Oxaliplatin, the lead DACH platinum, is currently registered in France for the treatment of colorectal cancer in combination with 5-fluorouracil *(47)*. In Japan, Kidani and colleagues *(48)* have synthesized platinum(IV) derivatives, like JM216, with lipophilic axial carboxylate ligands. One complex, C5-OHP with *bis*-valerato axial ligands, exhibited marginal oral antitumor activity when administered to mice bearing the murine L1210 leukemia (maximum T/C% of 148 with 20 mg/kg daily schedule for 5 d). More recently, a mono *n*-valerate

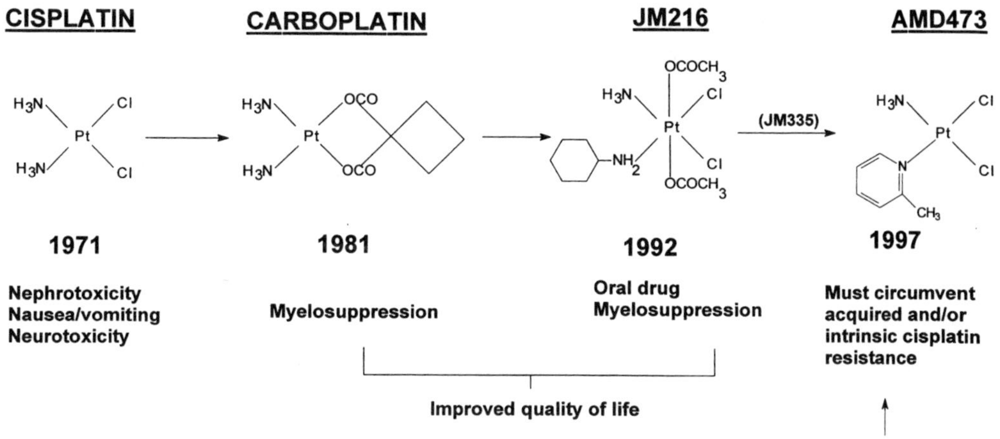

Fig. 6. Summary of the ICR/JM platinum drug discovery program: carboplatin to AMD473/ZD473.

derivative (C5-OHP-Cl; see Fig. 1 for structure) has been shown to possess improved absorption properties compared with C5-OHP and oral antitumor activity against the sc M5076 reticulosarcoma model using a daily schedule for 5 d in two cycles initiated on d 5 and 12 post implantation *(49)*.

5. SUMMARY

From its origins of about 20 years ago based around the Harrap, Connors, Cleare axis, the ICR/JM collaboration has made a significant contribution to platinum anticancer drug development. These achievements are summarized in chronologic order in Fig. 6. Three new platinum drugs have entered clinical trial: JM8 (carboplatin), still the only platinum analog to be widely registered for clinical use; JM216 (with Bristol Myers Squibb), the original orally active platinum drug; and, most recently, AMD473/ZD0473. A fourth agent, JM335, remains one of the most interesting and active of the class of *trans*-platinum complex. Since JM216, the focus has been on the need to circumvent acquired and/or intrinsic tumor resistance to cisplatin rather than quality of life issues. From several hundred compounds evaluated in the test cascade (Fig. 4), only AMD473 emerged as worthy of clinical study. The first in vitro cytotoxicity assessment of AMD473 was conducted in March, 1993 (poignantly, in the same week as one of the founder ICR "platinizers," George Abel, died). From the ICR/JM perspective, the search for additional novel platinum analogs has now ceased. Although a great deal has been elucidated concerning how tumors (especially cell lines) become resistant to cisplatin, circumventing resistance in the clinic remains a particularly challenging prospect. We await with great interest the clinical studies with AMD473 (and other recently introduced novel platinum structures targeted at cisplatin-resistant disease, such as BBR3464).

As we head into the new millennium, platinum drugs of reduced morbidity compared with cisplatin have become a reality for cancer patients. However, on a cautionary note, alternative strategies to platinum-containing analogs (e.g., drugs aimed at manipulating the underlying cell signaling pathways whereby large numbers of tumors possess resistance to cisplatin and carboplatin) may be required to produce significant long-term survival benefit in those high numbers of patients whose tumors fail on cisplatin/carboplatin. Therein lies the challenge for future chemistry/biology collaborations.

ACKNOWLEDGMENTS

Thanks are due to the many scientists at ICR and JM who worked on the platinum program for almost two decades, notably at ICR, the Director of Drug Development, Ken Harrap, postdoctoral scientists Prakash Mistry and Florence Raynaud, PhD students Sarah Morgan, Swee Sharp (née Loh), Kirste Mellish, Ciaran O'Neill, and Jeffrey Holford, Research Officers Mervyn Jones, Phyllis Goddard, Frances Boxall, George Abel, and Melanie Valenti, and clinicians Mark McKeage and Philip Beale with Ian Judson. Work at ICR was supported by grants, predominantly from the UK Cancer Research Campaign. At JM (and then AnorMED), thanks are due to Barry Murrer, Chris Barnard, Mike Abrams, Chris Giandomenico, Geoff Henson, Mike Cleare, and Don Picker.

REFERENCES

1. Harrap, K. R. (1985) Preclinical studies identifying carboplatin as a viable cisplatin alternative. *Cancer Treat. Rev.* **12,** 21–33.
2. Siddik, Z. H., Boxall, F. E., Goddard, P. M., Barnard, C. F. J., and Harrap, K. R. (1984) Antitumor, pharmacokinetic and toxicity studies with orally administered cisplatin, CBDCA and CHIP. *Proc. Am. Assoc. Cancer Res.* **25,** abstract no 1462.
3. Connors, T. A., Cleare, M. J., and Harrap, K. R. (1979) Structure-activity relationships of the antitumor platinum coordination complexes. *Cancer Treat. Rep.* **63,** 1499–1502.
4. Goddard, P. M., Valenti, M. R., and Harrap, K. R. (1991) The role of murine tumor models and their acquired platinum-resistant counterparts in the evaluation of novel platinum antitumor agents: a cautionary note. *Ann. Oncol.* **2,** 535–540.
5. Van Hennik, M. B., van der Vijgh, W. J. F., Klein, I., Vermorken, J. B., and Pinedo, H. M. (1989) Human pharmacokinetics of carboplatin after oral administration. *Cancer Chemother. Pharmacol.* **23,** 126–127.
6. Hills, C. A., Kelland, L. R., Abel, G., Siracky, J., Wilson, A. P., and Harrap, K. R. (1989) Biological properties of ten human ovarian carcinoma cell lines: calibration *in vitro* against four platinum complexes. *Br. J. Cancer* **59,** 527–534.
7. Harrap, K. R., Jones, M., Siracky, J., Pollard, L., and Kelland, L.R. (1990) The establishment, characterisation and calibration of human ovarian carcinoma xenografts for the evaluation of novel platinum anticancer drugs. *Ann. Oncol.* **1,** 65–76.
8. Giandomenico, C. M., Abrams, M. J., Murrer, B. A., Vollano, J. F., Rheinheimer, M. I., Wyer, S. B., et al. (1995) Carboxylation of kinetically inert platinum(IV) hydroxy complexes. An entrée into orally active platinum(IV) antitumor agents. *Inorg. Chem,* **34,** 1015–1021.
9. Giandomenico, C. M., Abrams, M. J., Murrer, B. A., Vollano, J. F., Barnard, C. F. J., Harrap,

K. R., et al. (1991) Synthesis and reactions of a new class of orally active Pt(IV) antitumor complexes, in *Platinum and Other Metal Coordination Complexes in Cancer Chemotherapy* (Howell, S. B., ed.), Plenum, New York, pp. 93–100.

10. Harrap, K. R., Murrer, B. A., Giandomenico, C., Morgan, S. E., Kelland, L. R., Jones, M., et al. (1991) Ammine/amine platinum IV dicarboxylates: a novel class of complexes which circumvent intrinsic cisplatin resistance, in *Platinum and Other Metal Coordination Complexes in Cancer Chemotherapy* (Howell, S. B., ed.), Plenum, New York, pp. 391–398.
11. Kelland, L. R., Jones, M., Gwynne, J. J., Valenti, M., Murrer, B. A., Barnard, C. F. J., et al. (1993) Antitumor activity of orally administered ammine/amine platinum(IV) dicarboxylate complexes against a panel of human ovarian carcinoma xenografts. *Int. J. Oncol.* **2,** 1043–1048.
12. Kelland, L. R., Abel, G., McKeage, M. J., Jones, M., Goddard, P. M., Valenti, M., et al. (1993) Preclinical antitumor evaluation of bis-acetato-ammine-dichloro cyclohexylamine platinum(IV): an orally active platinum drug. *Cancer Res.* **53,** 2581–2586.
13. Rose, W. C., Crosswell, A. R., Schurig, J. E., and Casazza, A. M. (1993) Preclinical antitumor activity of orally administered platinum(IV) complexes. *Cancer Chemother. Pharmacol.* **32,** 197–203.
14. McKeage, M. J., Morgan, S. E., Boxall, F. E., Murrer, B. A., Hard, G. C., and Harrap, K. R. (1994) Preclinical toxicology and tissue distribution of novel oral antitumor platinum complexes: ammine/amine platinum(IV) dicarboxylates. *Cancer Chemother. Pharmacol.*, **33,** 497–503.
15. McKeage, M. J., Morgan, S. E., Boxall, F. E., Murrer, B. A., Hard, G. C., and Harrap, K. R. (1993) Lack of nephrotoxicity of oral ammine/amine platinum(IV) dicarboxylates in rodents. *Br. J. Cancer* **67,** 996–1000.
16. McKeage, M. J., Boxall, F. E., Jones, M., and Harrap, K. R. (1994) Lack of neurotoxicity of oral bis-acetatoamminedichlorocyclohexylamine platinum(IV) in comparison to cisplatin and tetraplatin in the rat. *Cancer Res.* **54,** 629–631.
17. McKeage, M. J., Kelland, L. R., Boxall, F. E., Valenti, M. R., Jones, M., Goddard, P. M., et al. (1994) Schedule-dependency of orally administered bis-acetato-ammine-dichloro-cyclohexylamine-platinum(IV) (JM216) in vivo. *Cancer Res.* **54,** 4118–4122.
18. Rose, W. C. (1997) Combination chemotherapy involving orally administered etoposide and JM-216 in murine tumor models. *Cancer Chemother. Pharmacol.* **40,** 51–56.
19. Mellish, K. J., Kelland, L. R., and Harrap, K. R. (1993) *In vitro* platinum drug chemosensitivity of human cervical squamous cell carcinoma cell lines with intrinsic and acquired resistance to cisplatin. *Br. J. Cancer* **68,** 240–250.
20. Mellish, K. J., Barnard, C. F. J., Murrer, B. A., and Kelland, L. R. (1995) DNA-binding properties of novel *cis* and *trans* platinum-based anticancer agents in 2 human ovarian carcinoma cell lines. *Int. J. Cancer* **62,** 711–723.
21. Mellish, K. J. and Kelland, L. R. (1994) Mechanisms of acquired resistance to the orally active platinum-based anticancer drug Bis-acetato-ammine-dichloro-cyclohexylamine platinum(IV) (JM216) in two human ovarian carcinoma cell lines. *Cancer Res.* **54,** 6194–6200.
22. Poon, G. K., Raynaud, F. I., Mistry, P., Odell, D. E., Kelland, L. R., Harrap, K. R., et al. (1995) Metabolic studies of an orally active platinum anticancer drug by liquid chromatography-electrospray ionization-mass spectrometry. *J. Chromatogr.* **712,** 61–66.
23. Raynaud, F. I., Odell, D. E., and Kelland, L. R. (1996) Intracellular metabolism of the orally active platinum drug JM216: influence of glutathione levels. *Br. J. Cancer* **74,** 380–386.
24. Raynaud, F. I., Boxall, F. E., Goddard, P., Barnard, C. F., Murrer, B. A., and Kelland, L.R. (1996) Metabolism, protein binding and *in vivo* activity of the oral platinum drug JM216 and its biotransformation products. *Anticancer Res.* **16,** 1857–1862.
25. Raynaud, F. I., Mistry, P., Donaghue, A., Poon, G. K., Kelland, L. R., Barnard, C. F. J., Murrer, B. A., and Harrap, K. R. (1996) Biotransformation of the platinum drug JM216 following oral administration to cancer patients. *Cancer Chemother. Pharmacol.* **38,** 155–162.

26. McKeage, M. J., Mistry, P., Ward, J., Boxall, F. E., Loh, S., O'Neill, C., et al. (1995) A phase I and pharmacology study of an oral platinum complex, JM216: dose-dependent pharmacokinetics with single-dose administration. *Cancer Chemother. Pharmacol.* **36,** 451–458.
27. McKeage, M. J., Raynaud, F., Ward, J., Berry, C., Odell, D., Kelland, L. R., et al. (1997) Phase I and pharmacokinetic study of an oral platinum complex given daily for 5 days in patients with cancer. *J. Clin. Oncol.* **15,** 2691–2700.
28. Beale, P., Raynaud, F., Hanwell, J., Berry, C., Moore, S., Odell, D., et al. (1998) Phase I study of oral JM216 given twice daily. *Cancer Chemother. Pharmacol.* **42,** 142–148.
29. Judson, I. R., Cerny, T., Epelbaum, R., Dunlop, D., Smyth, J., Schaefer, B., et al. (1997) Phase II trial of the oral platinum complex JM216 in non-small cell lung cancer: an EORTC early clinical studies group investigation. *Ann. Oncol.* **8,** 604–606.
30. Groen, H. J. M., Smit, E. F., Bauer, J., Calvert, A. H., Weil, C., Crabeels, D., et al. (1996) A Phase II study of oral platinum JM-216 as first line treatment in small cell lung cancer (SCLC). *Proc. Am. Soc. Clin. Oncol.* **437,** abstract no. 1128.
31. Peereboom, D., Wood, L., Connell, C., Spisak, J., Smith, D., Vaughn, D., et al. (1998) Phase II trial of oral platinum (JM-216) in hormone refractory prostate cancer (HRPC) *Proc. Am. Soc. Clin. Oncol.* **439,** abstract no. 1210.
32. Johnson, S. W., Ferry, K. V., and Hamilton, T. C. (1998) Recent insights into platinum drug resistance in cancer. *Drug Res. Updates* **1,** 243–254.
33. Loh, S. Y., Mistry, P., Kelland, L. R., Abel, G., and Harrap, K. R. (1992) Reduced drug accumulation as a major mechanism of acquired resistance to cisplatin in a human ovarian carcinoma cell line: circumvention studies using novel platinum (II) and (IV) ammine/amine complexes. *Br. J. Cancer* **66,** 1109–1115.
34. Kelland, L. R., Mistry, P., Abel, G., Loh, S. Y., O'Neill, C. F., Murrer, B. A., et al. (1992) Mechanism-related circumvention of acquired *cis*-diamminedichloro platinum(II) resistance using two pairs of human ovarian carcinoma cell lines by ammine/amine platinum(IV) dicarboxylates. *Cancer Res.* **52,** 3857–3864.
35. Mistry, P., Kelland, L.R., Abel, G., Sidhur, S., and Harrap, K. R. (1991) The relationships between glutathione, glutathione-S-transferase and cytotoxicity of platinum drugs and melphalan in eight human ovarian carcinoma cell lines. *Br. J. Cancer* **64,** 215–220.
36. Kelland, L. R., Jones, M., Abel, G., and Harrap, K. R. (1992) Human ovarian carcinoma cell lines and companion xenografts: a disease oriented approach to new platinum anticancer drug development. *Cancer Chemother. Pharmacol.* **30,** 43–50.
37. Farrell, N., Ha, T. T. B., Souchard, J. P., Wimmer, F. L., Cros, S., and Johnson, N. P. (1989) Cytostatic *trans*-platinum(II) complexes. *J. Med. Chem.* **32,** 2240–2241.
38. Kelland, L. R., Barnard, C. F. J., Mellish, K. J., Jones, M., Goddard, P. M., Valenti, M., et al. (1994) A novel *trans*-platinum coordination complex possessing *in vitro* and *in vivo* antitumor activity. *Cancer Res.* **54,** 5618–5622.
39. O'Neill, C. F., Ormerod, M. G., Robertson, D., Titley, J. C., Cumber-Walseer, Y., and Kelland, L. R. (1996) Apoptotic and non-apoptotic cell death induced by *cis* and *trans* analogs of a novel ammine(cyclohexylamine)dihydroxodichloroplatinum(IV) complex. *Br. J. Cancer* **74,** 1037–1045.
40. Kelland, L. R., Barnard, C. F. J., Evans, I. G., Murrer, B. A., Theobald, B. R. C., Wyer, S. B., et al. (1995) Synthesis and *in vitro* and *in vivo* antitumor activity of a series of *trans* platinum antitumor complexes. *J. Med. Chem.* **38,** 3016–3024.
41. Holford, J., Sharp, S. Y., Murrer, B. A., Abrams, M., and Kelland, L. R. (1998) In vitro circumvention of cisplatin resistance by the novel sterically hindered platinum complex AMD473. *Br. J. Cancer* **77,** 366–373.
42. Raynaud, F. I., Boxall, F. E., Goddard, P. M., Valenti, M., Jones, M., Murrer, B. A., et al. (1997) cis-Amminedichloro(2-methylpyridine) platinum (II) (AMD473), a novel sterically hindered platinum complex: in vivo activity, toxicology, and pharmacokinetics in mice. *Clin. Cancer Res.* **3,** 2063–2074.

43. Raynaud, F. I., Boxall, F. E., Wong, T., Goddard, K., Nutley, B., Barnard, C. F. J., et al. (1998) Biotransformation of AMD473, a novel platinum analogue in plasma, cell culture and tissue. *Ann. Oncol.* **9(Suppl 2),** abstract no. 190.
44. Holford, J., Raynaud, F., Murrer, B. A., Grimaldi, K., Hartley, J. A., Abrams, M., et al. (1998) Chemical, biochemical and pharmacological activity of the novel sterically hindered platinum co-ordination complex, cis-[amminedichloro(2-methylpyridine)] platinum (II) (AMD473). *Anti-Cancer Drug Des.* **13,** 1–18.
45. Miner, C. B., Raynaud, F. I., Holford, J., Kelland, L. R., Hardcastle, A., and Aherne, G. W. (1997) Characterisation of a polyclonal antibody raised to DNA adducts of AMD473. *Br. J. Cancer* **75(Suppl 1),** abstract no. 10.
46. Dhara, S. C. (1970) A rapid method for the synthesis of cis-[$Pt(NH_3)_2Cl_2$]. *Indian J. Chem.* **8,** 193–194.
47. Machover, D., Diaz-Rubio, E., de Gramont, A., Schilf, A., Gastiaburu, J. J., Brienza, S., et al. (1996) Two consecutive phase II trials of oxaliplatin (L-OHP) for treatment of patients with advanced colorectal carcinoma who were resistant to previous treatment with fluoropyrimidines. *Ann. Oncol.* **7,** 95–98.
48. Kizu, R., Nakanishi, T., Miyazaki, M., Tashiro, T., Noji, M., Matsuzawa, A., et al. (1996) An orally active antitumor cyclohexanediamine-Pt(IV) complex: trans, cis, cis-bis(n-valerato) (oxalato) (1R,2R-cyclohexanediamine) Pt(IV) *Anti-Cancer Drugs* **7,** 248–256.
49. Kizu, R. and Kidani, Y. (1998) Preclinical development of orally antitumor active oxaliplatin derivative, trans-(n-valerato)chloro (1r,2r-cyclohexanediamine) (oxalato) platinum(IV). *Ann. Oncol.* **2(Suppl 2),** abstract no. 148.

14 Polynuclear Charged Platinum Compounds as a New Class of Anticancer Agents

Toward a New Paradigm

Nicholas Farrell

CONTENTS

1. INTRODUCTION

Throughout this monograph, all the chemical structures of platinum-based anticancer agents currently in clinical trials have been directly related to cisplatin. Thus, while leaving group (X) and carrier ligand (amine) may be varied, all the structures are described by the simple formula *cis*-$[PtX_2(amine)_2]$. Polynuclear platinum compounds as represented by the dinuclear and trinuclear examples of Fig. 1 comprise a further unique class of anticancer agents with distinct chemical and biologic properties discrete from their mononuclear counterparts. In June, 1998, the first drug from this class entered Phase I clinical trials. The structure of this novel trinuclear platinum agent, BBR3464, is best described as two *trans*-$[PtCl(NH_3)_2]$ units linked by a bridging tetra-amine *trans*-$[Pt(NH_3)_2\{H_2N(CH_2)_6NH_2\}_2]$ (Fig. 1). The compound is the first genuinely new clinical drug not based on the "classical" cisplatin structure. The structure is notable for the presence of the central coordination sphere, which contributes to DNA affinity only through electrostatic and H-bonding interactions and the overall 4+ charge. The presence of at least two Pt coordination

From: *Platinum-Based Drugs in Cancer Therapy*
Edited by: L. R. Kelland and N. Farrell © Humana Press Inc., Totowa, NJ

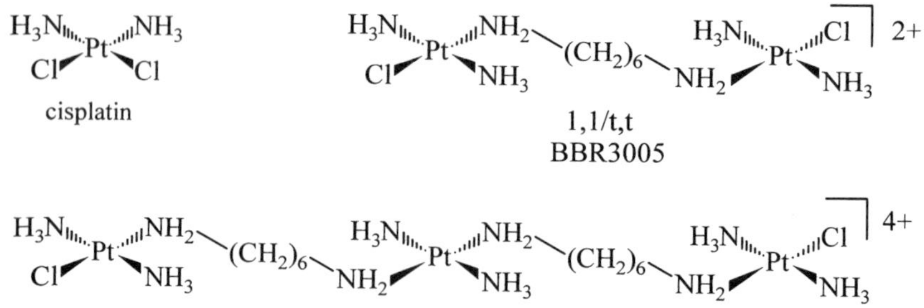

cisplatin

1,1/t,t
BBR3005

1,0,1/t,t,t
BBR3464

Fig. 1. Chemical structures of mononuclear (cisplatin), dinuclear (BBR3005), and trinuclear (BBR3464) anticancer agents. The abbreviation 1,1/t,t refers to the presence of 1 Cl on each Pt center *trans* to the diamine bridge. BBR numbers refer to codes from Boehringer Mannheim, Italy.

units capable of binding to DNA and the consequences of such DNA binding are further unique features of this class of drugs. With this advance the paradigm of cisplatin-based antitumor agents is altered.

The identification of BBR3464 as the lead compound, and eventually as the first clinical drug, arose from systematic studies on dinuclear and polynuclear compounds *(1)*. It was the initial hypothesis that development of platinum compounds structurally *dissimilar* to cisplatin may, by virtue of formation of different types of Pt-DNA adducts, lead to compounds with a spectrum of clinical activity genuinely complementary to the parent drug *(2,3)*. At time of writing, the only clinically used analog of cisplatin is carboplatin. It is still too early to say whether the promising preclinical profiles of other analogs will be reflected in clinical utility. Although there is still room for innovation within the basic cisplatin structure, it has been our repeated consideration that future discovery of clinically useful platinum agents is likely to arise from "nonclassical" structures. This chapter describes the studies leading to the choice of BBR3464 as clinical candidate.

2. HISTORY OF DEVELOPMENT

The dinuclear motif was first reported in 1988 and consisted of two *cis*-$[PtCl_2(NH_3)]$ units linked by a flexible diamine chain *(4)*. Thus, the ability to prepare two antitumor active moieties in the same molecule was shown (Fig. 2). Trinuclear compounds containing three cisplatin units were reported later in 1993 *(5)* (Fig. 2).

At the start of this work in 1988, the predominant goal for new drugs was activity in cisplatin-resistant cells and a broader profile of antitumor activity. Indeed, this goal remains essentially unchanged for any related drug devel-

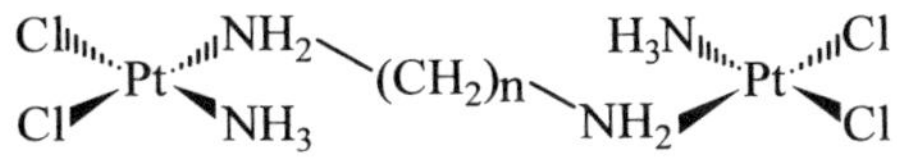

2,2/c,c

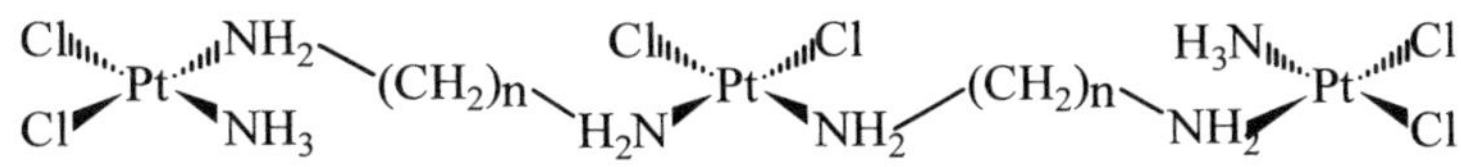

2,2,2/c,c,c

Fig. 2. Chemical structures of dinuclear and trinuclear platinum complexes containing cisplatin units.

opment project. The "original" 2,2 compounds showed high in vivo activity in cisplatin-resistant cells *(6)*. Mechanistic studies indicated that the compounds also produced a large percentage of DNA-DNA (Pt,Pt) interstrand crosslinks, by attachment of one Pt unit to each DNA strand *(7)*. Thus the structures of such adducts are expected to be significantly different from those of their mononuclear counterparts. The presence of two *cis*-$[PtCl_2(NH_3)]$ units in one compound means that the DNA binding is tetrafunctional, with concomitant increase in complexity. It is inherently obvious that only one Pt-Cl bond is necessary in each unit to produce (Pt,Pt) interstrand crosslinking. As a model, we therefore prepared the 1,1/t,t compound $[$*trans*-$\{PtCl(NH_3)_2\}_2H_2N(CH_2)_4NH_2]^{2+}$ *(8)*. Following the empirical structure-activity relationships for platinum, this compound would not be expected to be antitumor active, being charged and containing only one Pt-Cl bond in each coordination sphere. It was therefore very exciting that this compound also proved active in cisplatin-resistant cells *(9)*. Early unpublished results from a collaboration with Warner Lambert-Parke Davis showed in vivo activity. Representative values for murine L1210 leukemia (5.0 mg/kg, inj., ipip, d3,7,11) gave a median survival time of treated mice/median survival time of controls × 100 (T/C%) of 130 (L1210S) and 146 (L1210/DDP5) *(9)*. In B16 melanoma a T/C of 3.7 d with 1/10 survivors was achieved (4.0 mg/kg, inj., sc/iv, d1,5,9). With this remarkable finding of in vivo activity, we immediately realized that the structure represented a new class of compounds capable of bifunctional DNA-binding—except that the bifunctional binding came from the monofunctional substitution of both the coordination spheres (Fig. 3). Thus, we could compare the effects on chemical and biologic activity with the classical bifunctional DNA binding of the mononuclear *cis*- $[PtCl_2(NH_3)_2]$ *(10)*.

2.1. Structure-Activity Relationships in the 1,1/t,t Series

EARLY RELATIONSHIPS: CHAIN LENGTH AND STERIC EFFECTS

The basic dinuclear unit is open to many systematic changes, e.g., in the coordination sphere and the geometry around the platinum, as well as the nature of the ligands in the coordination sphere. Trifunctional, tetrafunctional, and bifunctional DNA binding agents are all easily accessible *(11,12)*. For the sake of brevity this discussion will be restricted to bifunctional agents, i.e., those containing only one Pt-Cl bond on each coordination unit. For equivalent coordination spheres, the overall structure is best given by the formula $[\{PtX_nL_{3-n}\}_2(diamine)]^{(2-n)+}$. (X is usually Cl and L usually NH_3; n = 1 or 2) *(9)*. The nature of the bridging group may also be changed and examined for steric effects and chain length. Thus, a very wide range of compounds is immediately available for evaluation. These systematic studies have been performed over the years and have now been summarized in a parallel review *(13)*. This survey revealed that the so-called 1,1/t,t series gave consistently high antitumor activity in cisplatin-resistant cells and so development concentrated on this series.

BBR3464, A NOVEL TRINUCLEAR AGENT

Fig. 3 shows the range of substitutions made on the basic structure. Antitumor activity is highly dependent on chain length. The 1,1/t,t $n = 6$ compound BBR3005 [*trans*-$\{PtCl(NH_3)_2\}_2\mu$-$H_2N(CH_2)_6NH_2]^{2+}$(Fig. 1) was initially selected for detailed evaluation. However, lung toxicity precluded its advancement. Models showed that the 1,1/t,t $n = 6$ compound could easily span a four-base pair segment of DNA. To improve water solubility and to improve DNA affinity further for long-range crosslinking, some H-bonding capacity in the backbone is desirable to react with the negatively charged DNA backbone. This has now been achieved in two ways—by use of a central platinum "tetraamine" coordination sphere and by use of polyamine linkers.

In fact, the chemical synthesis of dinuclear complexes automatically gives rise to some trinuclear species. The synthesis of a 1,1/t,t compound such as BBR3005 is achieved by monofunctional activation of *trans*-$[PtCl_2(NH_3)_2]$, followed by linking to free diamine *(14)*:

$$2\ trans\text{-}[PtCl(DMF)(NH_3)_2]^+ + H_2N(CH_2)_6NH_2 \rightarrow [\{trans\text{-}PtCl(NH_3)_2\}_2\mu\text{-}H_2N(CH_2)_6NH_2]^{2+}$$

In general, linear trinuclear platinum compounds are prepared by linking a precursor *central (c)* molecule, Pt(c) to two equivalents of a *target* terminal platinum coordination sphere, Pt(t):

$$2\ Pt(t) + Pt(c) \rightarrow Pt(t) - Pt(c) - Pt(t)$$

Thus, the general preparation involves synthesis of a suitable precursor containing two monoprotected diamines followed by treatment with acid to give

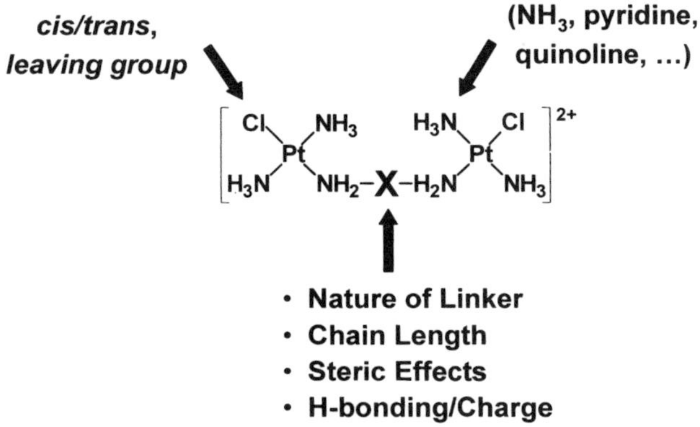

Fig. 3. Systematic modification of the 1,1/t,t structure to optimize antitumor activity. See ref. *13* for details.

the protonated amine $RNH_3^+Cl^-$ incorporated into Pt(c) followed by reaction with two equivalents of an appropriate target molecule Pt(t) to afford the desired product *(5)*. Specifically for BBR3464:

$$2\ trans\text{-}[PtCl(DMF)(NH_3)_2]^+ + trans\text{-}[Pt(NH_3)_2\{H_2N(CH_2)_6NH_3\}_2]^{4+}$$

$$\rightarrow trans\text{-}[\{trans\text{-}PtCl(NH_3)_2\}_2\mu\text{-}\{H_2N(CH_2)_6NH_2)\}_2Pt(NH_3)_2\}]^{4+}\ (BBR3464)$$

Much to our delight, further enhancement of antitumor activity was obtained with 3+ and 4+ charged compounds (Tables 1 and 13). A wide range of compounds is again available. The nature of the coordination spheres may be changed readily, and the homologs BBR3499 (1,0,1/t,c,t) and BBR3573 (1,0,1/c,t,c) are readily prepared (Fig. 4).

Polyamine-Linked Dinuclear Platinum Complexes

A second method of incorporating charge along a diamine backbone is to use polyamines as linkers. This was achieved through synthesis of *dinuclear* platinum complexes with hydrogen-bonding ligands spermine (total charge 4+) and spermidine (total charge 3+) linkers (Fig. 5 and 6). Platination to the terminal NH_2 group is achieved by selective blocking and deblocking of the secondary nitrogens. Designed synthesis of dinuclear platinum complexes in this manner mimics the essential biologic features of BBR3464 *(13,15)*. Note that in all chemical schemes the anions are omitted for clarity. Usually the compounds are prepared as nitrate or chloride salts. The total charges on the compounds reflect the need to neutralize not only the cationic Pt-Cl coordination spheres but also the central platinum (trinuclear compounds) or amine (dinuclear polyamine).

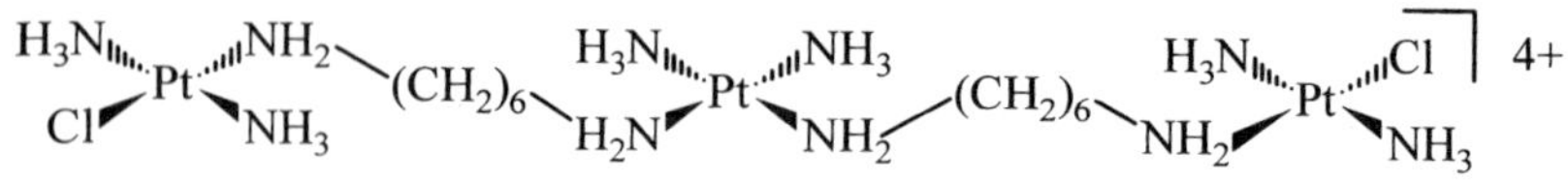

1,0,1/t,c,t
BBR 3499

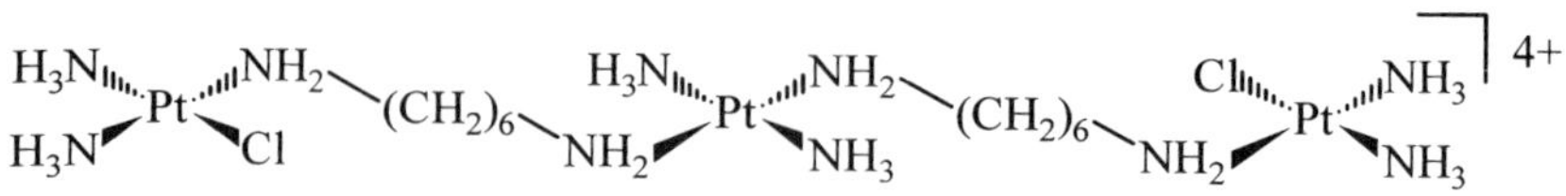

1,0,1/c,t,c
BBR 3573

Fig. 4. Chemical structures of the congeners of BBR3464, where geometry around the platinum centers is varied.

3. BIOLOGIC ACTIVITY

Table 1 shows selected but representative biologic activity for the dinuclear and trinuclear complexes of Figs. 4–6 *(16,17)*. The biologic testing was performed by Boehringer Mannheim Italia in Monza through licensing and sponsored research agreements. In May, 1997, Roche acquired Boehringer Mannheim. The Monza operation is now a spin-off company, Novuspharma, wholly owned by Roche. As of time of writing, all licensing arrangments are now the responsibility of F. Hoffmann-La Roche Ltd., whereas Novuspharma will continue to lead the clinical development.

The approach to drug evaluation in this project has been to obtain appropriate in vitro and in vivo pharmacologic data on effective and toxic doses in murine L1210 leukemia and its cisplatin-resistant subline. There is considerable historical precedent for cisplatin in both cases. A second phase involves a similar study in a human ovarian tumor line such as A2780 followed by in vivo studies on selected human solid tumors such as the LX-1 lung tumor. Finally, lead compounds undergo exhaustive testing on a range of common human xenografts. The LX-1 is a non-small cell lung cancer tumor characterized as mutant p53 and is historically insensitive to cisplatin. Table 1 shows that the charged compounds uniformly display a remarkable potency. Early empirical structure-activity relationships for cisplatin stressed the need for neutrality. This is clearly not necessary, and all the charged species show high activity at *lower* doses than cisplatin. Indeed, whereas the vast majority of direct cisplatin analogs require higher doses to achieve similar therapeutic effects, the polynuclear platinum complexes are distinguished as a class by the generally low doses required.

Table 1
Cytotoxicity and Antitumor Activity of Polynuclear Platinum Complexes in Murine Leukemia Sensitive (L1210) and Resistant to CDDP (L1210/CDDP) and in the LX-1 Human Tumor Xenograft[a]

	In vitro IC_{50} (μg/mL)		*In vivo (L1210/CDDP only)[b]*		*In vivo LX-1*	
Compound	*L1210*	*L1210/ CDDP*	*Dose (mg/kg/d)*	*T/C%*	*Dose (mg/kg/d)*	*TWI%*
BBR 3537	0.76	4.40	2	100	—	—
BBR 3571	0.042	0.0062	0.25	261	0.25	83
BBR 3535	0.55	1.1	1	161,178	0.7	85
BBR 3610	0.0012	0.0011	0.025	457 (3/7)	—	—
BBR 3611	0.0005	0.00041	0.006	256	—	—
BBR 3005	2.3	1.8	4.5	133	3	60
BBR 3464	0.116	0.093	0.25	239,389 (5/16)	0.3	73
Cisplatin[c]	0.9	8.3	6	110 (100–122)	4	38

[a]See Figs. 1, 4, 5, and 6 for structures. All compounds were dissolved in NaCl 0.9% and further diluted in complete culture medium. IC_{50}, inhibiting concentration 50% of cellular growth after 48 h of drug exposure; TWI, tumor weight inhibition.

[b]10^5 cells ip into CD2F1 male mice. Treatment ip on d 1, 5, and 9 tumor transplantation (d 0). All compounds were dissolved in saline just before use. T/C, median survival time of treated mice/median survival time of controls × 100. Long-term survivors are in parentheses.

[c]Mean of 198 experiments.

Data adapted from refs. *16–18*.

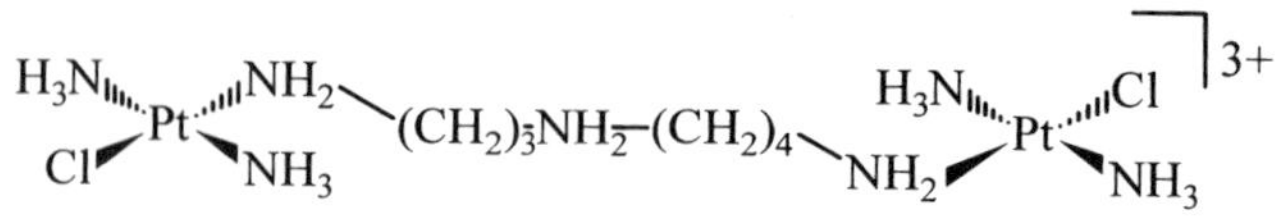

BBR3571

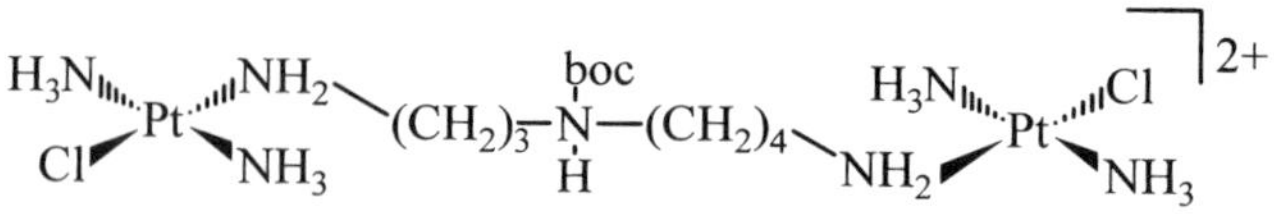

BBR3537

Fig. 5. Chemical structures of dinuclear spermidine-bridged derivatives. BOC = tert-butoxycarbonyl.

To summarize the data:

1. Geometry of coordination spheres in trinuclear compounds affects potency. The "expanded" BBR3464 (1,0,1/t,t,t) is more potent than either the 1,0,1/c,t,c or 1,0,1/t,c,t homologs. Interestingly, the central *cis* unit of BBR3499 results in substantially reduced cytotoxicity.

2. Designed synthesis of polyamine backbones gives a series of exceptionally potent compounds that successfully mimic the biologic activity of BBR3464. Activity within this series is affected by both overall charge and chain length of the polyamine linker. The presence of one or two central charged $-NH_2$- groups appears essential to give compounds with high cytotoxicity and potency. Compare the pair BBR3571/3537—in the latter case the blocking Boc group is still present on the central nitrogen. This causes a reduction in charge (Fig. 5) and also potency.

3. In the spermine family, overall chain length appears to be important—the long-chain compounds BBR3610 (5,4,5, where 5,4,5 represents the number of carbon atoms between each amine) and BBR3611 (6,2,6) were designed to present the same distance between Pt-Cl units as BBR3464. Both species are cytotoxic at *nanomolar* concentrations and significantly more potent than the "parent" (3,4,3) spermine BBR3535.

4. The biologic activity in human tumors such as LX-1 is nothing short of exceptional. Maximum tolerated doses parallel the in vitro cytotoxicity—the more cytotoxic, the lower the effective dose needed. In LX-1, both spermidine (BBR3571) and spermine (BBR3535) compounds show activity with maximal tumor weight inhibition (TWI%) of 83 and 85, respectively, at the maximum

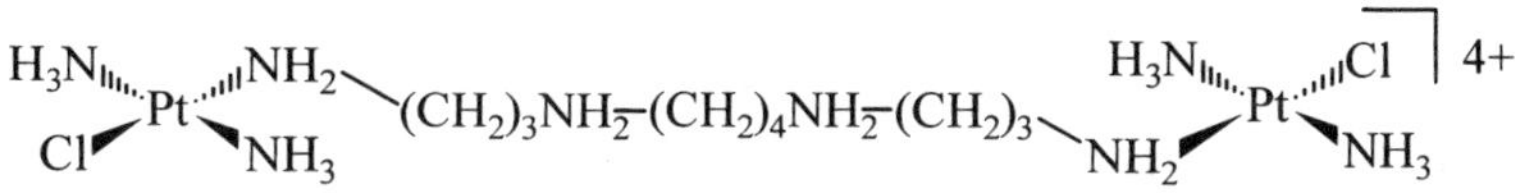

BBR 3535

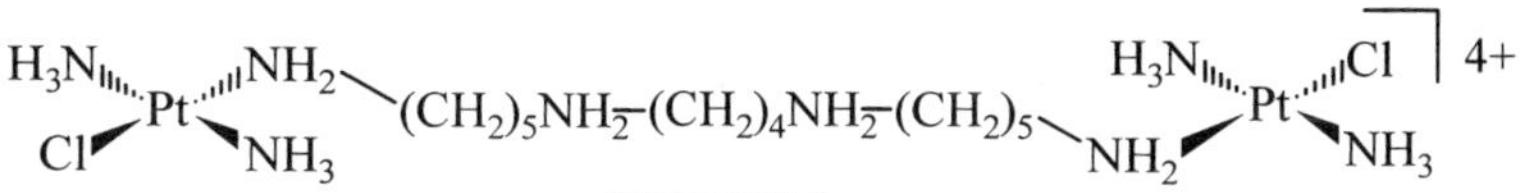

BBR 3610

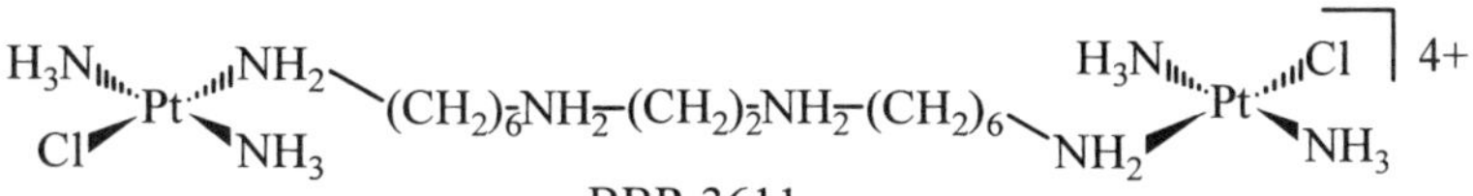

BBR 3611

Fig. 6. Chemical structures of spermine-bridged derivatives. BBR3610 and BBR3611 were designed to present the same distance between the terminal Pt-Cl units as in BBR3464.

tolerated doses. The LX-1 tumor is historically insensitive to cisplatin intervention (Table 1), yet the tumor is sensitive to all dinuclear and trinuclear compounds tested. So we can now use activity in LX-1 as a differentiator for further development of polynuclear complexes—a much more rigorous "cutoff" selection criterion than either L1210 or even A2780!

5. Introduction of charge in the linker backbone significantly improves potency over the "original" straight-chain diamines such as BBR3005. An important point to note is that in our examination, the *profile* of antitumor activity of a simple dinuclear compound such as BBR3005 (1,1/t,t $n = 6$; Fig. 1) is in general similar to that of BBR3464 (activity in cisplatin-resistant cell lines, enhanced activity in solid tumors classified as mutant p53 such as LX-1). What differs is the effective dose and potency—in general, BBR3005 is active at doses similar to cisplatin, a remarkable enough effect for a 2+ compound. The generation of 3+ and 4+ compounds results in effective doses of an order of magnitude less than that of cisplatin.

3.1. BBR3464, A Phase I Clinical Drug

The first compound to be selected for exhaustive tests was BBR3464. The profile of preclinical activity of BBR3464 is characterized by activity in human tumor (e.g., ovarian) xenografts resistant to cisplatin and alkylating agents; a high activity in a broad spectrum of human tumors commonly insensitive to

Table 2
Comparison at Maximum Tolerated Dose of BBR 3464 (0.2–0.4 mg/kg) and Cisplatin (3–6 mg/kg) After iv Repeated Treatment on Staged Tumors[a]

Clinical parameter[a]	*BBR 3464*	*Cisplatin*
Resistance, TWI < 50%	0	9 (4 NSCLC, 2 ovarian, 2 gastric, 1 prostatic)
Relative Resistance, TWI 50–70%	3 (1 NSCLC, 1 gastric, 1 prostatic)	7 (2 SCLC, 2 NSCLC, 2 ovarian, 1 bladder)
Sensitivity, TWI > 70%	15 (3 SCLC, 5 NSCLC, 5 ovarian, 1 gastric, 1 bladder)	2 (1 ovarian, 1 SCLC)

[a]TWI %, tumor weight inhibition compared with controls; SCLC, small cell lung cancer; NSCLC, non-small cell lung cancer. The clinical parameter refers to the fact that clinical resistance, relative resistance, and sensitivity are most likely to be seen at these TWI levels. Thus, BBR 3464 is significantly more potent than cisplatin—good tumor sensitivity was observed in 15/18 cases for BBR 3464.

Data from ref. *18*.

chemotherapeutic intervention (e.g., non-small cell lung, gastric) and characterized as p53-mutant. Table 2 summarizes the overall profile from 18 human tumors tested *(18)*. The data show a broad spectrum response of tumors to BBR3464, with 15/18 tumors indicative of a clinical response.

Table 3 shows the activity of a subset of the tumors evaluated by Dr. F. Zunino and selected for p53 status *(19)*. The p53 protein is recognized as an important cell regulatory element necessary for cell cycle arrest and apoptosis induction. Wild-type p53 function plays a critical role in cellular response to drug-induced DNA damage, although there is no simple relationship between DNA damage and p53 functional status *(20)*. The new effective agent displays remarkably high activity in all cases. In five of six cases the TWI is indicative of clinical sensitivity. So, not only is the agent in tumors with both acquired and inherent resistance to cisplatin but it also maintains activity in tumors with mutant p53. The activity data were sufficiently exciting that, on successful passage of regulatory safety tests on animals, BBR3464 was advanced to Phase I clinical trials.

4. CELLULAR PHARMACOLOGY OF BBR3464

The design and development of polynuclear platinum complexes has been predicated to a large degree on their different DNA binding profiles in comparison with that of cisplatin. Pharmacokinetic factors such as cellular uptake and cellular Pt-DNA binding also dictate to a large degree the efficacy of any drug in vivo. To understand better the cellular basis of the efficacy of BBR3464

Table 3
Activity and p53 Status of Human Tumors Treated with Platinum Compounds

Tumor model/type	*Drug[a] (mg/kg)*	*TWI%[b]*	*Resistance*	*p53 Status*
POVD/ DDP (SCLC)	Cisplatin 6	70	Acquired	Mutant
	3464 0.4	93		
Calu-3 (NSCLC)	Cisplatin 6	60	Intrinsic	Mutant
	3464 0.3	92		
LX-1 (NSCLC)	Cisplatin 4	38	Intrinsic	Mutant
	3464 0.3	73		
POCS (SCLC)	Cisplatin 6	56	Intrinsic	Mutant
	3464 0.4	92		
IGROV/DDP (Ovarian)	Cisplatin 6	68	Acquired	Mutant
	3464 0.3	80		

[a]Tumor fragments sc into CD1 nu/nu female mice (d 0). Treatment iv on d 1, 8, and 15 when tumor weight reached an average of 100 mg. All compounds were dissolved in saline before use.

[b]TWI% [tumor weight inhibition (on d 22)]: 100 − (mean relative tumor weight of treated mice/mean relative tumor weight of courses × 100). Relative tumor weight is determined as Tx/To where T is the tumor weight at the start of treatment (d 1), and Tx is the tumor weight at d X.

Adapted from ref. *19.*

against cisplatin-resistant tumors, cellular pharmacologic studies have been carried out on a series of cell lines. The cell lines studied to date include murine L1210 leukemia, human ovarian A2780 and SKOV-3, and the human osteosarcoma U2-OS cell lines. In all but SKOV-3, sublines have been rendered cisplatin resistant by continuous exposure. The SKOV-3 cell line is intrinsically insensitive to cisplatin. Common cellular pharmacology parameters that are easily measured include total platinum uptake, total Pt DNA binding, and the quantitation of DNA-DNA interstrand crosslinks. In this contribution we will summarize principally the data from the human osteosarcoma cell lines *(21)*. The conclusions, however, also apply to the other cell lines studied *(22)*, and a consistent picture of the cellular pharmacology of BBR3464 is emerging.

4.1. Cytotoxicity and Cellular Accumulation

Cytotoxicity of BBR 3464 and cisplatin on U2-OS and U2-OS/Pt cells was assessed after a 1-h drug exposure to allow comparison with other cellular uptake and DNA damage data. In the sensitive cell line, IC_{50} values were 13.6 ± 2.7 and 0.89 ± 0.57 μ*M* for cisplatin and BBR3464, respectively. A complete lack of cross-resistance was found for BBR3464 in the U2-OS/Pt cells, which presented a fivefold resistance to cisplatin. Comparison of cellular drug accumulation was performed following the same exposure time of the cytotoxicity experiments. Exposure of cells to drug concentrations ranging from 10 to 90 μg/mL indicated that cisplatin accumulation was linear in cisplatin-sensitive and -resistant cells. An approximate 1.5- to 2-fold decreased cisplatin accumulation was found in the U2-OS/Pt cells throughout the range of concentrations used for both cisplatin and BBR3464. The extent of BBR 3464 accumulation in cisplatin-resistant cells was substantially higher (four to fivefold) than that achieved by cisplatin. However, the order of magnitude of platinum accumulation was comparable when the two cell lines were exposed to equitoxic concentrations of BBR 3464 and cisplatin.

These results are mirrored by the dinuclear platinum-polyamine compounds and in other cell lines *(23)*. Table 4 shows data for two human ovarian cancer cell lines (A2780 and SKOV-3) for BBR3464 and the spermidine compound BBR3571. These cell lines were chosen because A2780 is wild-type p53 and SKOV-3 is p53 null (confirmed in our laboratories). The results are instructive. First, there is little difference between sensitivity of A2780 and SKOV-3 to the charged polynuclear complexes but a large differential in response to cisplatin. The results suggest that cytotoxic and therapeutic effects of BBR3464 may be independent of p53 function. Second, cellular uptake is again enhanced for the charged compounds, a dramatic rebuttal of the early concept that platinum agents should be neutral to enter cells. Note again the similarity between the trinuclear agent and the spermidine compound BBR3571. However, even though there is a a 5- to 10-fold enhanced uptake over cisplatin, this by itself does not explain the very improved cytotoxicity over cisplatin.

4.2. DNA-Bound Platinum and Formation of Interstrand Crosslinks

A further determinant of cytotoxicity is the amount of platinum actually bound to intracellular DNA, which reflects both the inherent affinity of the drug for DNA and the effect of competing metabolic processes such as binding to plasma proteins and intracellular thiols such as glutathione. Measurement of DNA-bound platinum after 1 h of drug exposure revealed that the amount of platination was higher in U2-OS and U2-OS/Pt cells exposed to BBR 3464 than in the same cell lines exposed to cisplatin.

Obviously, quantitation of DNA-bound platinum does not reflect the structural nature of the DNA adducts. The presence of DNA-DNA interstrand crosslinks can be easily assayed by the technique of alkaline elution. The profile for interstrand crosslink formation by BBR3464 is similar to that previously observed for dinuclear platinum compounds and is distinctly different from that of cisplatin *(12)*. It is well established that maximal interstrand crosslinking for cisplatin occurs from 6 to 8 h following drug incubation. In contrast, maximal interstrand crosslinking for BBR 3464 occurs immediately (i.e., $t = 0$ after drug removal) and remains consistent throughout the period studied. Most importantly, little difference in ICL frequency was found in

Table 4
Cytotoxicity and Cellular Uptake of Two Human Ovarian Tumor Cell Lines Treated with Platinum Compounds

	IC_{50}, μM (±SE) 2-h exposure		*2-h Accumulation 5-μM dose (attamol/cell/μM Pt compound)*	
Compound	*A2780*	*SKOV-3*	*A2780*	*SKOV-3*
Cisplatin	1.20 (0.38)	81 (15)	1.0	1.0
BBR3571	0.007 (0.002)	0.03	4.2	5.2
BBR3464	0.018 (0.007)	0.02 (0.01)	12	10.2

cisplatin-sensitive and -resistant cells exposed to BBR 3464. However, the amount of ICL relative to cisplatin did not match the in vitro experiments outlined in Section 5. Surprisingly, the amount of ICL is about the same for both agents. However, the interstrand crosslinks of BBR3464 persist longer than those of cisplain. This result is perfectly consistent with the structural differences expected for both types of interstrand crosslink and suggest that the (Pt,Pt) adducts are less susceptible to repair.

4.3. Biologic Properties of the U2-OS /Pt System

The cisplatin-resistant phenotype of U2-OS/Pt was associated with multiple alterations, including reduced cisplatin accumulation, reduced interstrand crosslink formation and DNA platination, microsatellite instability, and reduced expression of the DNA mismatch repair protein PMS2. A deficiency in some components of the mismatch repair system has been implicated in resistance to cisplatin since this system is capable of recognizing cisplatin-induced DNA lesions, probably functioning as a sensor for triggering apoptosis. The lack of cross-resistance of U2OS/Pt to BBR 3464 suggests that the integrity of mismatch repair systems is not a determinant of cellular sensitivity to the multinuclear platinum complex. The cellular pharmacology results obtained to date support the hypothesis that BBR 3464 overcomes multiple mechanisms of cisplatin resistance including alterations in DNA mismatch repair. The cellular pharmacology studies indicate that the cellular basis of lack of cross-resistance is related to a different mechanism of DNA interaction rather than the ability to overcome defects in accumulation or decreased adduct formation.

5. DNA BINDING OF BBR3464

The interactions of bifunctional polynuclear platinum complexes with target DNA are unlike those of any DNA-damaging agent in clinical use. The profile of antitumor activity is also different. The question remains—how are they

Table 5
Summary of DNA Binding of Trinuclear BBR3464 and Comparison with DNA Binding of Dinuclear BBR3005 and Mononuclear Cisplatin

	BBR3464	*BBR3005*	*Cisplatin*
DNA binding ($t_{1/2}$)	40 min	200–300 min	~240 min
Decrease of EtBr fluorescence	Strong	Strong	Medium
% Interstrand cross-links/adduct (after 48 h)	20	70–90	6
Unwinding angle/adduct	14°	10–14°	13°
Z-DNA induction	Yes	Yes	No
Inhibition of antibodies			
AB_{cis}	No	No	Yes
Ab_{trans}	Yes	Yes	No

Adapted from ref. *25* and references therein.

connected? The plausible explanation of the hypersensitivity of human tumors with mutant p53 to BBR3464 is that apoptosis induced by the drug is not mediated by p53. The "bypassing" of the p53 pathway may have its origin in the novel DNA binding modes of BBR3464. Likewise, the studies reported in the previous section also support the concept that the origins of the different biologic responses of cisplatin and BBR3464 lie in the different DNA binding of the two agents.

The general outline of BBR3464-DNA binding is shown in Table 5 and is similar to that previously described for dinuclear complexes *(10,24,25)*. The high charge on BBR3464 facilitates rapid binding to DNA with a $t_{1/2}$ of approx 40 min, significantly faster than the neutral cisplatin. The kinetics of DNA binding of charged platinum compounds is significantly greater than for cisplatin. For a 2-h incubation (20 μM compound) on calf thymus DNA the relative amounts of Pt bound are 7.3:1.8:1 for BBR3464 (4+ charge), BBR3005 (2+), and cisplatin, respectively (even after allowing for the 3:2:1 Pt ratio in the compounds). The rapid binding of BBR3464 could affect sequence specificity—the high charge could lead to initial electrostatic interactions very different from those in small molecules such as cisplatin and the alkylating agents, leading to enhanced sequence specificity. BBR3464 produces an unwinding angle of 14° in negatively supercoiled pSP73 plasmid DNA, indicative of bifunctional DNA binding. Quantitation of interstrand DNA-DNA crosslinking in plasmid pSP73DNA linearized by *Eco*R1 indicated that approximately 20% of the DNA was interstrand crosslinked. Although this is significantly higher than the value for cisplatin, it is, interestingly, lower than that for dinuclear platinum compounds such as BBR3005. Either the presence of charge in the linker backbone

5'-T G A A T T C $\mathbf{G_i}$ A G C T C G G T A-3'

3'-A C T T A A $\mathbf{G_{iii}}$ C T C $\mathbf{G_{ii}}$ A G C C A T-5'

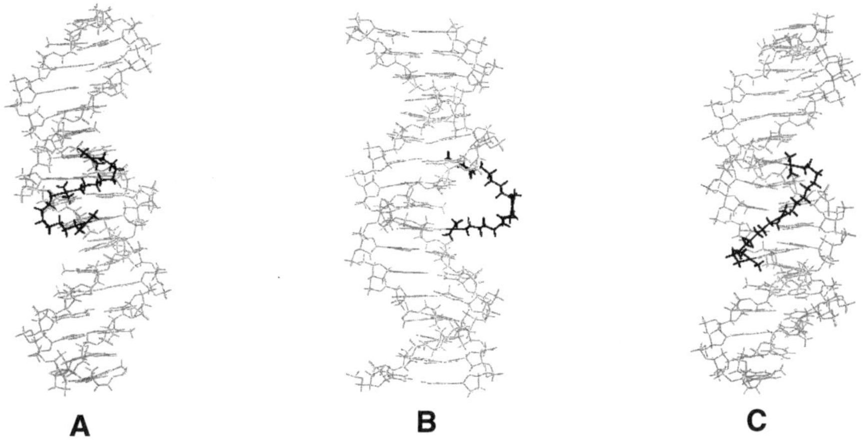

Figure 7. Models for long-range intrastrand and interstrand crosslinks by BBR3464 on DNA. **(A, B)** Two conformations of a 1,4 interstrand crosslink formed between $\mathbf{G_i}$ and $\mathbf{G_{ii}}$. **(C)** A 1,5 intrastrand crosslink formed between $\mathbf{G_{ii}}$ and $\mathbf{G_{iii}}$. See ref. *25* for details.

or the increased distance between platinating moieties may contribute to this relatively decreased ability of BBR3464 to induce DNA-DNA interstrand crosslinking. This result matches that from the cellular systems above.

The question of formation of interstrand vs intratrand crosslinks merits further attention. Sequence specificity studies *(25)* showed that a fragment of pSP73 plasmid contained polymerase stop sites at the guanine residues within the sequence indicated in Fig. 7. This is taken to mean that BBR3464 is bound in or at these sites. The sequence was analyzed considering only guanine-Pt bonding in the 5′-5′ direction, in agreement with previous studies *(26)*. The possible 1,4 interstrand (Fig. 7A and B) and 1,5-intrastrand crosslinks (Fig. 7C) were modeled. These initial calculations indicated that the long-range intrastrand and interstrand crosslinks are almost equally favored. Whether this is due to chain length of BBR3464 being so flexible or the charge along the backbone is yet to be determined. Fluorescence experiments with ethidium bromide were consistent with the formation of long-range delocalized lesions on DNA produced by BBR3464. Nevertheless, it is appropriate to consider how effects from both these limiting adduct structures may contribute to cytotoxicity.

The (Pt,Pt) interstrand crosslink is implicated in cytotoxicity and the ability to irreversibly induce the B $\rightarrow$ Z conformational change is also a feature of the most potent agents *(27)*. DNA sequences that have the potential to form

Z-DNA have been found within the mammalian cell genome including transcriptional regulatory regions and DNA replication origins. The induction of Z-DNA within the cell would have serious consequences with regard to transcription and DNA replication. Finally, immunochemical analysis confirmed the unique nature of the DNA adducts formed by BBR3464. Competitive ELISA showed that antibodies raised to cisplatin-adducted DNA (Ab_{cis}) did not recognize DNA modified by BBR3464. In contrast, DNA modified by BBR3464 inhibited the binding of antibodies raised to transplatin-adducted DNA (Ab_{trans}). In summary, the results point to a unique profile of DNA binding for BBR3464, strengthening the originial hypothesis that modification of DNA binding in manners distinct from that of cisplatin will also lead to a distinct and unique profile of antitumor activity.

6. SUMMARY

Chemotherapy for the treatment of cancer has its beginnings in the late 1940s with the introduction of the first DNA alkylating agent, nitrogen mustard. The most recent alkylating agent to enter clinical trials was ifosfamide, in 1990. Chemotherapy handbooks list the approximately dozen approved drugs and their recommended uses. It is also difficult to predict whether a similar array of platinum agents will be listed in 30 years. Many of the alkylating agents in the clinical armamentarium were developed before the advances of molecular biology and the increased sophistication of structure oriented drug design. The sequential development (described by Kelland in the previous chapter) of cisplatin, carboplatin, the orally active JM-216, and indeed ZO-473 is an excellent example of sustained development within a structural series.

The differences and similarities we will observe between the polynuclear platinum agents and the "classical" cisplatin compounds as they hopefully proceed through the clinic will add to our understanding of drug discovery and design for further rational approaches to the drug treatment of cancer. A prototypical new drug such as BBR3464 may well give rise to at least a "second-generation" less toxic derivative as well as an orally active agent. The results descibed here show that a family of dinuclear compounds similar to BBR3464 can be achieved through use of polyamine linkers. Just as a molecule of structure [*cis*-$PtX_2(amine)_2$] is now *expected* to be antitumor active with predictable DNA binding characteristics [high proportion of d(GpG) intrastrand crosslinks, few interstrand crosslinks, bending of DNA into major groove], the charged compounds described in this review are now *expected* to reproduce high antitumor activity, activity in p53 mutant tumors, and a predictable DNA binding profile.

The mechanistic importance of the polynuclear platinum drugs is that we must now reevaluate the classic structure-activity relationships. It has been possible by suitable coordination chemistry to develop a distinct new class of antitumor agents. It is yet feasible that further classes of platinum-based drugs with unique DNA binding characteristics and appropriate pharmacology may be developed as clinical agents. The ability to modify biologic response by suitable coordination chemistry on DNA is unmatched in organic chemistry and represents a significant contribution of inorganic chemistry to medicine.

ACKNOWLEDGMENTS

It is a great pleasure to recognize the excellent contributions of collaborators past and present. In particular, the group from Boehringer Mannheim Italy deserves tremendous credit for their successful clinical development of BBR3464. Collaborations with the groups of Dr. Franco Zunino and Viktor Brabec are also gratefully acknowledged.

REFERENCES

1. Farrell, N. (1996) DNA binding of dinuclear platinum complexes, in *Advances in DNA Sequence Specific Agents*, vol. 2 (Hurley, L. H., and Chaires, J. B., eds.), JAI, New Haven, CT, pp. 187–216.
2. Farrell, N. (1995) DNA binding and chemistry of dinuclear platinum complexes. *Comments Inorg. Chem.* **16,** 373–389.
3. Farrell, N. (1993) Non-classical platinum antitumor complexes. Perspectives for design and development of new drugs complementary to cisplatin. *Cancer Invest.* **11,** 578–589.
4. Farrell, N. P., de Almeida, S. G., and Skov, K. A. (1988) Bisplatinum complexes containing two *cis*-Pt(amine)$_2$ units. Synthesis and initial DNA-binding studies. *J. Am. Chem. Soc.* **110,** 5018–5019.
5. Qu, Y., Appleton, T. G., Hoeschele, J. D., and Farrell, N. (1993) Cisplatin as synthon. Synthesis and characterization of triplatinum complexes containing three cis-Pt(amine)$_2$ units linked in a linear fashion. *Inorg. Chem.* **32,** 2591–2593.
6. Kraker, A. J., Hoeschele, J. D., Elliott, W. L., Showalter, H. D. H., Sercel, A. D., and Farrell, N. (1992) Anticancer activity in murine and human tumor cell lines of bis(platinum) complexes incorporating straight-chain aliphatic diamine linker groups. *J. Med. Chem.* **35,** 4526–4532.
7. Roberts, J. D. van Houten, B., Qu, Y., and Farrell, N. P. (1989) Interaction of novel bis(platinum) complexes with DNA. *Nucleic Acids Res.* **17,** 9719–9733.
8. Farrell, N., Qu, Y., Feng, L., and Van Houten, B. (1990) A comparison of chemical reactivity, cytotoxicity, interstrand cross-linking and DNA sequence specificity of bis(platinum) complexes containing monodentate or bidentate coordination spheres with their monomeric analogues. *Biochemistry* **29,** 9522–9531.
9. Hoeschele, J. D., Kraker, A. J., Qu, Y., Van Houten, B., and Farrell, N. (1990) Bis(platinum) complexes, in *Chemistry, Antitumor Activity and DNA-Binding: Molecular Basis of Specificity in Nucleic Acid-Drug Interactions* (Pullman, B. and Jortner, J., eds.), Kluwer Academic, Dordrecht, pp. 301–321.
10. Farrell, N., Appleton, T. G., Qu, Y., Roberts, J. D., Soares Fontes, A. P., Skov, K. A., et al. (1995) Effects of geometric isomerism and ligand substitution in bifunctional dinuclear platinum complexes on binding properties and conformational changes in DNA. *Biochemistry* **34,** 15480–15486.
11. Farrell, N. (1997) DNA binding of non-classical platinum antitumor complexes, in *Interaction of Anticancer Agents with Nucleic Acids*, vol. 3 (Palumbo, M., ed.), JAI, New Haven, CT, pp. 179–199.

12. Farrell, N., Qu, Y., and Roberts, J. D. (1999) Multifunctional DNA-binding metal complexes, in *Topics in Biological Inorganic Chemistry* (Clarke, M. J., and Sadler, P. J. eds.), New York, Springer, pp. 100–115.
13. Farrell, N., Bierbach, U., Qu, Y., Valsecchi, M., and Menta, E. (1999) Structure activity relationships in bifunctional dinuclear and trinuclear platinum anticancer agents, in *Cisplatin: Chemistry and Biochemistry of a Leading Anticancer Drug* (Lippert, B., ed.), Verlag, Basel, pp. 479–496.
14. Qu, Y. and Farrell, N. (1992) The product of the reaction of trans-diamminedichloroplatinum(II) with diamines is dependent on chain length. Example of a bridging ethylenediaminc and formation of a novel trans-chelated structure with 1,5-pentanediamine. *Inorg. Chem.* **31,** 930–932.
15. Rauter, H., Di Domenico R., Menta, E., Oliva, A., Qu, Y., and Farrell, N. (1997) Selective platination of biologically relevant polyamines. Linear coordinating spermidine and spermine as amplifying linkers in dinuclear platinum complexes. *Inorg. Chem.* **36,** 3919–3927.
16. Rauter, H., DiDomenico, R., Menta, E., Da Re, G., De Cillis, G., Conti, M., et al. (1998) Chemistry and biological activity of polyamines as amplifying linkers in dinuclear platinum complexes. *Proc. AACR* **39,** 1096.
17. Menta, E., Farrell, N., Valsecchi, M., Conti, M., Piazzoni, L., Randisi, E., et al. (1999) Antitumor evaluation of linker-modified trinuclear platinum complexes congeners of the phase I clinical agent BBR3464, in *Proceedings of the 8th ISPCCC, Meeting,* Oxford, UK. Abstract 1.P13
18. Manzotti, C., Torriani, D., Randisi, E., De Giorgi, M., Pezzoni, G., Menta, E., et al. (1997) Antitumor activity profile of a novel charged trinuclear platinum complex endowed with efficacy against human and murine tumor models with acquired or intrinsic cisplatin resistance. *Proc. AACR* **38,** 2080
19. Pratesi, G., Righetti, S. C., Supino, R., Polizzi, D., Manzotti, C., Giuliania, F. C., et al. (1999) High antitumor activity of a novel multinuclear platinum complex against cisplatin-resistant p53 mutant human tumors. *Br. J. Cancer*, **80,** 1912–1919.
20. Harris, C. C. and Hollstein M. (1993) Clinical implications of the p53 tumor suppressor gene *N. Engl. J. Med.* **88,** 1318–1327.
21. Perego, P., Caserini, C., Gatti, L., Carenini, N., Romanelli, S., Supino, R., et al. (1999) A novel trinuclear platinum complex overcomes cisplatin resistance in an osteosarcoma cell system. *Mol. Pharmacol.,* **55,** 528–534.
22. Roberts, J. D., Peroutka, J., and Farrell, N. (1999) Cellular Pharmacology of Di and Trinuclear Platinum Complexes. *J. Inorg. Biochem.,* in press; DiBlasi, P., Bernareggi, A., Begiolin, G., Piazoni, L., Menta, E., Formento, M. L. (1998) Cytotoxicity, cellular uptake and DNA binding of the novel trinuclear platinum complex BBR3464 in sensitive and cisplatin resistant murine leukemia cells. *Anticancer Res.* **18,** 3113–3116.
23. Roberts, J. D., Rauter, H., Peroutka, J., and Farrell (1998) Activity of a polyamine-linked dinuclear platinum complex in cisplatin-resistant L1210 is due in part to preserved accumulation. *Proc. AACR* **39,** 1098.
24. Zaludová, R., Zakovská, A., Kašpárková, J., Balcarová, Z., Kleinwächter V., Vrána, O., et al. (1997) DNA interactions of bifunctional dinuclear platinum(II) antitumor agents. *Eur. J. Biochem.*, **246,** 508–516.
25. Brabec, V., Kašpárková, J., Vrána, O., Nováková, O., Cox, J., Qu, Y., et al. (1999) DNA modifications by a novel bifunctional trinuclear platinum phase I anticancer agent. *Biochemistry,* **38,** 6781–6790.
26. Zou, Y., Van Houten, B., and Farrell, N. (1994) Sequence specificity of DNA-DNA interstrand cross-link formation by cisplatin and dinuclear platinum complexes. *Biochemistry*, **33,** 5404–5410.
27. Wu, P., Kharatishvili, M., Qu, Y., and Farrell, N. (1996) A circular dichroism study of ethidium bromide binding to Z-DNA induced by dinuclear platinum complexes. *J. Inorg. Biochem.* **63,** 9–16.

Index